AF839619

Nanotechnology for Biomedical Applications

This book explores the intersection of nanotechnology and biomedicine, presenting cutting-edge innovations that are transforming healthcare delivery worldwide. This book examines how materials engineered at the nanoscale address complex biological challenges previously considered insurmountable.

Nanotechnology for Biomedical Applications: Innovations in Diagnostics, Therapeutics, and Biosafety bridges fundamental nanoscience principles with practical clinical applications, providing readers with both theoretical frameworks and actionable insights for implementation. Featuring insights from global experts, it offers a diverse and multidisciplinary perspective on nanotechnology and provides actionable strategies and real-world examples in various scopes of applications. Readers will gain an understanding of advanced biosensors and drug delivery systems to radioisotope enhancement and food safety technologies. Each chapter balances technical depth with accessibility, making complex concepts understandable without sacrificing scientific rigor. It uniquely emphasizes both innovation and responsibility, with dedicated sections on nanotoxicology and regulatory frameworks, ensuring readers develop a complete understanding of both capabilities and considerations in this rapidly evolving field.

This book is intended for graduate and postgraduate students, research fellows, and experts in nanotechnology, biotechnology, nanomedicine, and bioengineering. It also targets industry professionals in pharmaceuticals, medical devices, and food technology and clinicians using nanotechnology for diagnostics and treatment.

Ankan Dutta Chowdhury is Associate Professor of Nanotechnology at Amity Institute of Biotechnology, Kolkata, India. He earned his PhD in Chemical Sciences from Saha Institute of Nuclear Physics, Kolkata, in 2015. He spent six years doing postdoctoral work at National Chiao Tung University, Taiwan, and Shizuoka University, Japan, where he spent two years as an assistant professor and supervised several master's and PhD students. His research interests include nanomaterials, biosensors, bioimaging, and drug delivery.

Ruey-An Doong earned his PhD in Environmental Engineering from National Taiwan University, Taiwan, in 1992. He is currently the Chair Professor at the Institute of Analytical and Environmental Sciences, National Tsing Hua University (NTHU), Taiwan. He is also the Dean of Tsing Hua International College. He is internationally known for his research in environmental nanotechnology, energy materials, and biosensors/nanosensing devices.

Nanotechnology for Biomedical Applications

Innovations in Diagnostics, Therapeutics, and Biosafety

Edited by

Ankan Dutta Chowdhury and Ruey-An Doong

CRC Press
Taylor & Francis Group
Boca Raton London New York

CRC Press is an imprint of the
Taylor & Francis Group, an **informa** business

Designed cover image: © Getty Images

First edition published 2027
by CRC Press
2385 NW Executive Center Drive, Suite 320, Boca Raton FL 33431

and by CRC Press
4 Park Square, Milton Park, Abingdon, Oxon, OX14 4RN

CRC Press is an imprint of Taylor & Francis Group, LLC

© 2027 selection and editorial matter, Ankan Dutta Chowdhury and Ruey-An Doong; individual chapters, the contributors

Reasonable efforts have been made to publish reliable data and information, but the author and publisher cannot assume responsibility for the validity of all materials or the consequences of their use. The authors and publishers have attempted to trace the copyright holders of all material reproduced in this publication and apologize to copyright holders if permission to publish in this form has not been obtained. If any copyright material has not been acknowledged please write and let us know so we may rectify in any future reprint.

Except as permitted under U.S. Copyright Law, no part of this book may be reprinted, reproduced, transmitted, or utilized in any form by any electronic, mechanical, or other means, now known or hereafter invented, including photocopying, microfilming, and recording, or in any information storage or retrieval system, without written permission from the publishers.

For permission to photocopy or use material electronically from this work, access www.copyright.com or contact the Copyright Clearance Center, Inc. (CCC), 222 Rosewood Drive, Danvers, MA 01923, 978-750-8400. For works that are not available on CCC please contact mpkbookspermissions@tandf.co.uk

For Product Safety Concerns and Information please contact our EU representative GPSR@taylorandfrancis.com. Taylor & Francis Verlag GmbH, Kaufingerstraße 24, 80331 München, Germany.

Trademark notice: Product or corporate names may be trademarks or registered trademarks and are used only for identification and explanation without intent to infringe.

ISBN: 978-1-041-21175-4 (hbk)
ISBN: 978-1-041-21179-2 (pbk)
ISBN: 978-1-003-72593-0 (ebk)

DOI: 10.1201/9781003725930

Typeset in Times
by codeMantra

Contents

Preface

Nanotechnology represents one of the most transformative frontiers in modern science and engineering. Nanomaterials exhibit different physical, chemical, and biological properties compared with their bulk counterparts, enabling control over matter and function. These unique properties have opened new pathways for innovation across multiple disciplines, including medicine, diagnostics, food technology, environmental remediation, and advanced materials science. As research in this field continues to expand rapidly, there is an increasing need for comprehensive resources that bridge fundamental concepts with emerging applications.

The inspiration for this book arose from the growing demand for nanotechnology in biomedical applications and our decade-long research experience in this field. Researchers, students, and professionals often encounter fragmented information spread across specialized literature. This book was therefore conceived to bring together diverse perspectives in a single resource, highlighting both the foundational principles and practical applications that are shaping the future of nanotechnology. A distinctive feature of this book is the international collaboration behind it. The 11 chapters were contributed by authors representing eight different countries, reflecting the truly global nature of nanotechnology research. This multinational authorship provides a broad range of scientific viewpoints and expertise, enriching the discussion and ensuring that the topics presented reflect both regional research priorities and worldwide scientific developments.

The structure of this book moves systematically from fundamental principles to advanced applications. Chapter 1 introduces the basic concepts and historical development of nanotechnology, providing readers with essential background knowledge. Subsequent chapters explore specialized topics including nanocatalysts, biomedical applications, biosensors, virus detection technologies, gas sensing systems, drug delivery platforms, and emerging nanomaterials for food technology. In addition to scientific advances, the later chapters also consider practical challenges associated with translating laboratory discoveries into real-world applications, including safety considerations, regulatory frameworks, and technological scalability. By integrating theoretical foundations with contemporary research developments, this book aims to serve as a valuable reference for students, researchers, and professionals working in nanoscience and nanotechnology. It is designed not only to provide an overview of current progress but also to highlight emerging opportunities where nanotechnology can address pressing global challenges in healthcare, environmental sustainability, and food security. This textbook is intended as a gateway rather than a final destination. We hope that it will inspire readers to explore new research directions and contribute to the next-generation applications in nanotechnology.

Contributors

Tamara V. Basova
Department of Structural Chemistry
Nikolaev Institute of Inorganic Chemistry, SB RAS
Nikolaev, Russia

Sneha Bhatta
Amity Institute of Nanotechnology
Amity University Kolkata
Kolkata, West Bengal, India

Avik Chakraborty
Bhabha Atomic Research Centre
Mumbai, India

Ankan Dutta Chowdhury
Amity Institute of Nanotechnology
Amity University Kolkata
Kolkata, West Bengal, India

Uddipan Dasgupta
Amity Institute of Nanotechnology
Amity University Kolkata
Kolkata, West Bengal, India

Ruey-An Doong
Institute of Analytical Chemistry & Environmental Sciences
National Tsing Hua University
Hsinchu, Taiwan

Akhilesh Babu Ganganboina
International Center for Young Scientists
National Institute of Materials Sciences
Tsukuba, Japan

Malabika Ghosh
Amity Institute of Nanotechnology
Amity University Kolkata
Kolkata, West Bengal, India

Indra Memdi Khoris
Chungnam National University
Daejeon, South Korea

Purvi Kishore
Amity Institute of Biotechnology
Amity University Kolkata
Kolkata, West Bengal, India

Darya Klyamer
Department of Structural Chemistry
Nikolaev Institute of Inorganic Chemistry SB RAS
Nikolaev, Russia

Jaebeom Lee
Chungnam National University
Daejeon, South Korea

Amit Ranjan Maity
Amity Institute of Biotechnology
Amity University Kolkata
Kolkata, West Bengal, India

Siew Suan Ng
Department of Biomedical Engineering & Environmental Sciences/Department of Electrical Engineering & Electronics
National Tsing Hua University
Hsinchu, Taiwan

David Nugroho
Khon Kaen University
Khon Kaen, Thailand

Enoch Y. Park
Shizuoka University
Shizuoka, Japan

Petar Ristivojevic
Faculty of Chemistry
University of Belgrade
Belgrade, Serbia

Anushka Roy
Amity Institute of Biotechnology
Amity University Kolkata
Kolkata, West Bengal, India

Aphinya Thinthasit
Khon Kaen University
Khon Kaen, Thailand

Petar Todorovic
Faculty of Chemistry
University of Belgrade
Belgrade, Serbia

Doddy Irawan Setyo Utomo
National Research and Innovation Agency (BRIN)
Jakarta, Indonesia

Jasmina Vidic
Université Paris-Saclay
INREA
Paris, France

1 Nanotechnology in Biomedical Applications

Uddipan Dasgupta, Malabika Ghosh, Sneha Bhatta, and Ankan Dutta Chowdhury

1.1 INTRODUCTION TO NANOTECHNOLOGY

Nanotechnology represents one of the most transformative frontiers of modern science, encompassing the understanding, manipulation, and control of matter at dimensions typically below 100 nm, where the classical rules of bulk materials give way to unique quantum, surface, and size-dependent effects. At this scale, atoms and molecules can be engineered with exquisite precision to display properties that differ dramatically from their macroscopic counterparts. Electrical conductivity, magnetism, optical absorption, catalytic activity, and mechanical strength all become tunable simply by altering particle size, geometry, or surface chemistry. The conceptual roots of nanotechnology trace back to Richard Feynman's visionary 1959 lecture, "There's Plenty of Room at the Bottom," which imagined a world where scientists could directly manipulate individual atoms. This vision matured when Norio Taniguchi introduced the term "nanotechnology" in 1974, referring to the engineering of materials at atomic precision. The invention of the scanning tunneling microscope and atomic force microscope in the early 1980s turned this imagination into reality by allowing researchers to observe and move atoms one by one. These innovations gave rise to the modern era of nanoscience, bridging disciplines as diverse as condensed matter physics, surface chemistry, molecular biology, and materials engineering.

In biomedicine, nanotechnology occupies a privileged position because the nanoscale overlaps precisely with the dimensions of fundamental biological structures, DNA's double helix (~2 nm in width), proteins (5–50 nm), viruses (20–200 nm), and cell membranes (5–10 nm thick). This size compatibility enables engineered nanomaterials to communicate seamlessly with biomolecules, cells, and tissues, allowing interventions that were once impossible using conventional tools. At the same time, the nanoscale environment accentuates surface phenomena: a single nanoparticle can have up to half of its atoms on the surface, dramatically amplifying reactivity and allowing high-density functionalization with biomolecules such as antibodies, peptides, or nucleic acids. These characteristics make nanostructures exceptionally useful for controlled drug delivery, precision imaging, biosensing, and regenerative medicine.

The scale of nanotechnology allows for precise control over disease mechanisms (Figure 1.1). Many pathological processes such as viral infection, genetic mutation, oxidative stress, and uncontrolled cell proliferation originate or propagate at the molecular level. Nanoscale engineering provides tools to recognize and bind disease

DOI: 10.1201/9781003725930-1

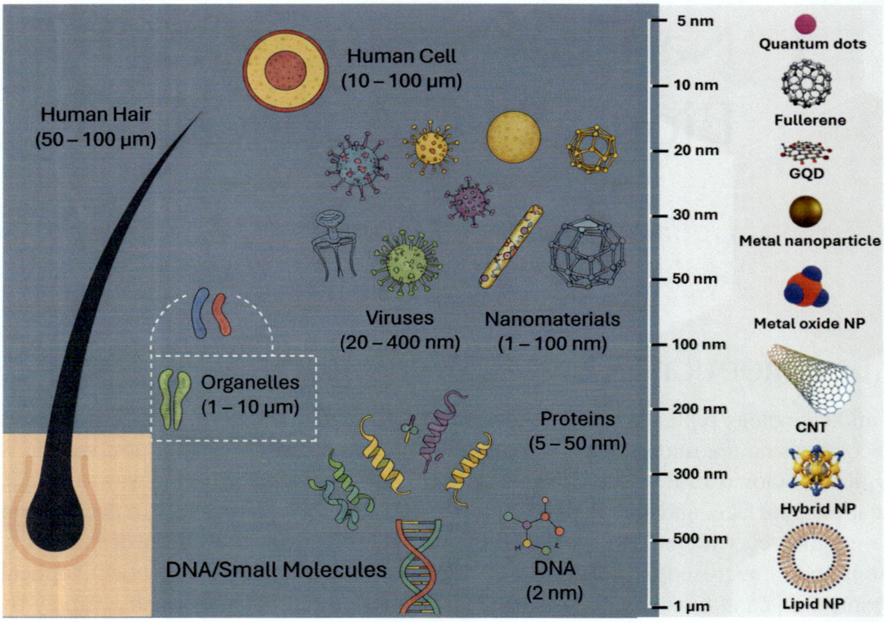

FIGURE 1.1 Illustration of comparative size scale of nanomaterials, viruses, proteins, and cells.

biomarkers with molecular precision. It can help to deliver therapeutic molecules selectively to diseased cells, minimizing side effects and generate high-resolution diagnostic signals through optical, magnetic, or electrochemical transduction. Thus, nanotechnology forms the basis of precision medicine, enabling personalized diagnostics and targeted interventions tailored to individual patients' molecular profiles.

The coming decades will see nanotechnology increasingly intertwined with artificial intelligence (AI), synthetic biology, and quantum computing, enabling adaptive, intelligent nanomedicines that respond to dynamic biological environments. By combining nanoscale precision with data-driven design, the next generation of biomedical technology will achieve outcomes once considered science fiction, real-time disease monitoring, self-regulated therapeutic release, and molecular-level tissue regeneration [1–3].

1.2 HISTORICAL EVOLUTION AND MILESTONES

The progress of nanotechnology from a theoretical concept to a transformative discipline has followed several landmark developments. Early foundations were laid in the mid-20th century with advances in electron microscopy that allowed visualization of atomic structures.

Key milestones are as follows:

- 1985: Discovery of Fullerenes (C_{60}): Buckminsterfullerene opened new avenues in carbon nanostructures [4].

- 1991: Carbon Nanotubes (CNTs): Sumio Iijima's discovery led to ultrahigh-strength and conductive nanomaterials.
- 1993–2000: Quantum Dots and Nanoshells: These introduced tunable optical properties for imaging and diagnostics.
- 2000s: Rise of Nanomedicine: Food and Drug Administration-approved liposomal drugs (e.g., Doxil®) and polymeric nanocarriers validated clinical translation [5].
- 2010s: Nanobiosensors and Gene Nanocarriers: Integration with bioelectronics and molecular diagnostics expanded rapidly.
- 2020s: mRNA-Lipid Nanoparticle Vaccines: The COVID-19 pandemic showcased the real-world impact of nanotechnology in global healthcare [6].

Each breakthrough reinforced the convergence of nanoscale science with biological and medical innovation, making nanotechnology indispensable for future healthcare paradigms.

1.3 TYPES OF NANOMATERIALS AND THEIR PROPERTIES

Nanomaterials can be broadly categorized by composition and dimensionality, each imparting distinct physicochemical behavior relevant to biomedical functions.

a. Metal and Metal-Oxide Nanoparticles: Metal-based nanoparticles are among the most extensively studied nanomaterials due to their remarkable optical, electrical, and catalytic properties. Gold (Au) and silver (Ag) nanoparticles exhibit localized surface plasmon resonance, enabling high-sensitivity colorimetric biosensing, photothermal therapy, and imaging applications. Iron oxide (Fe_3O_4 or γ-Fe_2O_3) nanoparticles display superparamagnetism, making them ideal for magnetic resonance imaging (MRI), targeted drug delivery, and hyperthermia-based cancer therapy. Similarly, zinc oxide (ZnO) and titanium dioxide (TiO_2) nanoparticles are valued for their photocatalytic and antimicrobial activities, serving in wound healing, disinfection, and photodynamic therapy. Metal-oxide nanostructures can also act as enzyme mimetics ("nanozymes") that catalyze specific biochemical reactions for biosensing applications.
b. Carbon-Based Nanostructures: Graphene, graphene oxide, CNTs, and graphene quantum dots (QDs) exhibit extraordinary electrical conductivity, mechanical strength, and biocompatibility. Their large surface area allows for high-density functionalization with biomolecules, making them suitable for electrochemical biosensors, gene delivery, and regenerative scaffolds. Fullerenes (C_{60}) and their derivatives possess antioxidant properties and are being explored for photodynamic therapy and neuroprotection. Furthermore, carbon QDs provide versatile fluorescence properties, enabling bioimaging and cellular tracking.
c. Polymeric and Lipid Nanocarriers: Polymeric nanomaterials, including poly(lactic-co-glycolic acid), polyethylene glycol (PEG), chitosan, and polylactic acid, offer biodegradability, low immunogenicity, and controlled drug

release capabilities. These polymers can be engineered into nanoparticles, micelles, or nanogels to encapsulate drugs, proteins, or nucleic acids. Surface modification with targeting ligands, antibodies, or aptamers enhances cell-specific recognition and therapeutic precision. Lipid-based systems such as liposomes, solid lipid nanoparticles, and nanostructured lipid carriers mimic biological membranes and have been successfully translated into several FDA-approved formulations, including mRNA vaccines and anticancer therapeutics.

d. Inorganic and Hybrid Nanomaterials: This category encompasses a wide array of nanostructures integrating inorganic, organic, or hybrid frameworks with tunable physicochemical characteristics. Mesoporous silica nanoparticles provide large surface area and adjustable pore sizes, facilitating high drug loading capacity and stimuli-responsive release. Metal–organic frameworks (MOFs), composed of metal ions interconnected by organic linkers, exhibit exceptional porosity, modular chemistry, and high surface area, allowing for enzyme immobilization, gas storage, and co-delivery of therapeutic agents. Emerging organic framework analogues, Covalent Organic Frameworks (COFs) and Hydrogen-Bonded Organic Frameworks (HOFs) have recently attracted attention for biomedical use. COFs are crystalline, porous polymers formed by strong covalent linkages (e.g., boronate ester, imine, or triazine bonds), and offer robust thermal stability, chemical tunability, and biocompatibility. Their ordered porosity and designable structure allow precise control over drug encapsulation, photosensitizer loading, and stimuli-responsive release. In contrast, HOFs, constructed via non-covalent hydrogen bonding interactions, exhibit solution processability, reversible self-assembly, and low cytotoxicity, making them promise for bioimaging, controlled drug release, and biosensing. Additionally, QDs, such as CdSe, ZnS, and carbon-based QDs, display tunable fluorescence, making them valuable for multiplexed optical imaging. Core–shell nanostructures (e.g., $Au@SiO_2$, $Fe_3O_4@Au$, or polymer-coated metals) combine the features of multiple materials, improving stability, biocompatibility, and multimodal imaging capabilities.

e. Ceramic and Dendrimer Nanomaterials: Ceramic nanoparticles, typically based on alumina (Al_2O_3), zirconia (ZrO_2), and calcium phosphate (CaP), are chemically inert, thermally stable, and suitable for bone regeneration, tissue engineering, and dental applications. Hydroxyapatite nanoparticles exhibit structural similarity to natural bone minerals and promote osteointegration and biocompatibility. Dendrimers, highly branched polymeric nanostructures with precise molecular architecture, provide well-defined surface functionalities for drug and gene delivery. Their multivalent surface allows conjugation with targeting ligands, fluorescent dyes, and therapeutic agents, ensuring high payload capacity and targeted transport. The internal cavities of dendrimers can encapsulate hydrophobic molecules, improving solubility and bioavailability.

At the nanoscale, large surface-to-volume ratios, surface charge, and functional groups govern biocompatibility and interaction with cellular membranes, dictating pharmacokinetics and therapeutic efficacy. Conventional nanoparticle synthesis methods often involve toxic reagents, organic solvents, and high-energy conditions, leading to environmental hazards and cytotoxic by-products. To overcome these limitations, biogenic or green synthesis approaches have emerged as sustainable alternatives. These utilize plant extracts, bacteria, fungi, algae, and biomolecules (proteins, amino acids, polyphenols, and polysaccharides) as natural reducing, stabilizing, and capping agents. Such biosynthetic methods operate under mild reaction conditions, producing nanoparticles with biocompatible organic coatings and controlled physicochemical features. The naturally derived capping molecules not only prevent aggregation but also impart surface passivation, reducing reactive oxygen species (ROS) generation and cellular toxicity. Additionally, these bio-functional coatings can enhance cellular internalization, pharmacokinetic stability, and target specificity. Hence, biogenic synthesis not only contributes to environmental sustainability but also promotes the safe clinical translation of nanomaterials by minimizing their inherent toxicological risks.

1.4 MECHANISMS OF INTERACTION WITH BIOLOGICAL SYSTEMS

The interaction between engineered nanomaterials and biological systems lies at the heart of biomedical nanotechnology. Once a nanoparticle enters a living system whether in a cell culture, bloodstream, or tissue, it does not remain chemically or physically "naked." Instead, it becomes dynamically modified by its biological environment. Understanding this complex interface is fundamental to predicting biological outcomes such as biodistribution, therapeutic efficiency, and toxicity.

Immediately upon contact with biological fluids such as blood plasma, lymph, or intracellular surroundings, nanoparticles become coated by an ensemble of biomolecules such as proteins, lipids, polysaccharides, and nucleic acids. This dynamic coating, known as the protein corona, defines the true biological identity of the nanoparticle. The corona forms through a rapid and reversible process governed by surface charge, hydrophobicity, curvature, and chemical functionality of the nanoparticle surface. A hard corona is composed of tightly bound proteins with slow exchange rates, whereas a soft corona contains loosely bound biomolecules that exchange rapidly with the environment. The composition of this corona determines how the immune system perceives the particle either as "self" or "foreign." For example, opsonins such as immunoglobulins and complement proteins can tag nanoparticles for clearance by macrophages, while the adsorption of albumin or apolipoproteins may enhance circulation time and cellular compatibility [7]. Hence, the engineering of "stealth" nanoparticles often involves surface modifications (e.g., PEGylation, zwitterionic coatings) that modulate corona formation to evade immune recognition.

The next stage of nano–bio interaction is cellular internalization, where nanoparticles cross the plasma membrane barrier to reach intracellular targets. This process is highly dependent on physicochemical parameters such as particle size, surface charge, shape, and ligand functionalization.

Mechanisms of nanoparticle uptake can be carried out by various routes:

- Clathrin-Mediated Endocytosis: Typically involves nanoparticles of 50–150 nm functionalized with receptor-targeting ligands (e.g., transferrin, folate).
- Caveolin-Mediated Endocytosis: Common for smaller, rigid, and hydrophobic nanoparticles (e.g., gold or silica), avoiding lysosomal degradation.
- Macropinocytosis: A nonselective engulfment mechanism allowing uptake of larger particles or clusters (>200 nm).
- Phagocytosis: Predominantly occurs in immune cells (macrophages, dendritic cells), facilitating clearance, but also exploitable for immune modulation or antigen delivery.

After endocytosis, nanoparticles are trafficked through endosomal compartments, where environmental conditions (acidic pH, redox potential, enzymatic activity) determine the release or degradation of their payload. Smart nanocarriers exploit these conditions such as pH-sensitive linkers or enzyme-cleavable coatings to ensure site-specific drug or gene release in the cytosol or nucleus. Understanding these trafficking routes is essential for designing effective and predictable nanotherapeutics.

Once in systemic circulation, nanoparticles encounter a hierarchy of biological barriers that control their biodistribution. Key determinants include size, surface charge, hydrophobicity, and shape:

- Nanoparticles smaller than ~10 nm can undergo rapid renal clearance through glomerular filtration, minimizing accumulation but limiting retention.
- Particles between 10 and 100 nm typically exhibit optimal circulation times, exploiting the enhanced permeability and retention effect in tumors or inflamed tissues.
- Larger particles (>200 nm) are prone to uptake by the mononuclear phagocyte system especially in the liver and spleen, reducing systemic half-life.
- PEGylation and other hydrophilic coatings prevent opsonization and aggregation, extending plasma half-life and improving pharmacokinetics.

While nanotechnology offers transformative medical potential, improper engineering can trigger adverse biological responses. Nanoparticles may generate ROS through redox reactions or surface catalysis, leading to oxidative stress, lipid peroxidation, and DNA damage. They can also disrupt cell membranes, alter ion homeostasis, or interfere with signaling pathways.

Common toxicity mechanisms include:

- Inflammatory Responses: Activation of macrophages and cytokine release.
- Genotoxicity: DNA strand breaks or chromosomal aberrations caused by oxidative stress.
- Mitochondrial Dysfunction: Interference with cellular respiration and apoptosis pathways.
- Long-Term Accumulation: Persistence in organs such as the liver, spleen, or brain for nondegradable nanomaterials.

Therefore, comprehensive physicochemical characterization including surface charge, aggregation behavior, zeta potential, and degradation kinetics is mandatory before biomedical application.

Recent advances in computational biology, in silico modeling, and AI are allowing researchers to simulate these interactions, predict nanoparticle behavior across tissues, and design optimized systems with minimal adverse effects. This system-level understanding represents the next phase of predictive nanomedicine where nano–bio interactions are not merely studied but actively engineered for desired biological responses.

1.5 CURRENT APPLICATIONS IN HEALTHCARE, DIAGNOSTICS, AND THERAPY

Nanotechnology has fundamentally transformed the practice of modern biomedical science, bridging the gap between molecular-scale design and clinical-scale solutions. From disease detection to personalized therapy and regenerative medicine, engineered nanomaterials now serve as the cornerstone of next-generation healthcare. Their ability to interact precisely with biomolecules, cells, and tissues has accelerated the translation of innovations from laboratory prototypes to real-world medical technologies. Today, the impact of nanotechnology is not confined to any single domain. Instead, it forms a continuum of interconnected disciplines that together constitute the landscape of biomedical nanotechnology. The present volume explores these interlinked areas through ten specialized chapters, each addressing a critical dimension of nanoscale science and its biomedical implications. The conceptual organization of this book, illustrated in Figure 1.2, positions "Nanotechnology in Biomedical Applications" at the core, surrounded by multiple thematic modules that reflect how nanoscale principles extend into diagnostics, therapeutics, catalysis, food safety, sensing, and biocompatibility.

Chapter 2 discusses how nanotechnology has revolutionized viral diagnostics, prevention, and therapeutic strategies. It explains the development of nanoparticle-based biosensing systems such as gold, QD, and magnetic nanoprobe platforms for the rapid and ultrasensitive detection of viral pathogens. The chapter also details nanocarrier-based antiviral drug delivery systems and the use of lipid nanoparticles (LNPs), virus-like particles, and polymeric nano vaccines in controlling viral infections. Furthermore, it highlights nanotechnology's critical role in pandemic preparedness and in developing scalable, portable diagnostic technologies for global virus surveillance.

Chapter 3 explores catalytic nanomaterials and their biomedical applications. It introduces the principles of nanocatalysis, emphasizing the enhanced surface activity and electron transfer properties that arise at the nanoscale. The chapter examines the development of nanozymes, artificial enzyme mimics derived from metallic or oxide nanostructures that drive biochemical reactions relevant to disease treatment, biosensing, and drug synthesis. It further links biomedical catalysis to environmental sustainability through green nano-chemistry, demonstrating how catalytic nanoparticles bridge chemical engineering and biological function.

Chapter 4 integrates the principles of nanotechnology with radiochemistry. It outlines the synthesis, functionalization, and characterization of nanoparticles labeled

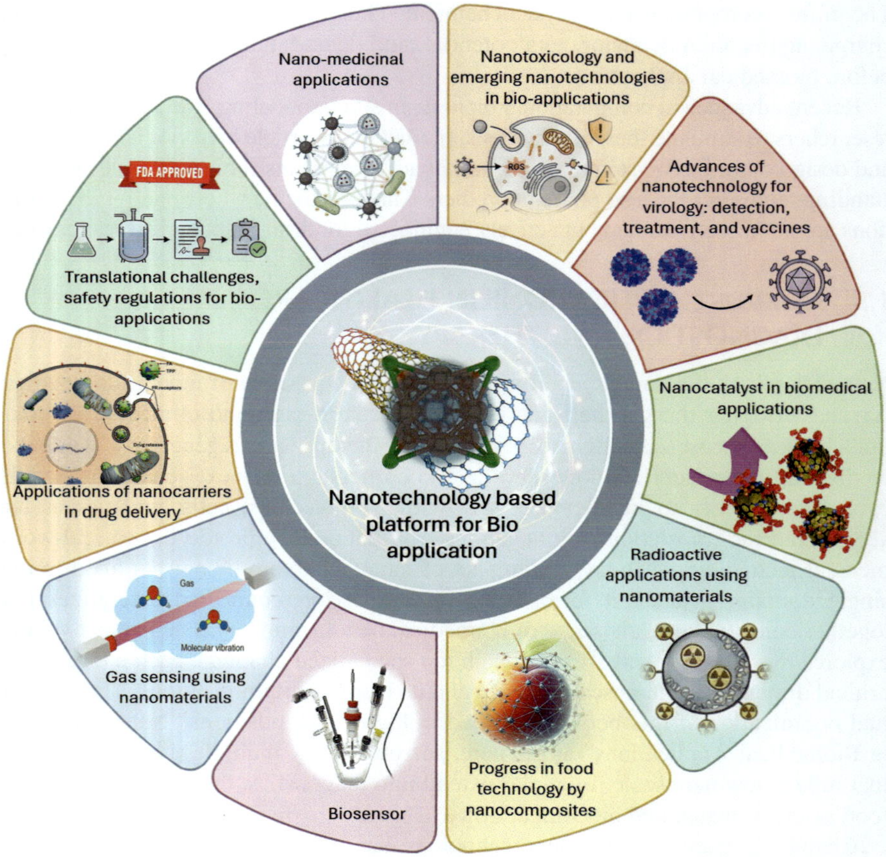

FIGURE 1.2 Graphical overview of nanotechnology as an enabling platform, highlighting key biomedical, environmental, and translational applications covered in this volume.

with isotopes for targeted imaging and radiotherapy. The chapter discusses how these hybrid systems enable both diagnostic and therapeutic functions within a single platform, underpinning the emerging field of radio-nanomedicine. Applications in nuclear imaging techniques such as positron emission tomography and single-photon emission computed tomography are presented alongside discussions on biosafety, radiation control, and clinical translation.

Chapter 5 extends nanoscience beyond medicine to food preservation, pathogen detection, and quality control. This chapter examines the development of nanomaterials for antimicrobial packaging, oxygen barrier coatings, and nutrient encapsulation to enhance shelf life and bioavailability. It also explores nanosensor-based foodborne pathogen detection systems and addresses ethical, regulatory, and environmental issues surrounding nanotechnology in food and agriculture. The chapter underscores how nanocomposites protect public health by ensuring food safety and sustainability.

Chapter 6 focuses on the integration of nanomaterials into biosensing technologies for medical and environmental diagnostics. It explains how nanostructures such as graphene, CNTs, and gold nanoparticles enhance the sensitivity, selectivity, and response time of biosensors. The chapter elaborates on various transduction mechanisms, including optical, electrochemical, and piezoelectric modes, and reviews recent advancements in wearable sensors, lab-on-chip devices, and multiplexed platforms. Together, these developments illustrate how nanoscale interfaces convert biochemical recognition events into measurable diagnostic signals.

Chapter 7 explores the application of nanotechnology in detecting toxic and bio-relevant gases. It outlines the use of metal oxide and two-dimensional nanomaterials in monitoring gases such as carbon monoxide, ammonia, and nitrogen oxides, as well as volatile organic compounds relevant to medical diagnostics. The chapter emphasizes nanomaterials' high surface area and tunable conductivity, which enable sensitive and selective gas detection. It also discusses their utility in breath-based disease diagnostics, air quality monitoring, and wearable environmental sensors.

Chapter 8 examines the design and clinical application of nanocarrier systems for controlled and targeted drug delivery. It describes liposomes, dendrimers, polymeric nanoparticles, and inorganic nanostructures used for site-specific drug release. The mechanisms of ligand-mediated targeting and stimuli-responsive systems such as triggered by pH, temperature, or redox gradients are discussed in detail. The chapter highlights how such platforms minimize systemic toxicity, improve pharmacokinetics, and form the basis of modern precision medicine.

Chapter 9 discusses the growing field of regenerative nanotechnology, where nanostructured scaffolds and hydrogels are engineered to mimic natural extracellular matrices. It focuses on the role of nanomaterials in modulating stem cell behavior, promoting differentiation, and facilitating the regeneration of bone, vascular, and neural tissues. Additionally, it examines nano-enabled therapeutics for neurological repair and tissue restoration, illustrating how nanotechnology contributes to healing and organ reconstruction.

Chapter 10 explores how nanoscale physicochemical properties govern biological interactions and safety outcomes. It discusses key toxicity mechanisms, including oxidative stress, inflammation, immune modulation, and long-term bioaccumulation, while highlighting emerging nanoplatforms for biomedical use. The chapter reviews advanced in vitro, in vivo, and computational assessment strategies, underscoring nanotoxicology as a foundational discipline for the safe and responsible development of next-generation bio-applications.

Chapter 11 examines the critical barriers that hinder the clinical translation of nanomedicines. It highlights challenges related to reproducibility, scalable manufacturing, and interspecies variability in biological responses. The chapter reviews international regulatory frameworks, including FDA, European Medicines Agency, OECD, and ISO guidance, and illustrates approval pathways through key case studies. Collectively, it emphasizes the need for integrated, standardized, and proactive approaches to ensure safe and effective nanotechnology-based bio-applications.

1.5.1 Summary of Learning Perspective

Each chapter of this book provides an integrated learning experience from the atomic design of nanomaterials to their systemic behavior in living organisms. By the end of the volume, students will have the following benefits:

- A comprehensive understanding of nanoscale materials and their biomedical relevance.
- A multidisciplinary perspective spanning chemistry, biology, physics, and engineering.
- An appreciation for translation and ethics, ensuring that technological progress aligns with safety and societal needs.

Thus, Nanotechnology in Biomedical Applications serves not merely as a collection of topics, but as a unified educational pathway guiding readers from fundamental principles to real-world innovations shaping the future of healthcare.

1.6 EMERGING TRENDS IN NANOBIOTECHNOLOGY

Nanobiotechnology continues to evolve rapidly through the integration of molecular biology, data science, and materials engineering, creating a transformative impact on the way diseases are diagnosed, treated, and prevented. The convergence of nanotechnology with genomics, AI, bioinformatics, and systems biology is propelling the field toward a new era of precision and sustainability. The following emerging trends illustrate how these synergies are shaping the future of biomedical innovation.

1.6.1 Smart and Stimuli-Responsive Nanoplatforms

Modern nanocarriers are no longer passive drug containers but intelligent systems capable of responding to physiological or pathological stimuli within the human body. These stimuli-responsive nanoplatforms are engineered to react to environmental changes such as variations in pH, temperature, enzyme concentration, redox potential, or even the presence of viral or cancer-specific biomarkers. For instance, pH-sensitive liposomes release anticancer drugs selectively in the acidic tumor microenvironment, while enzyme-triggered polymeric nanoparticles degrade specifically in inflamed or infected tissues [8,9]. Such spatiotemporal control minimizes off-target toxicity and maximizes therapeutic efficacy. Emerging designs also integrate dual- or multi-responsive behavior, where light, magnetic fields, or ultrasound act as external triggers for controlled release, marking the evolution toward advanced nanotherapy.

1.6.2 Hybrid and Multifunctional Nanosystems

The next generation of biomedical nanomaterials is built on hybrid architectures that combine the advantages of different material classes like organic, inorganic, and biological. Lipid–polymer hybrids, silica-coated magnetic nanoparticles, and MOFs exemplify multifunctional systems capable of simultaneous drug delivery, bioimaging, and therapeutic monitoring [10,11]. These systems are central to theranostics, enabling real-time tracking of drug distribution and therapeutic response through integrated imaging modalities such as fluorescence, MRI, or photoacoustics. The incorporation of catalytic or plasmonic cores further allows photothermal or photodynamic therapy, uniting diagnosis, and treatment within a single nanoscale platform. Hybrid nanostructures are expected to become the backbone of future personalized medical technologies due to their modularity and tunability.

1.6.3 CRISPR, RNA Therapeutics, and Gene-Editing Nanocarriers

The integration of nanotechnology with molecular genetics is reshaping the treatment of viral and hereditary diseases. Nanoparticle-assisted delivery systems provide protection and targeted transport for fragile biomolecules such as siRNA, mRNA, and CRISPR-Cas gene-editing complexes [12,13]. LNPs, polymeric nanocapsules, and gold nanocarriers enable these nucleic acids to cross cellular membranes and reach their intracellular targets with high efficiency. The global success of mRNA-LNP vaccines during the COVID-19 pandemic has demonstrated the real-world potential of RNA nanomedicine [14]. Future directions involve developing tissue-specific gene delivery, CRISPR activation and silencing nanocarriers, and combination therapies that integrate gene correction with immunomodulation. These advances mark the transition from symptom management to molecular-level disease correction.

1.6.4 Nano-Bioelectronics and Wearable Diagnostics

The fusion of nanomaterials with microelectronics has given rise to nano-bioelectronic devices–flexible, miniaturized systems capable of continuous health monitoring and real-time biosensing. Graphene, CNTs, and conducting polymers form the core of flexible electronic circuits that detect minute biochemical signals such as glucose levels, neurotransmitters, or oxygen saturation. Wearable and implantable nanosensors now enable the measurement of physiological parameters without invasive sampling, paving the way for personalized and preventive healthcare. Integration with wireless communication and data analytics further allows remote diagnostics and early disease intervention [15,16].

1.6.5 AI-Driven Nanomaterial Design and Predictive Nanomedicine

AI and machine learning are redefining how nanomaterials are designed, optimized, and tested. Traditional trial-and-error approaches are being replaced by data-driven predictive modeling, where algorithms analyze vast experimental datasets to forecast nanoparticle behavior, stability, and biocompatibility. AI assists in identifying optimal compositions, particle sizes, and surface modifications for specific biomedical tasks such as drug delivery or biosensing. In silico simulations of nano–bio interactions reduce the need for extensive animal testing, accelerating translational research. Beyond material design, AI also aids in personalized nanomedicine by correlating patient genomic or metabolomic profiles with nanoparticle performance, leading to individualized treatment strategies with higher success rates [17,18].

1.6.6 Green and Sustainable Nanotechnology

With the rapid expansion of nanomaterial production, environmental and ethical sustainability have become central considerations. Green nanotechnology emphasizes eco-friendly synthesis methods using plant extracts, microorganisms, or biodegradable precursors that eliminate toxic reagents and minimize waste. Biogenic synthesis routes for gold, silver, and metal-oxide nanoparticles provide not only safer but also more cost-effective alternatives for biomedical use. Moreover, lifecycle assessment and sustainable material recovery are being integrated into nanomanufacturing to reduce environmental burden. The alignment of nanomedicine with green chemistry principles ensures that technological progress is harmonized with environmental stewardship and societal responsibility.

1.7 FUTURE PERSPECTIVES AND CHALLENGES

As nanotechnology continues to redefine the landscape of biomedicine, the next stage of progress must balance rapid innovation with safety, scalability, and social responsibility. The unprecedented potential of nanoscale science in diagnosis, therapy, and regenerative medicine is accompanied by equally significant challenges that must be addressed before its full translation into routine clinical practice can be achieved. One of the foremost challenges is the lack of standardization and reproducibility across the synthesis, characterization, and biological evaluation of nanomaterials. Even minor variations in particle size, shape, surface chemistry, or synthesis routes can drastically alter biological interactions and therapeutic outcomes. The absence of universal protocols for evaluating toxicity, pharmacokinetics, and efficacy often leads to inconsistent data, complicating the regulatory approval process. Establishing globally harmonized guidelines for nanoparticle characterization and performance testing will therefore be crucial to ensure reproducibility and foster international collaboration in nanomedicine research. Equally important is the issue of long-term safety and toxicological evaluation. Although many nanomaterials demonstrate remarkable biocompatibility in short-term studies, their chronic effects, biodegradation pathways, and cumulative toxicity remain insufficiently understood. Prolonged exposure can lead to bioaccumulation, oxidative stress, or immunogenic reactions that may only become apparent over extended periods. Comprehensive nanotoxicology research integrating molecular biology, computational modeling, and in vivo imaging is essential to trace biodistribution and clearance in real time, ensuring that therapeutic benefits do not come at the cost of biological harm.

Another pressing concern lies in scalability and manufacturing. Laboratory-scale synthesis methods often yield highly controlled nanoparticles with precise physicochemical properties, but replicating these features during large-scale production presents substantial challenges. Maintaining uniformity, purity, and stability while achieving cost-effective mass manufacturing remains a major technological bottleneck. The future of nanomedicine depends on innovations in green synthesis, microfluidic fabrication, and automated process control to ensure reproducible, industrial-grade nanomaterial production suitable for clinical translation. The integration of nanotechnology into healthcare also raises complex regulatory and ethical questions. The use of nanomedicines involves sensitive data on genetic and molecular profiles, demanding stringent frameworks to protect patient privacy and informed consent. Moreover, ethical oversight must govern the use of nanomaterials in gene editing, neural modulation, and human enhancement to prevent misuse. Transparent communication between scientists, clinicians, policymakers, and the public will be necessary to build societal trust and establish coherent international policies that guide the safe and responsible development of nanoscale therapeutics.

Looking ahead, the future trajectory of nanotechnology points toward deep integration with emerging scientific frontiers. The convergence of nanoscale engineering with quantum computing, synthetic biology, and bio-AI will give rise to adaptive and self-regulating therapeutic systems capable of real-time decision-making within the human body. Intelligent nanocarriers, guided by biosensing feedback loops, may autonomously adjust drug dosage or diagnostic signals according to the patient's physiological state. At the same time, the merging of nanotechnology with tissue engineering and regenerative biology will enable the creation of biohybrid materials that mimic, repair, or even enhance natural biological functions. Ultimately, the future of nanobiomedicine will depend not only on technological ingenuity but also on our ability to integrate safety, ethics, and sustainability into every stage of research and development. As nanoscale science evolves from a laboratory curiosity into an indispensable component of healthcare infrastructure, it will serve as both a tool and a paradigm for understanding, manipulating, and engineering life at its most fundamental level.

1.8 CONCLUSION

Nanotechnology has emerged as a cornerstone of modern biomedical science, offering unprecedented control over materials and biological processes at the molecular scale. By bridging physics, chemistry, and biology, it has enabled significant advancements in diagnostics, targeted therapy, and regenerative medicine, laying the groundwork for precision and personalized healthcare. The integration of AI, computational modeling, and sustainable synthesis methods continues to enhance the design, efficiency, and safety of nanosystems. However, realizing the full potential of nanotechnology requires overcoming critical challenges related to large-scale reproducibility, long-term biocompatibility, and regulatory compliance. Addressing these issues through standardized frameworks and ethical governance will ensure responsible clinical translation. Ultimately, nanotechnology represents more than a technological innovation; it signifies a transformative shift in the way we understand, diagnose, and treat diseases, redefining the future of healthcare through precision, intelligence, and sustainability.

REFERENCES

1. I.S. Pretorius, T.A. Dixon, M. Boers, I.T. Paulsen, D.L. Johnson, The coming wave of confluent biosynthetic, bioinformational and bioengineering technologies, *Nature Communications*, 16(2025) 2959.
2. S.N. Faraji, S. Masjoodi, S. Azmand, Biotechnology, nanotechnology, and AI: Transformative convergence in healthcare (a mini-review), *Advances in Applied NanoBio-Technologies*, 5(2024) 23–28.

3. X. Ju, C. Chen, C.M. Oral, S. Sevim, R. Golestanian, M. Sun, et al., Technology roadmap of micro/nanorobots, *ACS Nano*, 19(2025) 24174–334.
4. H.W. Kroto, J.R. Heath, S.C. O'Brien, R.F. Curl, R.E. Smalley, C60: Buckminsterfullerene, *Nature*, 318(1985) 162–3.
5. J. Patel, Liposomal doxorubicin: Doxil®, *Journal of Oncology Pharmacy Practice*, 2(1996) 201–10.
6. B. Wilson, K.M. Geetha, Lipid nanoparticles in the development of mRNA vaccines for COVID-19, *Journal of Drug Delivery Science and Technology*, 74(2022) 103553.
7. D.E. Owens III, N.A. Peppas, Opsonization, biodistribution, and pharmacokinetics of polymeric nanoparticles, *International Journal of Pharmaceutics*, 307(2006) 93–102.
8. S. Mura, J. Nicolas, P. Couvreur, Stimuli-responsive nanocarriers for drug delivery, *Nature Materials*, 12(2013) 991–1003.
9. Y. Lee, D. Thompson, Stimuli-responsive liposomes for drug delivery, *Wiley Interdisciplinary Reviews: Nanomedicine and Nanobiotechnology*, 9(2017) e1450.
10. K. Lu, T. Aung, N. Guo, R. Weichselbaum, W. Lin, Nanoscale metal–organic frameworks for therapeutic, imaging, and sensing applications, *Advanced Materials*, 30(2018) 1707634.
11. J. Liu, J. Huang, L. Zhang, J. Lei, Multifunctional metal–organic framework heterostructures for enhanced cancer therapy, *Chemical Society Reviews*, 50(2021) 1188–218.
12. M.W. Ghani, A. Iqbal, H. Ghani, S. Bibi, Z. Wang, R. Pei, Recent advances in nanocomposite-based delivery systems for targeted CRISPR/Cas delivery and therapeutic genetic manipulation, *Journal of Materials Chemistry B*, 11(2023) 5251–71.
13. H.-J. Kim, N.D. Le, H.-J. Oh, B. Kim, E. Yoo, J. Kim, et al., Lipid nanoparticle-assisted mRNA therapy for cancer treatment, *Applied Physics Reviews*, 12(2025) 031328.
14. X. Huang, N. Kong, X. Zhang, Y. Cao, R. Langer, W. Tao, The landscape of mRNA nanomedicine, *Nature Medicine*, 28(2022) 2273–87.
15. J.V. Vaghasiya, C.C. Mayorga-Martinez, M. Pumera, Wearable sensors for telehealth based on emerging materials and nanoarchitectonics, *npj Flexible Electronics*, 7(2023) 26.
16. C.D. Flynn, D. Chang, A. Mahmud, H. Yousefi, J. Das, K.T. Riordan, et al., Biomolecular sensors for advanced physiological monitoring, *Nature Reviews Bioengineering*, 1(2023) 560–75.
17. L. Rao, Y. Yuan, X. Shen, G. Yu, X. Chen, Designing nanotheranostics with machine learning, *Nature Nanotechnology*, 19(2024) 1769–81.
18. S. Chakroborty, N. Nath, S. Sahoo, B.P. Singh, T. Bal, K. Tiwari, et al., A review of emerging trends in nanomaterial-driven ai for biomedical application, *Nanoscale Advances*, 7(2025) 3619–30.

2 Advances of Nanotechnology for Virology

Detection, Treatment, and Vaccines

Enoch Y. Park

2.1 INTRODUCTION

Virology, the study of viruses and their interactions with hosts, has undergone a significant shift in recent decades, driven by the emergence of nanotechnology as a transformative tool. Traditional virological methods, while powerful, often face limitations in sensitivity, speed, and specificity when detecting, monitoring, or combating viral pathogens. The advent of nanoscale science has opened new frontiers by enabling precise manipulation of matter at molecular and atomic levels, offering unprecedented opportunities for viral diagnostics, prevention, and therapeutics (Figure 2.1). Nanotechnology provides a versatile platform for addressing challenges across the entire spectrum of virology, from early and ultra-sensitive detection of viral particles to the development of targeted antiviral delivery systems and next-generation vaccines. Nanomaterials such as gold nanoparticles (AuNPs), quantum dots (QDs), liposomes, polymeric nanocarriers, carbon-based nanostructures, and metal–organic frameworks have demonstrated remarkable capabilities in enhancing the signal transduction, biocompatibility, and stability of virological tools. Their tunable physicochemical properties, high surface-to-volume ratios, and ease of functionalization with biomolecules such as antibodies, aptamers, or nucleic acids make them ideal candidates for interacting with viruses at the same size scale.

The recent global outbreaks of emerging and re-emerging viruses, including SARS-CoV-2, Zika, Ebola, and influenza, have underscored the urgent need for rapid, accurate, and cost-effective strategies in virology. Nanotechnology-driven innovations have already accelerated the development of point-of-care diagnostic devices, real-time viral imaging platforms, and nanoparticle-based vaccine adjuvants. Moreover, the convergence of nanotechnology with molecular biology, synthetic biology, and computational modeling is enabling integrated approaches for virus tracking, early-stage infection diagnosis, and precise antiviral therapy with minimal off-target effects. This chapter provides a comprehensive overview of recent progress in virology through the lens of nanotechnology, highlighting advances in

DOI: 10.1201/9781003725930-2

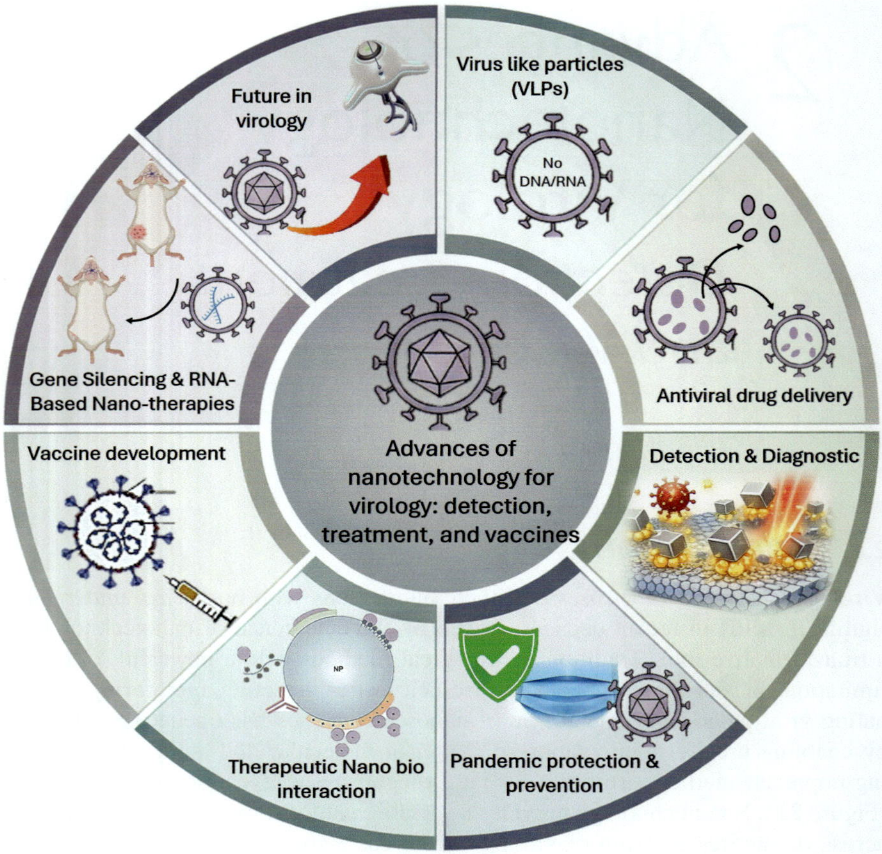

FIGURE 2.1 An illustration of virus-linked applications involving nanotechnology.

nano-enabled viral diagnostics, therapeutics, and preventive strategies. It also examines current challenges, translational opportunities, and the future goal for nanotechnology-driven virology in addressing public health threats. By bridging the nanoscale design of materials with the complexities of viral pathogenesis, this interdisciplinary domain promises to redefine how viral diseases are detected, understood, and treated in the coming decades.

2.2 ESSENTIAL ROLE OF NANOMATERIALS FOR VIRUS DETECTION

Nanomaterials have revolutionized viral diagnostics by enhancing sensitivity, reducing assay time, enabling point-of-care formats, and facilitating multiplexed readouts. Their unique physical properties, localized surface plasmon resonance (LSPR) in noble metal nanoparticles, size-tunable fluorescence in QDs, high surface area and conductivity in graphene and other two-dimensional (2D) materials, magnetic responsiveness of iron oxide nanoparticles, and the electromagnetic hotspots of surface-enhanced Raman scattering (SERS) substrates, are routinely explored to convert a biomolecular recognition event into a measurable optical, electrical, or other spectral signals (Figure 2.2). Over the past decade, these platforms have advanced from proof-of-concept studies to field-deployable tests and clinical prototypes, notably during the SARS-CoV-2 pandemic, where rapid, sensitive, and mass-deployable tests were urgently required.

2.2.1 Gold Nanoparticles (AuNPs) in Colorimetric Assays

AuNPs are among the earliest and most widely used nanomaterials in diagnostic assays because of easy synthesis, robust surface chemistry (thiol-gold linkage), strong LSPR that produces intense colors, and a visible color change when particles

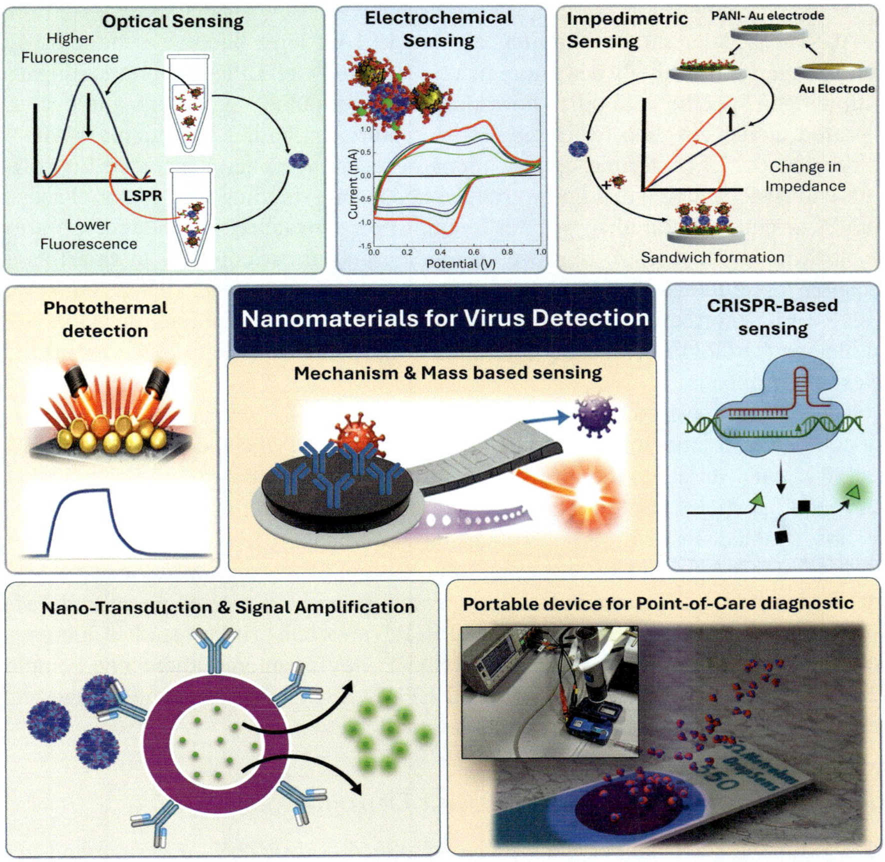

FIGURE 2.2 Various sensing applications using emerging nanomaterials.

aggregate or change size. Monodisperse spherical AuNPs of ~10–40 nm appear red in colloidal suspension due to LSPR; upon aggregation (e.g., caused by crosslinking via target-mediated bridging or by salt-induced destabilization), the plasmon band red-shifts and broadens, producing a purple/blue color. Simple aggregation-based assays exploit this effect: probes (antibodies, oligonucleotides, or aptamers) are bound to AuNPs so that, in the presence of the viral target (antigen or nucleic acid), crosslinking causes immediate aggregation and a visible color change detectable by eye or quantified by spectrophotometry. This mechanism underlies many rapid, low-cost colorimetric tests and has been widely applied in the development of SARS-CoV-2 assays. Colorimetric assays are inexpensive, rapid (minutes), and do not always require instrumentation, making them ideal for resource-limited settings. They are flexible (detect proteins, nucleic acids, or whole particles) and work well in lateral flow formats and microfluidic strips when integrated with membranes and control lines. However, their sensitivity can be limited by the detection threshold for observable color changes; signal amplification strategies and dual-mode readouts (colorimetric + fluorescence/electrochemical) have thus been developed to further lower the detection limits.

AuNP-based lateral flow immunoassays (LFIAs) have become a standard for rapid antigen and antibody detection. In a typical sandwich LFIA, AuNPs conjugated with antigen-specific antibodies flow along a nitrocellulose membrane and become captured at the test line by immobilized capture antibodies, producing a visible colored stripe. LFIA format optimizations in recent years have included improved AuNP surface functionalization to reduce nonspecific binding, the use of clustered AuNPs or nanostructured aggregates to amplify the visual signal, the incorporation of blocking chemistries to improve specificity, and direct coupling to smartphone imaging for semiquantitative readout. During the COVID-19 pandemic, numerous AuNP LFIAs were developed for either viral antigen (rapid antigen tests) or host antibodies (serology), with design iterations improving sensitivity toward clinically relevant viral loads.

However, in most colorimetric assays, key limitations include reduced sensitivity compared to laboratory RT-PCR for low viral loads and the potential for false negatives early or late in the infection. Innovations to overcome these issues include dual-mode particles (colorimetric + fluorescent), enzymatic or nucleic acid amplification coupled upstream (e.g., isothermal amplification feeding into LFIA), and integration of sample preconcentration steps. Recent papers also describe engineered AuNP clusters that enhance colorimetric response without sacrificing colloidal stability, improving visual detection thresholds. Reviews and primary studies document AuNP LFIAs for influenza, dengue, and SARS-CoV-2, among others; one comprehensive review summarizes AuNP-based LFIAs in COVID-19 diagnosis and suggests improvements for robustness and variant detection.

2.2.2 Quantum Dots for Fluorescent Detection

QDs, semiconductor nanocrystals such as CdSe/ZnS, InP/ZnS, or carbon and graphene QDs, exhibit size-tunable, bright fluorescence with high quantum yields and narrow emission spectra. Their resistance to photobleaching and potential for surface functionalization make them well suited to sensitive fluorescent immunoassays and nucleic acid detection. QDs are particularly advantageous for multiplexed assays because different-sized QDs can be excited with a single wavelength but emit at spectrally distinct wavelengths, allowing for the simultaneous detection of multiple viral targets in a single assay channel.

QD-based LFIAs and microarray formats exploit the narrow emission peaks of QDs to label different antibodies or probes, each with a QD of distinct emissions. When combined with a spectrally resolving reader (portable fluorimeter or smartphone with filters), the presence and relative abundance of multiple antigens or antibodies can be read from a single test. This is especially useful in respiratory panels, where differentiating between influenza, respiratory syncytial virus (RSV), and SARS-CoV-2 in a single test is clinically advantageous. QDs can be coupled with signal-amplifying chemistries, such as time-resolved fluorescence to suppress background, Förster resonance energy transfer arrangements for target-dependent quenching/recovery, or enzymatic amplification driving cumulative fluorescent product formation, achieving detection limits that rival or approach those of nucleic acid amplification tests in some formats.

Carbon QDs and doped QDs are also being explored for safer, heavy metal–free options for clinical use. Toxicity concerns regarding heavy-metal QDs (e.g., cadmium, lead) have driven the development of indium phosphide and carbon QDs; however, regulatory acceptance for human diagnostics requires comprehensive biocompatibility data. Integrating low-cost readers is another challenge, as spectral-resolving readers are available; broad deployment requires simplified optics or smartphone-based solutions. The commercialization of QD LFIAs has been slower than that of AuNP LFIAs; however, ongoing advances in QD chemistry and miniaturized optics make clinical translation a promising prospect. QD-based multiplexed LFIAs have been developed for COVID-19 antigen/antibody panels, dengue/arbovirus panels, and simultaneous detection of different influenza strains.

2.2.3 Graphene and 2D Nanomaterials for Electrochemical Sensing

Voltametric and electrochemical impedance spectroscopy (EIS) have emerged as highly effective transduction techniques for virus biosensors based on graphene and other 2D nanomaterials. In a typical EIS biosensor, viral recognition elements, such as antibodies, aptamers, or nucleic acid probes, are immobilized onto the surface of graphene or a 2D material. The binding of viral antigens or nucleic acids induces measurable changes in charge transfer resistance or double-layer capacitance at the electrode–electrolyte interface. This label-free detection approach enables real-time monitoring with high sensitivity, often down to femtomolar concentrations, and is compatible with portable, low-power instrumentation. For example, graphene oxide– or molybdenum disulfide–modified electrodes have been developed for detecting SARS-CoV-2 spike proteins and influenza RNA, achieving rapid response times and strong specificity through optimized surface functionalization. Despite challenges such as nonspecific adsorption and device reproducibility, the integration of EIS-based graphene/2D material biosensors with microfluidic sample handling is making them increasingly viable for point-of-care viral diagnostics.

2.2.3.1 Field-Effect Transistor (FET) Biosensors

Graphene and related 2D materials (graphene oxide, molybdenum disulfide, etc.) are excellent transducer materials for label-free electrical biosensors because of their exceptional charge carrier mobility, large surface area, and atomically thin channels (making them exquisitely sensitive to surface charge changes). In a graphene-based FET biosensor, biomolecular recognition elements (antibodies, aptamers, or receptor proteins) are immobilized on the graphene channel. The binding of charged viral particles or proteins modulates the local electrostatic environment, altering the current–voltage characteristics and producing an electrical signal. FETs have demonstrated ultralow detection limits in some reports, down to single-virus or femtomolar antigen concentrations, and rapid, real-time detection without the need for labels.

The functionalized FET biosensor demonstrated rapid detection in clinical matrices (saliva, nasopharyngeal swabs) with sensitivity and response times superior to those of many optical assays. Advances include laser-induced graphene platforms and surface chemistries that improve reproducibility and minimize nonspecific adsorption. FETs offer label-free, real-time measurements and can be miniaturized into multiplexed arrays. Challenges include device-to-device variability, drift in clinical matrices, fouling, and the need for stable, reproducible functionalization chemistries. Precise surface engineering (blocking layers, antifouling polymers) and microfluidic sample handling have been shown to overcome some of these practical issues.

2.2.3.2 Label-Free Detection Approaches Using Other 2D Materials

Beyond graphene, transition metal dichalcogenides and MXenes (a 2D nanosheet material composed of transition metals such as titanium (Ti) and vanadium (V), along with carbon (C) and nitrogen (N), with a thickness of several nanometers) have been explored for electrochemical and impedimetric sensing; their semiconducting behavior and tunable bandgaps provide alternative electronic transduction methods for label-free viral detection. Electrochemical sensors based on nanostructured 2D films also exhibit rapid response and compatibility with low-cost potentiostats, making them attractive for decentralized testing when paired with suitable biorecognition elements.

2.2.4 Magnetic Nanoparticles for Viral Enrichment

Magnetic nanoparticles (MNPs, typically iron oxide cores with polymer or silica shells) are widely used for sample preparation, target enrichment, and as transducers in magnetic biosensing. Their principal utility in viral diagnostics stems from two functions: (i) magnetic separation/enrichment of low-abundance targets from complex matrices (blood, saliva, wastewater) by functionalizing MNPs with capture ligands (antibodies, lectins, aptamers), and (ii) transduction in magnetic sensors (magnetoresistive sensors, magnetic relaxation switches) that detect the presence of bound targets. Magnetic enrichment concentrates viral antigens or nucleic acids from large volumes, improving sensitivity and reducing interference from matrix components. A common workflow uses MNPs to capture and magnetically pellet the virus or viral RNA, wash away inhibitors, and then elute material for downstream amplification (RT-PCR, isothermal amplification) or direct detection via magnetoresistive sensors. Magnetic relaxation switches (where clustering alters relaxation times) and giant magnetoresistance sensors have been applied to detect viral particles with high sensitivity in miniaturized formats.

2.2.5 Surface-Enhanced Raman Scattering (SERS) Nanostructures

SERS relies on large electromagnetic field enhancements produced near metallic nanostructures, such as typically roughened Au or Ag nanostructures, nanoparticle aggregates, or specifically designed nanogap substrates. Molecules in the enhanced near-field experience greatly amplified Raman scattering, often enabling single-molecule detection. For viral detection, SERS can provide a highly specific spectral "fingerprint" of viral proteins, nucleic acids, or reporter molecules labeled with SERS-active agents. Because Raman spectra are rich in vibrational information, SERS can discriminate closely related biomarkers and, when combined with chemometric or machine learning (ML) analysis, can classify viruses or strains. Label-free SERS aims to detect intrinsic viral signatures, but complex biological matrices can mask weak signals.

In contrast, labeled SERS, where analyte binding brings tagged-reporter molecules, called nanotags, into SERS-active hotspots, offers higher sensitivity and more robust readouts. Polymeric cocoon and stimuli-responsive properties of nanotags have been used to encapsulate SERS nanotags containing plasmonic molybdenum trioxide QDs (MoO_3-QDs). The pH-controlled release of the encapsulated nanotags and their subsequent localization by maleimide-functionalized MNPs facilitated the creation of hotspot regions with catalyzed SERS activities (Figure 2.3). This approach led to the development of a biosensing platform for ultra-sensitive immunoassays of hepatitis E virus (HEV) and norovirus (NoV) with detection limits of 6.5 and 8.2 fg/mL, respectively [1]. The signal enhancement factor of the SERS-based technique reached up to $\sim 10^8$ due to the combined electromagnetic and chemical mechanisms of the employed dual-SERS substrate, consisting of MoO_3-QDs/2D hexagonal boron nitride (h-BN) nanosheets [2].

SERS-based assays have been used to detect influenza, SARS-CoV-2 [3], and other respiratory viruses with rapid turnaround and high specificity. Coupling SERS with microfluidics and automated spectral analysis has produced portable systems capable of differentiating multiple viral species in clinical samples. However, challenges remain regarding substrate reproducibility and cost for widescale commercial deployment.

2.2.6 Challenges, Regulatory, and Future Directions

While nanomaterial-enabled diagnostics offer technical advantages, challenges must be addressed for routine clinical use. Standardization of nanomaterial synthesis and functionalization to ensure batch-to-batch reproducibility is a major challenge for biosensors to replace standard PCR or ELISA-based analyses. Ongoing efforts in engineered, reproducible nanofabrication (for SERS substrates and FETs) and integrated sample-to-answer systems (magnetic enrichment + isothermal amplification + LFIA/GFET readout) promise to broaden adoption in both high- and low-resource

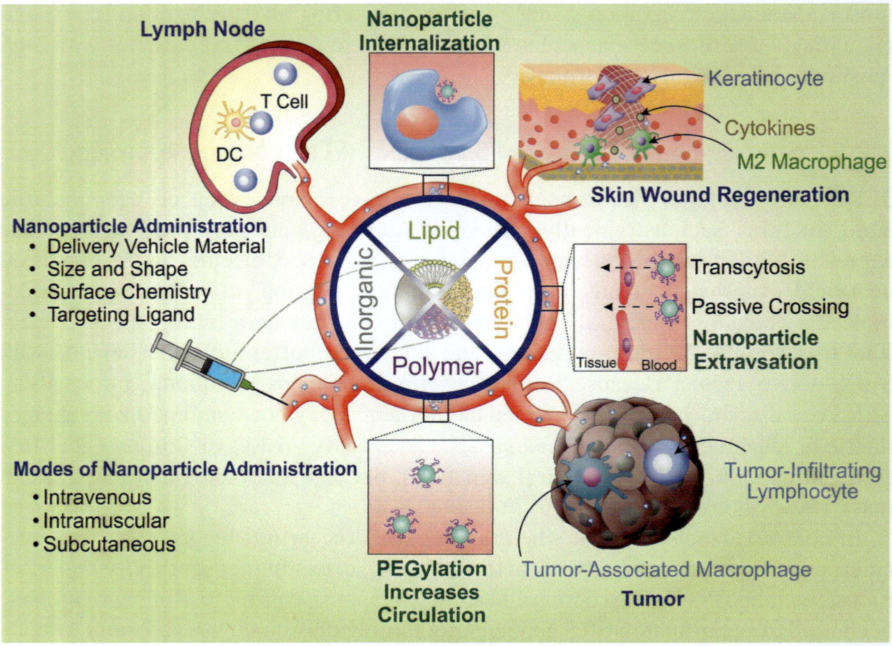

FIGURE 2.3 Nanotechnology-enabled immunoengineering approaches to advance therapeutic applications. (Adapted from Ref. [6] (CC BY).)

settings. The next wave of devices will likely be hybrid platforms that combine the speed and accessibility of LFIAs with the sensitivity of electrical or spectral readouts, packaged in manufacturable, low-cost formats that meet regulatory and safety standards for clinical use deployment.

2.3 NANOTECHNOLOGY IN VIRAL THERAPEUTICS

Conventional small-molecule antivirals, although effective, often suffer from low bioavailability, poor tissue targeting, and a requirement for high systemic doses, which can lead to increased off-target effects. Nanotechnology offers solutions through engineered platforms that improve drug delivery, enable nucleic acid-based therapeutics, and enhance vaccine efficacy through novel nanoformulations. These include liposomes, polymeric nanoparticles, dendrimers, RNA nanocarriers, CRISPR-nanoplatforms, nanoadjuvants, and virus-like particles (VLPs). Over the past decade, many of these technologies have advanced from concept to preclinical or even clinical stages.

2.3.1 Nanocarriers for Antiviral Drug Delivery

Liposomes: These spherical vesicles, composed of lipid bilayers surrounding aqueous cores, have long been exploited for drug delivery due to their biocompatibility and customizable properties. Liposomal formulations shield drugs from degradation, improve pharmacokinetics, enable encapsulation of both hydrophilic and lipophilic antivirals, and permit passive and active targeting (e.g., PEGylation or ligand conjugation). Notably, liposomal formulations of interferon-α and acyclovir show improved biodistribution and efficacy in herpesvirus infections. During the COVID-19 pandemic, lipid nanoparticle (LNP) delivery systems played a crucial role in the success of mRNA vaccines. Although mRNA vaccine delivery overlaps with vaccine development, LNPs are also being explored for delivering small-molecule antivirals and RNA-based therapeutics.

Polymeric Nanoparticles: Composed of biodegradable materials such as poly(lactic-co-glycolic acid) (PLGA), can encapsulate drugs for sustained release. Functionalized with targeting ligands (e.g., antibodies, peptides) or surface-modified with polyethylene glycol (PEG) for stealth properties, polymeric nanoparticles can enhance the delivery of antivirals such as remdesivir and ribavirin to infected tissues, including the lungs. Preclinical trials demonstrate improved viral clearance and reduced inflammation in animal models.

Dendrimers: These are highly branched, tree-like macromolecules with tunable surface groups, that enable multivalent binding and precise molecular architecture. Antiviral dendrimers (e.g., SPL7013, astodrimer sodium) can bind viral envelope proteins and block virus–cell interactions, functioning as entry inhibitors. Dendrimer-based formulations are particularly explored for topical prophylaxis against Herpes simplex virus type 2 and SARS-CoV-2 in mucosal applications.

VLPs: VLPs derived from various viruses have been used for gene and drug delivery systems. Since VLPs possess properties similar to intact viruses but lack the genomic DNA or RNA that encodes viral proteins, safety concerns associated with the use of inactivated or attenuated viruses can be mitigated, particularly for in vivo applications of VLPs. Additionally, VLPs have an empty interior that can be filled with various materials, including nucleic acids and nanoparticles, for gene and drug delivery.

VLPs can be functionalized using various methods to confer nanoparticle specificity. The surface and interior of VLPs can be tailored for specific functions, including cell specificity, antigen display, and stabilization via chemical and genetic modifications. The surface of VLPs can be functionalized via covalent binding of amino acid residues, such as lysine and cysteine, which is an irreversible reaction that promotes long-term binding to targets. Alternatively, peptides and proteins can be displayed on the surface of non-enveloped VLPs via fusion with viral capsid proteins. Fusion of a foreign protein with the full-length or transmembrane domain of a viral envelope protein enables its display on the surface of VLPs. Additionally, foreign transmembrane proteins can be displayed on enveloped VLPs through co-expression in host cells, enabling the creation of multifunctional VLPs. To provide the specific binding to cancer cells, a single-chain variable fragment (scFv) of humanized CC49 antibody (hCC49), specifically binding to tumor-associated glycoprotein 72 of cancer cells, was displayed on the surface of Rous sarcoma virus-like particles (RSV-LPs) by the fusion of the transmembrane and cytoplasmic domains of hemagglutinin of influenza A (H1N1). Additionally, doxorubicin (DOX) was incorporated into hCC49 scFv-displaying RSV-LPs, enabling specific targeting of LS174T cancer cells. The DOX-loaded hCC49 scFv-displaying RSV-LPs effectively killed LS174T cells through targeted delivery, but HEK293 cells remained alive even in the presence of the DOX-loaded carriers [4]. Chimeric VLPs composed of two capsid proteins, gag and M1, from the influenza virus have shown potential as drug delivery systems. These chimeric VLPs displayed a glycosylphosphatidylinositol-anchored scFv region that targeted colon carcinoma cells and were packaged with doxorubicin [5]. These functionalized VLPs demonstrated high specificity for cancer cells and successfully delivered the drug to them.

2.3.2 Gene Silencing and RNA-Based Nanotherapies

2.3.2.1 siRNA Delivery Using Nanocarriers

RNA interference, using small interfering RNA (siRNA), enables the selective degradation of viral RNA, providing a potent means of inhibiting replication. However, naked siRNA is unstable, immunogenic, and poorly taken up by cells; nanocarriers address these issues by protecting siRNA and facilitating its delivery to target cells. LNPs have emerged as the leading vectors for siRNA delivery. They encapsulate siRNA within ionizable lipids that bind RNA in acidic liposomal cores and release it in the cytosol after endosomal escape. LNP-mediated siRNA delivery demonstrated proof of concept against Zika virus, influenza, and RSV in animal models, resulting in a significant reduction in viral titers.

Polymeric carriers such as polyethyleneimine (PEI), chitosan, and dendrimeric polymers have also been used to condense siRNA into polyplexes. Surface functionalization with targeting ligands (e.g., transferrin or viral receptor mimics) enhances tissue specificity. Toxicity concerns with PEI are being addressed using biodegradable, modified polymers (e.g., PEG-PEI copolymers). Animal models show siRNA nanocarriers reduce viral loads and improve survival in lethal viral infections. For example, an inhalable LNP platform delivering siRNA against influenza A decreased viral titers and lung pathology in mice.

2.3.2.2 CRISPR-Cas Systems with Nanoplatforms

CRISPR diagnostics and therapeutics have expanded rapidly. CRISPR systems, such as Cas13, have been repurposed for direct cleavage of viral RNA. Delivery of CRISPR-Cas components (Cas protein + guide RNA) via nanocarriers offers potential for antiviral or rapid therapeutic interventions. Analogous to mRNA vaccines, LNPs deliver Cas13 mRNA and guide RNA; upon expression, Cas13 cleaves viral RNA selectively. In vitro and animal studies targeting SARS-CoV-2 and influenza show robust reduction in viral titers without host genome editing. Researchers are also exploring polymeric nanoparticles and engineered extracellular vesicles to deliver CRISPR components to respiratory epithelial cells, thereby enabling noninvasive, inhalable therapy. These approaches aim for organ-specific delivery, reduced immunogenicity, and multiplex targeting of viral variants.

2.3.3 Nanoadjuvants for Enhanced Immune Response

To enhance the immunogenicity of subunit or inactivated vaccines, adjuvants are used to improve antigen display, stimulate immune activation, and modulate immune polarization. Nanoadjuvants, which serve as both antigen delivery vehicles and immunostimulatory agents, are gaining prominence as nanoparticle carriers.

Traditional aluminum (alum) adjuvants, such as oil-in-water emulsions (MF59), liposomes, ISCOMs (immune-stimulating complexes), and polymeric nanoparticles, augment immunogenicity with reduced side effects. For example, influenza vaccines formulated with MF59 or liposomal adjuvants generate robust neutralizing antibody and T-cell responses, often at reduced antigen doses.

Recent developments include nanoparticle platforms that co-deliver antigen and immunostimulatory molecules (e.g., TLR agonists) within the same particle, achieving localized activation of antigen-presenting cells. Nanoadjuvants designed for mucosal (intranasal) vaccination have shown promise in stimulating mucosal immunity, which is especially crucial for respiratory viruses.

2.3.3.1 Virus-Like Particles

VLPs are the most promising vaccine platforms, as they closely mimic the native structural organization of viruses while lacking the viral genome, thereby eliminating the risk of infection or replication. VLPs are derived from animal viruses, bacteriophages, or plant viruses and are actively studied and developed for various applications [7]. The viral genome infects host cells and is transcribed in the nucleus. The resulting mRNAs are translated, forming capsid or coat protein (1 of Figure 2.4), and membrane proteins are produced through the same process. After post-translational modification, these proteins are transported to the cell membrane (2 of Figure 2.4). Capsids self-assembled inside the cell membrane and bud off, forming VLPs enveloped by the cell membrane (3 of Figure 2.4), called an enveloped VLP (4 and a of Figure 2.4). Occasionally, these VLP acquire multiple layers, becoming multilayered VLPs (b of Figure 2.4). In contrast, capsid proteins are self-assembled into icosahedral structures, forming non-enveloped VLPs (5 and c of Figure 2.4).

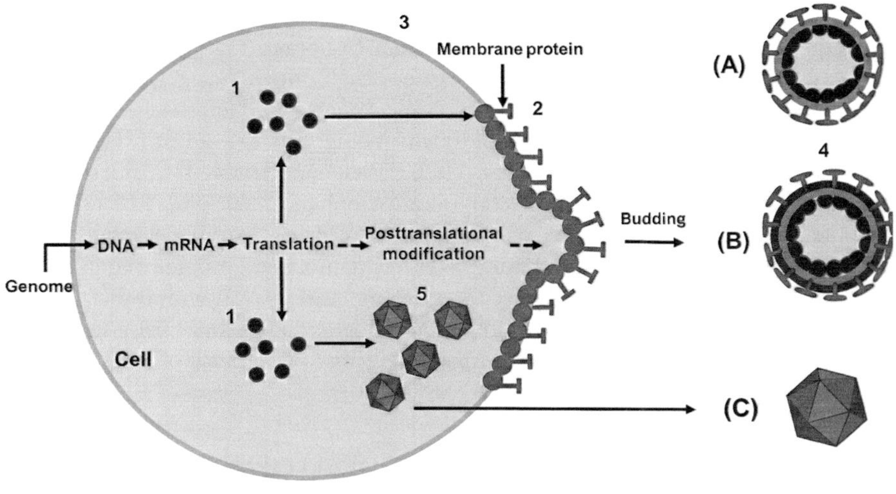

FIGURE 2.4 Schematic representation of the process of enveloped VLP (a), multilayered VLP (b), and non-enveloped VLP (c). 1 and 2, capsid and membrane proteins; 3, cell membrane; 4 and 5, enveloped VLP and non-enveloped VLP. (Adapted from Ref. [7] with permission from Elsevier.)

Composed of self-assembling viral structural proteins, VLPs present repetitive conformational epitopes on their surface that strongly stimulate the immune system, efficiently activating both B-cell and T-cell responses, often without the need for additional adjuvants. Their high immunogenicity has been validated by licensed vaccines against the hepatitis B virus (HBV) and human papillomavirus (HPV), which remain among the most successful examples of VLP technology in clinical use.

2.3.3.2 Hybrid Systems Combine Features Across Nanotechnology

Hybrid nanotechnology platforms are emerging as next-generation antiviral strategies by combining complementary modalities into a single system to achieve synergistic therapeutic effects. One promising approach involves LNPs co-loaded with siRNA and conventional antiviral drugs, where siRNA silences viral gene expression at the genetic level. In contrast, the drug simultaneously disrupts viral replication or assembly pathways. This dual-action mechanism has demonstrated superior efficacy in animal models of influenza and Zika virus infection, with enhanced viral clearance and reduced drug doses compared with monotherapies, thereby minimizing toxicity. Another innovative strategy under development involves engineering VLPs to encapsulate CRISPR-Cas components, such as Cas proteins and guide RNAs, within their protein shells. By mimicking the structure and cell-targeting properties of natural viruses, these CRISPR-loaded VLPs can selectively deliver gene-editing machinery to infected cells, enabling precise cleavage of viral genomes while avoiding off-target effects in healthy tissues. Although still in the early stages of preclinical exploration, such hybrid systems illustrate the potential of integrating delivery efficiency, immune stimulation, and precision editing into unified nanoplatforms. Collectively, these multifunctional designs represent a paradigm shift in antiviral therapy, moving beyond single-modality treatments toward combinatorial, highly adaptable platforms tailored to counter both existing and emerging viral threats.

Nanotechnology has transformed viral therapeutics by enabling advanced delivery and treatment strategies. Nanocarriers, including liposomes, biodegradable polymers, and dendrimers, enhance antiviral efficacy by improving targeting, sustaining release, and reducing toxicity. Meanwhile, nucleic acid–based approaches, including siRNA and CRISPR therapies, are rapidly advancing with the aid of LNP delivery systems and novel targeting mechanisms. In parallel, nano-enabled vaccines, including those leveraging nanoadjuvants for immune enhancement and VLPs for safe yet potent antigen display, represent the forefront of next-generation vaccine development. Together, these nanotechnology-driven approaches provide modular and adaptable platforms for rapid response to emerging viral threats, with future translation relying on the continued integration of targeting ligands, stimuli-responsive features, enhanced stability, and scalable manufacturing to accelerate clinical adoption and pandemic preparedness.

2.4 NANOPARTICLE-BASED VACCINE DEVELOPMENT

Vaccine development is a complex, multistage process that begins with identifying the pathogen and its key antigens, the molecular structures that trigger an immune response. Once a suitable antigen is selected, researchers design a vaccine platform, which may include traditional approaches such as inactivated or live-attenuated pathogens, or modern technologies like protein subunits, VLPs, DNA, or mRNA. Preclinical studies follow this in cell cultures and animal models to evaluate safety, immunogenicity, and potential efficacy.

Promising candidates then progress to clinical trials, conducted in three phases: Phase I tests safety and dosage in small groups of healthy volunteers, Phase II evaluates immune responses in larger populations, and Phase III involves thousands of participants to confirm efficacy and monitor rare side effects. Regulatory agencies review the results before approving public use. Even after approval, post-marketing surveillance (Phase IV) ensures the long-term safety and effectiveness of a product in real-world populations. Throughout this process, advances in biotechnology, nanotechnology, and computational modeling have accelerated vaccine development, exemplified by the rapid creation of mRNA-based vaccines against COVID-19.

The emergence of nanotechnology as a transformative platform in vaccinology has fundamentally altered how vaccines are designed, manufactured, and delivered. Nanoparticle-based vaccines, encompassing LNPs, VLPs, polymeric carriers, inorganic nanostructures, and hybrid systems, offer distinct advantages over conventional vaccine formats in terms of antigen stability, targeted delivery, controlled release, and enhanced immunogenicity. Unlike traditional vaccines that rely on attenuated or inactivated viruses, nanoparticle vaccines often focus on presenting purified antigens, recombinant proteins, or nucleic acids in a way that mimics natural infection without introducing pathogenic genetic material. This design reduces safety concerns while preserving or even amplifying the immune-stimulating properties of the antigen. Nanoparticle systems also enable the integration of adjuvant properties directly into the delivery vehicle. The result is a combined antigen–adjuvant package capable of inducing robust humoral and cellular immune responses. This synergistic approach is particularly useful against viruses with high mutation rates or complex immune evasion strategies, such as influenza, HIV, and SARS-CoV-2. Furthermore, nanoparticle-based vaccines allow for flexible antigen display geometries, enabling precise spatial orientation and density of epitopes, which are known to influence B-cell receptor crosslinking and subsequent immune activation strongly. The following subsections examine major nanoparticle vaccine strategies and platforms, focusing on VLPs, nanoadjuvants, LNP delivery for mRNA vaccines, and multivalent antigen display. Case studies of real-world applications, including those for COVID-19, HPV, and RSV vaccines, are integrated to illustrate the translational impact of the findings.

2.4.1 VLPs and Their Engineering

VLPs can be engineered by modifying their surface, allowing for the exploration of various vaccine applications. The enveloped VLPs and non-enveloped VLPs will be modified for the most popular vaccine applications. In the case of enveloped VLPs, a desired antigen can be displayed by fusing it to a viral membrane protein or a transmembrane domain [4,5,8] (Figure 2.5a), or by co-expressing it in the same cells (Figure 2.5b) [9–11]. Non-enveloped VLPs lack an outer envelope, making it difficult to display antigens through co-expression with structural proteins. To display

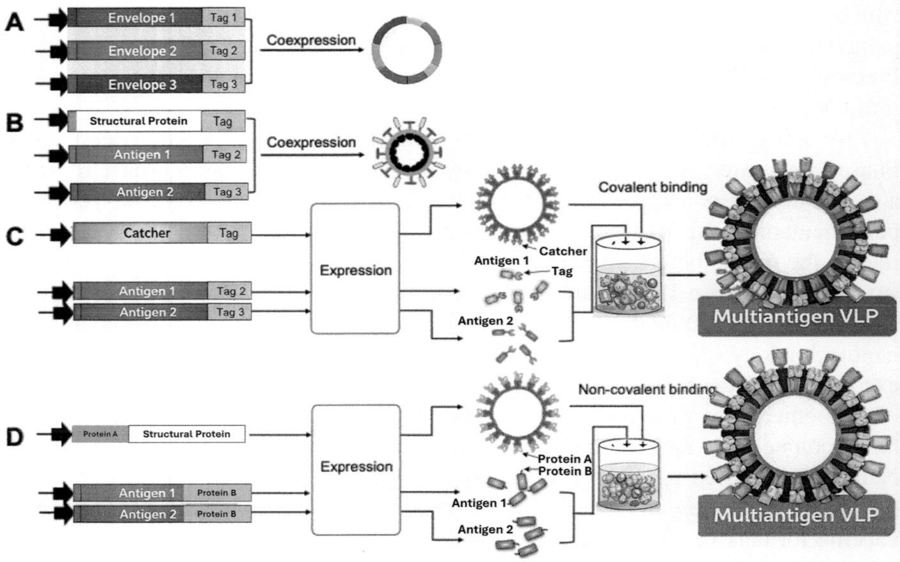

FIGURE 2.5 Antigens display concepts on the VLP surface modified from (a) co-expression of multiple envelope proteins to create multivalent enveloped VLPs. (b) Display of tagged antigens on enveloped VLP surfaces. (c) Catcher-fused scaffold VLPs and tagged antigens are expressed, purified individually, and conjugated via tag–catcher covalent binding to display multiple antigens on non-enveloped VLPs. (d) Protein A-fused scaffold VLPs and protein B-fused antigens are expressed, purified individually, and conjugated via protein A and protein B interaction to display multiple antigens on the non-enveloped VLPs. (Adapted from Ref. [7] with permission from Elsevier.)

antigens on their surface, binding interactions between antigens and structural proteins are necessary. This can be achieved through covalent or non-covalent binding. In covalent binding, "Catcher" and "Tag" are fused to either the structural protein's N-terminus or the antigen's C-terminus (Figure 2.5c) [12–15]. One significant "Catcher" and "Tag" is the isopeptide bond discovered in the fibronectin-binding protein (FbaB) of the Gram-positive pathogen *Streptococcus pyogenes* [16]. The second immunoglobulin-like collagen adhesin domain (CnaB2) of FbaB plays a crucial role in the phagocytosis-like uptake of *S. pyogenes* by endothelial cells [17]. The CnaB2 can be split into two components: a C-terminal peptide with 13 amino acids (SpyTag) and an N-terminal protein fragment with 138 amino acids (15 kDa) (SpyCatcher) [18]. The SpyTag (SpT) peptide contains a reactive Asp^{117} that quickly forms a covalent isopeptide bond with a Lys^{31} residue in SpyCatcher (SpC), a protein partner derived from the CnaB2. In this reaction, Glu^{77} of the SpC and Asp^{117} of SpT are essential for the formation of the covalent isopeptide bond. In *Streptococcus pneumoniae*, the D4 immunoglobulin-like domain of RrgA also forms the isopeptide bond between Lys^{742} and Asn^{854} residues. The D4 domain in the loop following the N-terminal β-strand was split into two partners: the peptide tag containing residues 734–745 (SnoopTag) and the protein partner containing residues 749–860

(SnoopCatcher) [19]. Non-covalent binding involves protein–protein interactions or affinity binding, in which "Protein A" is fused to the N-terminus of the structural protein and "Protein B" to the C-terminus of the antigen (Figure 2.5d). A particularly exciting innovation is the development of engineered, or "mosaic," VLPs that display antigens from multiple viral strains or variants on a single particle, broadening protective efficacy and addressing viral diversity. For instance, multivalent VLPs displaying spike proteins from different SARS-CoV-2 variants have been shown to elicit cross-neutralizing antibody responses, thereby paving the way for more effective vaccine strategies. Their high immunogenicity has been validated by licensed vaccines against the HBV and HPV, which remain among the most successful examples of VLP technology in clinical use. Experimental VLP vaccines against influenza, Zika virus, and SARS-CoV-2 have advanced to clinical trials, where they have demonstrated favorable safety profiles and strong immunogenicity.

Scalable production methods, such as molecular farming in plants like *Nicotiana benthamiana* and baculovirus-based expression in insect cells, have further expanded the feasibility of VLP-based therapeutics by reducing costs and enabling a rapid response to emerging outbreaks. Alternatively, silkworms are recognized as promising hosts for the mass production of VLPs. They have been utilized to meet human needs for over 5,000 years, with silk derived from silkworms holding significant economic importance for centuries. More recently, silkworms have gained attention in biopharmaceuticals for their ability to express eukaryotic recombinant proteins that require post-translational modifications. In 1985, silkworm larvae became the first in the world to demonstrate the ability to produce recombinant protein [20,21]. Since then, various approaches have been developed to express recombinant proteins in silkworms. Silkworm (*Bombyx mori*) larvae, which undergo modifications similar to those in mammalian cells, offer a cost-effective method for high-yield protein production [7,22,23]. With their excellent safety, adaptability, and potent immunogenicity, VLPs are positioned as a versatile vaccine platform capable of addressing both current viral threats and future pandemic challenges.

2.4.2 Multivalent Nanoparticle Vaccine Platforms

Viruses with high mutation rates or multiple serotypes pose challenges for traditional vaccines, and multivalent nanoparticle platforms address this by combining multiple antigens into a single construct. These vaccines can be engineered through surface conjugation, where distinct antigens are physically displayed on the nanoparticle; genetic fusion, where multiple antigenic sequences are encoded within a protein that self-assembles on a nanoparticle scaffold; or layer-by-layer assembly, where alternating antigen and adjuvant coatings are applied around a core.

SpT/SpC chemical conjugation is very convenient for preparing multivalent VLPs. In a malaria vaccine, target antigens of multiple lifecycle stages are required to prevent infection by *Plasmodium* parasites. Bivalent VLPs displaying *Plasmodium yoelii* Merozoite surface protein-1 p19 (PyMSP1-19) and Circumsporozoite protein (PyCSP) as antigens for the erythrocytic blood stage and the hepatocyte invasion stage, respectively, were developed [24]. PyMSP1-19 and PyCSP were fused to SpCΔNΔC, which lacks VTTLSGLSGEQGPSGDMTTEE at the N-terminus and

EATKGDAHT at the C-terminus of the SpC, resulting in SpCΔNΔC-PyMSP1-19 and SpCΔNΔC-CSP, respectively. The C-terminus of VP1 of the NoV was genetically fused with the SpT using two linkers (EAAAK), resulting in the construction of NoV L2(c-SpT) [25]. These three proteins were expressed in silkworms, purified individually, and conjugated to produce a bivalent malaria vaccine. In the case of the dengue virus (DENV), four different serotype antigens should be displayed on the VLPs to improve vaccine efficacy. Recently, Muthuraman et al. successfully displayed DENV serotype envelope domain III 1, 2, 3, and 4 (1EDIII–4EDIII, tetEDIII) on the surface of VLPs [15,26]. Dengue virus capsid-like particles (DENV C-LPs) and canine parvovirus-like particles (CPV-LPs) served as scaffolds for displaying these antigens. The SpC-fused 1, 2, 3, and 4EDIIIs, SpT-fused-CPV-LPs, and -DENV C-LPs are individually expressed in silkworms and subsequently purified. Through in vitro SpT/SpC covalent ligation, the EDIIIs were exhibited on the surfaces of both CPV-LPs and DENV C-LPs (Figure 2.6). Two types of tetravalent CPV-LPs (tetCPV-LPs) and DENV C-LPs (tetDENV C-LPs) were found to elicit neutralizing antibodies in BALB/c mice. Notably, the immunogenicity of tetDENV C-LPs for anti-IgG EDIIIs was higher than that of tetCPV-LPs for serotypes 1 and 3 [27]. Specifically, tetDENV C-LPs exhibited higher neutralization activity than tetCPV-LPs for serotype 1. These results demonstrate that both engineered homologous tetDENV C-LPs and heterologous tetCPV-LPs can serve as effective tetravalent VLP vaccines. These designs promote broad-spectrum immunity capable of neutralizing multiple strains or subtypes, reduce immune escape by combining conserved

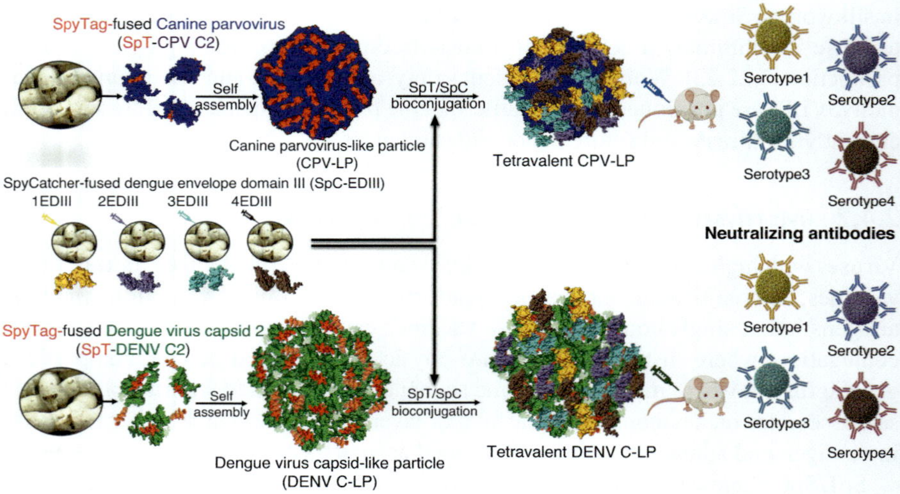

FIGURE 2.6 Schematic diagram of four dengue serotype EDIIIs-displaying tetVLPs SpT-fused DENV C-LPs and CPV-LPs as scaffolds were expressed in silkworms and purified. Also, SpC-fused tetEDIII was expressed in silkworms. Equimolar tetEDIII and scaffold were bioconjugated in vitro through the SpT/SpC system. tetCPV-LPs and tetDENV C-LPs were used for immunogenicity and neutralizing activity. (Adapted from Ref. [27] with permission from American Chemical Society.)

regions with variable epitopes, and improve dose efficiency by achieving multivalent protection with fewer injections. Illustrative applications include influenza nanoparticles displaying diverse hemagglutinin subtypes, SARS-CoV-2 nanoparticles incorporating spike proteins from multiple variants, and prototype pan-coronavirus candidates that aim for cross-family coverage.

2.4.3 Nanoadjuvants

Nanoadjuvants enhance vaccine efficacy through multiple interconnected mechanisms. They create a depot effect by prolonging antigen retention at the injection site or within lymphoid tissues, thereby extending the duration of immune exposure. Their nanoscale properties also enable efficient uptake by antigen-presenting cells, such as dendritic cells and macrophages, thereby facilitating improved antigen processing and display. In addition, certain nanomaterials act as danger signal amplifiers by stimulating pattern recognition receptors and mimicking pathogen-associated molecular patterns, which strengthens the immune response. Nanoadjuvants offer significant advantages in vaccine development due to their tunable degradation rates, which enable controlled, sustained antigen release. This property reduces the need for repeated booster doses while promoting more effective and durable immunity. Various nanomaterial platforms enhance these capabilities. Lipid-based nanoadjuvants, such as cationic lipids, serve dual roles as both carriers and immune stimulators. Polymeric nanoadjuvants, such as those made from biodegradable PLGA, offer controlled antigen release and are biocompatible. Inorganic nanoadjuvants, including gold, silica, and alum-based nanoparticles, are used to stabilize antigens and elicit immune activation. Furthermore, nanoadjuvants can be engineered to bias the immune response toward either Th1-type (cell-mediated) or Th2-type (antibody-mediated) immunity, depending on the target pathogen. This immunomodulation is particularly critical for viruses, where cellular immunity is predominant.

2.4.4 mRNA Vaccine Delivery

The mRNA vaccine platform relies heavily on efficient delivery systems to protect fragile nucleic acids and ensure effective expression in target cells, with LNPs emerging as the most successful technology to date. LNPs are typically composed of ionizable cationic lipids that bind and encapsulate negatively charged mRNA while promoting endosomal escape, phospholipids that stabilize the bilayer structure, cholesterol that enhances membrane fluidity and stability, and PEGylated lipids that prolong circulation time and minimize aggregation. Once administered, LNPs shield the mRNA from degradation by extracellular RNases and enter cells primarily via endocytosis. Within the acidic environment of endosomes, ionizable lipids become positively charged, destabilizing the endosomal membrane and enabling release of mRNA into the cytoplasm, where host ribosomes translate it into viral antigens that trigger immune recognition (Figure 2.7). Compared to conventional approaches, LNP-based mRNA vaccines enable rapid development in response to emerging viral threats, avoid the risks of genomic integration, and can be manufactured on a large

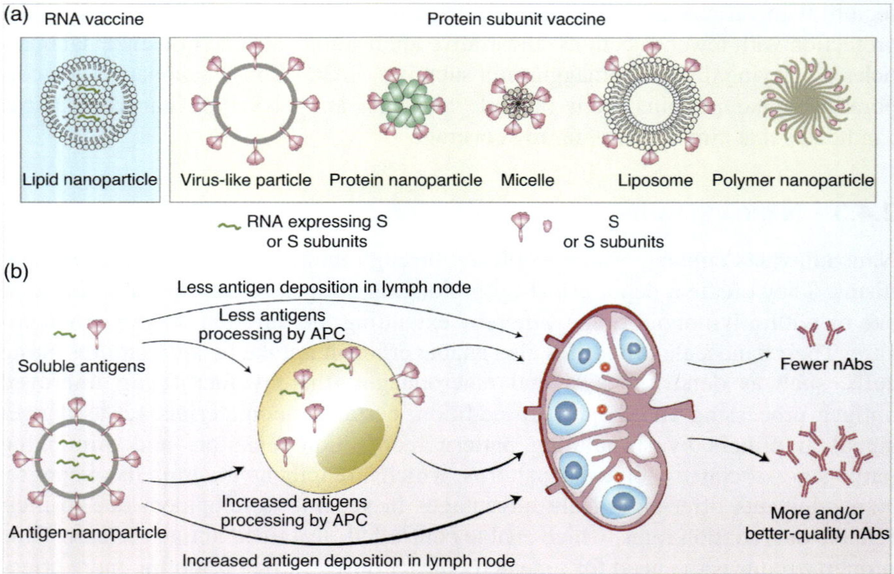

FIGURE 2.7 Vaccine development by nanoparticles. (Adapted from Ref. [28] with permission from Elsevier.)

scale. The clinical success of COVID-19 mRNA vaccines has confirmed the effectiveness of this platform, demonstrating strong T- and B-cell responses, high efficiency, and favorable safety profiles, making LNPs a key element of future vaccine technologies.

2.4.5 Challenges and Future Directions

Despite remarkable advances, the development of nanoparticle-based vaccines continues to face several hurdles. Cold chain requirements remain a significant limitation, particularly for LNP-based mRNA vaccines, which require stringent storage conditions. Scaling up manufacturing while maintaining consistent nanoparticle size, stability, and composition poses another significant challenge at the industrial level. In addition, long-term safety data are still limited for many emerging nanomaterial platforms, raising concerns about their clinical translation. Global accessibility also remains a pressing issue, as high production costs and distribution complexities hinder equitable access in low-resource settings. Looking ahead, future research is likely to focus on thermostable formulations that can decrease reliance on cold chains, developing self-amplifying RNA platforms to reduce dosage needs, and creating universal multivalent vaccines capable of providing broad protection against various viral strains. Progress in artificial intelligence (AI) is also expected to accelerate nanoparticle design, enabling rapid and flexible responses to future pandemics.

2.5 NANOTECHNOLOGY FOR PANDEMIC PREPAREDNESS AND CONTROL

Global health systems have faced repeated stress tests over the last two decades due to viral outbreaks such as SARS, Influenza, Ebola, Zika, and, most notably, the COVID-19 pandemic. These crises have underscored the urgent need for technologies that enable faster detection, scalable intervention, and coordinated responses to outbreaks. Nanotechnology offers solutions across the entire spectrum of outbreak management, from early warning to mass immunization.

2.5.1 Point-of-Care Nanobiosensors for Early Outbreak Detection

Early detection of outbreaks is critical for containment before widespread transmission, and nanobiosensors offer near-instantaneous detection of pathogens at the point of care. These devices utilize nanomaterials, such as AuNPs, QDs, carbon nanotubes, and graphene, which offer enhanced sensitivity due to their high surface reactivity. They enable signal amplification through surface plasmon resonance or fluorescence and facilitate rapid binding kinetics due to their nanoscale interfaces. Different diagnostic formats include colorimetric assays, where AuNPs change color upon aggregation for visual detection; electrochemical sensors, which transduce molecular binding into electrical signals within seconds; and optical sensors, which utilize QD fluorescence or plasmon resonance shifts for high sensitivity and specificity. With advantages such as on-site testing, minimal sample preparation, and low-cost materials, nanobiosensors enable detection within minutes to hours of patient presentation, thereby significantly reducing diagnostic delays and allowing health authorities to begin contact tracing and isolation earlier in the outbreak curve.

2.5.2 Nanoparticle Synthesis for Mass Vaccine/Drug Production

Once a pathogen is identified, rapid production of vaccines and therapeutics is essential, and nanotechnology-based manufacturing offers major advantages in scalability. High-throughput synthesis methods such as microfluidics, continuous flow reactors, and self-assembly platforms enable precise size control, automated quality assurance using inline sensors, and consistent large-scale production of nanoparticles. The COVID-19 pandemic demonstrated the scalability of LNP-mRNA vaccines, where microfluidic mixing systems produced reproducible batches at millions of doses per week. Stabilization strategies, including formulation science for extended shelf life at ambient temperatures, reduce reliance on ultra-cold storage and facilitate delivery to remote areas. Furthermore, modular nanoparticle production lines allow reconfiguration for new pathogens, reducing the lag between sequencing and vaccine distribution, thereby supporting a rapid global response.

2.5.3 Nanoparticle-Enabled Detection of Viruses in Water and Air

Pandemic preparedness extends beyond clinical diagnostics to include environmental surveillance, where nanotechnology enables sensitive detection of pathogens in wastewater, air, and surface swabs. Wastewater monitoring, for example, can serve as an early warning system by detecting the spread of viruses within a community. Functionalized MNPs can bind to viral RNA or capsid proteins, enabling efficient on-site preconcentration and reducing the need for large-scale sample transportation. Airborne surveillance technologies, including nanoporous filters and electrostatic nanoparticle collectors, capture viral particles for real-time analysis using nanosensors, proving especially valuable in airports, hospitals, and other high-risk zones. By detecting pathogens in the environment before symptoms appear, nanotechnology-based surveillance allows for proactive public health actions, such as targeted testing, disinfection efforts, and timely public alerts.

2.5.4 Smartphone-Connected Nanoparticle-Based Tests for Field Use

Portable diagnostic devices that incorporate nanobiosensors, combined with smartphones, offer decentralized outbreak monitoring and real-time epidemiological tracking. These systems use compact formats, such as handheld devices or lateral-flow strips, in which nanoparticles generate detectable signals that are captured by the smartphone's camera, microphone, or other sensors. Cloud connectivity enables the immediate, encrypted upload of results, allowing for centralized outbreak mapping. The workflow typically includes sample collection (e.g., nasal swab, saliva, or environmental swab), on-device processing using nanoparticle-based cartridges, smartphone-based signal analysis, and data transmission to health dashboards. Such platforms are particularly beneficial in rural areas, conflict zones, or developing countries with limited centralized laboratory infrastructure, as they provide rapid, user-friendly, and field-deployable solutions for early outbreak detection.

2.5.5 Combining Detection, Treatment, and Data Analytics for Outbreak Control

Effective pandemic control requires the integration of diagnostics, therapeutics, and data analytics, with nanotechnology providing a unifying platform to achieve this. Theragnostic nanoparticles can combine diagnostic agents with antiviral drugs, allowing for simultaneous detection and treatment. AI-driven nanodiagnostics further enhance outbreak management by processing sensor data in real time to predict infection patterns. At the same time, smart drug delivery systems release therapeutics in response to viral enzymes or changes in pH. Together, these technologies enable closed-loop outbreak management, starting with nanosensor detection, immediate data upload to surveillance systems, targeted deployment of therapeutics or vaccines, and feedback-based adjustments to intervention strategies. This approach reduces transmission through rapid isolation, optimally allocates medical resources, and supports adaptive strategies that evolve in response to outbreak dynamics.

2.6 FUTURE DIRECTIONS IN VIROLOGY FOR NANOPARTICLES

Nanoparticles have emerged as powerful tools in virology, enabling breakthroughs in detection, imaging, drug delivery, and vaccine development. While current applications already demonstrate considerable clinical and public health benefits, the next generation of nanoparticle technologies will further expand these capabilities through precision, adaptability, and integration with advanced computational systems. These future directions will transform how viral infections are diagnosed, treated, and monitored, shifting from generalized, population-wide strategies to personalized, real-time, and data-driven interventions.

2.6.1 Smart Nanoparticles: Stimuli-Responsive Systems for Targeted Release

Smart nanoparticles represent a significant evolution from passive drug carriers to intelligent therapeutic agents that can respond to specific environmental triggers within the host or viral microenvironment. Unlike conventional nanoparticle systems, these advanced platforms can detect and respond to both intrinsic stimuli, such as pH changes, enzyme activity, and redox potential, as well as extrinsic triggers, including temperature fluctuations, light exposure, and magnetic fields. This responsiveness enables precise control over drug-release kinetics and spatial distribution, transforming nanomedicine from a broad-spectrum approach to a highly targeted therapeutic strategy.

The use of stimuli-responsive nanosystems offers several significant advantages over traditional drug delivery methods. Targeted delivery mechanisms significantly reduce systemic side effects by directing therapeutic agents specifically to infection sites, while also increasing local drug concentrations to effective therapeutic levels. This specific delivery approach also plays a crucial role in minimizing the emergence of drug resistance, as it maintains consistently high local drug concentrations that prevent viral adaptation and mutation. These benefits collectively address some of the most urgent challenges in antiviral therapy, particularly the balance between therapeutic efficacy and patient safety.

pH-responsive nanoparticles utilize the acidic microenvironments generated during viral infection processes. Many viruses enter host cells via endocytosis, during which the pH inside the endosomal compartments becomes acidic. These specialized nanoparticles remain stable under physiological conditions (pH ~7.4) but disassemble rapidly when exposed to the acidic environment of endosomes, releasing their antiviral payload directly at the site of viral uncoating. A particularly promising example involves polymeric micelles engineered with acid-labile linkages that selectively degrade in low-pH environments, enabling the targeted release of siRNA molecules designed to silence viral genes at the precise location where viral replication initiates.

Temperature-responsive nanoparticles use fever responses as biological triggers for drug activation. Since fever is a key symptom of many viral infections, thermo-responsive polymers can be designed to undergo controlled phase transitions at slightly elevated body temperatures, enabling fever-activated drug release. This method is especially useful for infections such as influenza or dengue fever, where febrile episodes coincide with periods of intense viral replication, ensuring that peak drug levels align with the highest therapeutic need.

Viral enzyme-responsive nanoparticles function as sophisticated "molecular tripwires" by incorporating enzyme-cleavable linkers that specifically respond to viral proteases or polymerases produced during active replication [29]. These systems remain inert in healthy tissues but are activated only upon exposure to virus-specific enzymes, thereby ensuring highly targeted drug release. HIV protease-sensitive liposomes exemplify this approach by releasing antiviral agents exclusively within HIV-infected cells, where the specific protease is present, thereby significantly reducing off-target toxicity while maximizing therapeutic impact at sites of active viral replication.

2.6.2 Combining Detection, Imaging, and Therapy in a Single Nanostructure

The next frontier in antiviral nanotechnology lies in the development of theragnostic nanoparticles, multifunctional systems capable of diagnosing, imaging, and treating infections within a single platform. The core–shell architecture represents a key design principle, where core materials, such as iron oxide or gold, provide imaging contrast, and outer shells composed of polymers or lipids carry therapeutic payloads. Surface functionalization with ligands, aptamers, or antibodies enables precise targeting of virus-infected cells, while integrated nanosensors detect molecular markers of infection and transmit real-time diagnostic feedback. For example, gold nanorods functionalized with viral antigen-specific antibodies can detect infections via plasmon resonance shifts, locate infected tissues through near-infrared photoacoustic imaging, and provide therapy through photothermal ablation upon laser irradiation. QDs conjugated with antiviral drugs are capable of both visualizing infected cells and delivering treatment simultaneously. These multifunctional nanoplatforms combine diagnostic and therapeutic functions, potentially enabling more integrated patient management and in vivo monitoring of therapeutic response.

2.6.3 AI/ML Integration for Nanoparticle–Virus Interactions

AI and ML are accelerating antiviral nanotechnology by enabling predictive modeling of nanoparticle–virus and nanoparticle–host interactions. ML models trained on large datasets can predict binding affinities, informing the design of optimal surface chemistries for targeting specific viral or cellular receptors. Algorithms also optimize formulation parameters, such as nanoparticle size, charge, and composition, to predict pharmacokinetics and biodistribution. Meanwhile, AI-driven resistance prediction simulates viral evolution to anticipate mutations that may alter the efficacy of nanoparticles. Beyond design, integrating nanoparticle-based sensors with AI-enabled outbreak monitoring systems supports real-time surveillance, continuous epidemiological modeling, and rapid identification of emerging high-risk viral strains. This framework enables the swift redesign of nanoparticle vaccines or therapeutics in response to evolving pathogens, thereby shortening the research and development cycle from years to months, increasing adaptability, and reducing trial-and-error experimentation in nanoparticle development.

2.6.4 Personalized Nanomedicine: Tailoring Nanotherapeutics to Patient-Specific Viral Strains and Immune Profiles

Personalized nanomedicine seeks to optimize antiviral treatments by tailoring nanoparticle-based therapies to patient-specific viral genotypes and immune profiles. For viruses with high genetic diversity, such as HIV and hepatitis C, sequencing patient-specific viral genomes can inform the design of nanoparticles loaded with genotype-targeted siRNA, CRISPR-Cas components, or inhibitors. In parallel, immune profile optimization considers host variability in cytokine levels, T-cell exhaustion markers, and pre-existing immunity to design nanoparticles that modulate immune responses for maximum therapeutic effect. Furthermore, nanoparticles can deliver patient-specific antiviral cocktails in optimized ratios, enabling precision treatment against resistant or rare viral strains. By aligning therapeutic strategies with individual host and viral characteristics, personalized nanomedicine reduces adverse reactions, enhances efficacy, and provides solutions for patients who are unresponsive to conventional therapies.

2.6.5 Regulatory Frameworks: Global Guidelines for Nanoparticle Use in Virology

The rapid expansion of nanotechnology in virology underscores the urgent need for harmonized global regulatory frameworks to ensure safety, efficacy, and equitable distribution of nanotechnology-based products. Current gaps include the absence of standardized definitions and testing protocols for nanomaterials across jurisdictions, limited availability of long-term toxicity data, and ethical challenges associated with the potential misuse of NP-enabled surveillance systems. Proposed regulatory strategies emphasize the creation of international standards, potentially led by the WHO, for nanoparticle characterization, preclinical assessment, and clinical trial protocols. Risk–benefit assessment models must balance the urgency of pandemic response with robust safety evaluations. At the same time, post-market surveillance should monitor long-term outcomes to ensure the safety of the intervention. Ethical considerations, including data privacy and responsible deployment of NP-based surveillance tools, are equally essential. Harmonized regulation would facilitate global collaboration, reduce redundant review processes, and ensure the timely yet safe deployment of nanoparticle-based diagnostics and therapeutics during health crises.

REFERENCES

1. O.J. Achadu, F. Abe, T.C. Li, I.M. Khoris, D. Lee, J. Lee, et al., Molybdenum trioxide quantum dot-encapsulated nanogels for virus detection by surface-enhanced Raman scattering on a 2D substrate, *ACS Appl Mater Interfaces*, 13(2021) 27836–44.
2. E.Y. Park, S. Maehata, I.M. Khoris, O.J. Achadu, Signal-amplified surface-enhanced Raman scattering using core/shell satellite nanoparticles for norovirus detection, *Microchim Acta*, 191(2024) 560.
3. O.J. Achadu, N. Nwaji, D. Lee, J. Lee, E.M. Akinoglu, M. Giersig, et al., 3D hierarchically porous magnetic molybdenum trioxide@gold nanospheres as a nanogap-enhanced Raman scattering biosensor for SARS-CoV-2, *Nanoscale Adv*, 4(2022) 871–83.

4. T. Kato, M. Yui, V.K. Deo, E.Y. Park, Development of Rous sarcoma virus-like particles displaying hCC49 scFv for specific targeted drug delivery to human colon carcinoma cells, *Pharm Res*, 32(2015) 3699–707.
5. V.K. Deo, T. Kato, E.Y. Park, Chimeric virus-like particles made using GAG and M1 capsid proteins providing dual drug delivery and vaccination platform, *Mol Pharm*, 12(2015) 839–45.
6. S.T. Chuang, B. Conklin, J.B. Stein, G. Pan, K.-B. Lee, Nanotechnology-enabled immunoengineering approaches to advance therapeutic applications, *Nano Converg*, 9(2022) 19.
7. E.Y. Park, From Silkroad to Bioroad-Silkworm Biotechnology, *Protein Expr Purif*, 234(2025) 106762.
8. Y. Tsuji, V.K. Deo, T. Kato, E.Y. Park, Production of Rous sarcoma virus-like particles displaying human transmembrane protein in silkworm larvae and its application to ligand-receptor binding assay, *J Biotechnol*, 155(2011) 185–92.
9. D.I.S. Utomo, I. Hirono, T. Kato, E.Y. Park, Formation of virus-like particles of the dengue virus serotype 2 expressed in silkworm larvae, *Mol Biotechnol*, 61(2019) 852–9.
10. D.I.S. Utomo, S. Pambudi, E.Y. Park, Humoral immune response induced with dengue virus-like particles serotypes 1 and 4 produced in silkworm, *AMB Express*, 12(2022) 8.
11. D.I.S. Utomo, S. Pambudi, F. Sjatha, T. Kato, E.Y. Park, Production of dengue virus-like particles serotype-3 in silkworm larvae and their ability to elicit a humoral immune response in mice, *AMB Express*, 10(2020) 147.
12. J. Boonyakida, D.I.S. Utomo, F.N. Soma, E.Y. Park, Two-step purification of tag-free norovirus-like particles from silkworm larvae (*Bombyx mori*), *Protein Expr Purif*, 190(2022) 106010.
13. J. Boonyakida, M. Matsuda, R. Suzuki, K.R. Muthuraman, E.Y. Park, Virus-like particle-based multiserotype quartet vaccine of dengue envelope protein domain III elicited potent anti-dengue responses, *Biomacromolecules*, 26(2025) 4449–63.
14. K.R. Muthuraman, J. Boonyakida, M. Matsuda, R. Suzuki, T. Kato, E.Y. Park, Tetravalent virus-like particles engineered to display envelope domain IIIs of four dengue serotypes in silkworm as vaccine candidates, *Biomacromolecules*, 26(2025) 2003–13.
15. K.R. Muthuraman, J. Boonyakida, M. Matsuda, R. Suzuki, T. Kato, E.Y. Park, Comparative immunogenicity study of quartet and bifurcated tetravalent dengue virus envelope domain III displayed virus-like particle vaccine candidates in BALB/c mice, *Vaccine*, 63(2025) 127670.
16. H.J. Kang, F. Coulibaly, F. Clow, T. Proft, E.N. Baker, Stabilizing isopeptide bonds revealed in gram-positive bacterial pilus structure, *Science*, 318(2007) 1625–8.
17. S. Amelung, A. Nerlich, M. Rohde, B. Spellerberg, J.N. Cole, V. Nizet, et al., The FbaB-type fibronectin-binding protein of *Streptococcus pyogenes* promotes specific invasion into endothelial cells, *Cell Microbiol*, 13(2011) 1200–11.
18. B. Zakeria, J.O. Fierera, E. Celikb, E.C. Chittocka, U. Schwarz-Linekc, V.T. Moyb, et al., Peptide tag forming a rapid covalent bond to a protein, through engineering a bacterial adhesin, *Proc Natl Acad Sci USA*, 109(2012) E690–7.
19. G. Veggiani, T. Nakamura, M.D. Brenner, R.V. Gayet, J. Yan, C.V. Robinson, et al., Programmable polyproteams built using twin peptide superglues, *Proc Natl Acad Sci USA*, 113(2016) 1202–7.
20. S. Maeda, T. Kawai, M. Obinata, H. Fujiwara, T. Horiuchi, Y. Saeki, et al., Production of human alpha-interferon in silkworm using a baculovirus vector, *Nature*, 315(1985) 592–4.
21. S. Maeda, Expression of foreign genes in insect cells using baculovirus vectors, *Insect Cell Biotechnology*, G.D.O. Maramorosch (ed.), CRC Press (2018) 1–42.

22. T. Motohashi, T. Shimojima, T. Fukagawa, K. Maenaka, E.Y. Park, Efficient large-scale protein production of larvae and pupae of silkworm by *Bombyx mori* nuclear polyhedrosis virus bacmid system, *Biochem Biophys Res Commun*, 326(2005) 564–9.
23. E.Y. Park, R. Minkner, A systematic approach for scalable purification of virus-like particles, *Protein Expr Purif*, 228(2025) 106664.
24. J. Boonyakida, K. Nakayama, K. Kusakisako, H. Ikadai, E.Y. Park, Modular display of *Plasmodium yoelii* circumsporozoite surface protein and merozoite surface protein-1 on norovirus-like particles, *Bioconjug Chem*, 35(2024) 1933–43.
25. J. Boonyakida, I.M. Khoris, F. Nasrin, E.Y. Park, Improvement of modular protein display efficiency in SpyTag-implemented norovirus-like particles, *Biomacromolecules*, 24(2022) 308–18.
26. K.R. Muthuraman, D.I.S. Utomo, M. Matsuda, R. Suzuki, E.Y. Park, Expression of dengue capsid-like particles in silkworm and display of envelope domain III of dengue virus serotype 2, *Protein Expr Purif*, 222(2024) 106543.
27. K.R. Muthuraman, J. Boonyakida, M. Matsuda, R. Suzuki, T. Kato, E.Y. Park, Tetravalent virus-like particles engineered to display envelope domain IIIs of four dengue serotypes in silkworm as vaccine candidates, *Biomacromolecules*, 26(2025) 2003–13.
28. M.N. Vu, H.G. Kelly, S.J. Kent, A.K. Wheatley, Current and future nanoparticle vaccines for COVID-19, *EBioMedicine*, 74(2021) 103699.
29. J. Xu, T. Nakanishi, T. Kato, E.Y. Park, In vivo enzymatic digestion of HRV 3C protease cleavage sites-containing proteins produced in a silkworm-baculovirus expression system, *Biosci Rep*, 42(2022) BSR20220739.

3 Nanocatalysts in Biomedical Applications

Siew Suan Ng and Ruey-An Doong

3.1 INTRODUCTION

Nanocatalysis has become one of the most dynamic areas of nanoscience, transforming traditional concepts of catalysis by replacing unique physicochemical properties of nanomaterials. At the nanoscale, materials possess an exceptionally high surface area-to-volume ratio, abundant active sites, and altered electronic band structures that are not observed in their bulk counterparts. These features collectively enhance catalytic efficiency, reaction selectivity, and stability under diverse conditions. Such characteristics are particularly important in biomedical science, where controlled catalytic reactions are required to modulate complex biological processes [1].

3.1.1 Nanozymes: Artificial Enzyme Mimics

Nanocatalysts can mimic or surpass the activity of natural enzymes, leading to the emergence of "nanozymes." Unlike natural enzymes, which are often constrained by narrow ranges of pH or temperature, limited stability, and high production costs, nanozymes can be engineered with desired size, morphology, surface chemistry, and functional groups, making them robust and versatile for clinical and industrial applications, as presented in Figure 3.1. The mechanisms that support nanocatalysis are diverse and closely tied to the material composition and nanoscale design. In many systems, electron transfer plays a central role, with nanoparticles facilitating the transfer of charges between substrates and intermediates, thereby lowering reaction barriers. Transition metal oxides with multiple valencies such as cerium oxide or manganese dioxide exhibit catalytic activity through continuous redox cycling, switching between their oxidation states to sustain multiple rounds of catalysis. Another important mechanism involves the generation of reactive oxygen species (ROS), including hydroxyl radicals, hydrogen peroxide, and superoxide anions. While excessive ROS can damage healthy tissues, their controlled production by nanocatalysts has been exploited for therapeutic purposes, particularly in cancer treatment and antimicrobial therapies. Expanding on these catalytic capabilities, the concept of catalysis-based drug-free therapeutics has emerged; nanocatalysts function under near-infrared (NIR) irradiation to generate oxidative holes and hydrogen molecules. This approach synergistically consumes intratumoral glutathione (GSH) and disrupts cellular energy metabolism, enabling inexhaustible therapeutic efficacy without the toxicity associated with traditional drugs [2]. Adsorption–desorption dynamics further contribute to catalytic activity, as the high-energy crystal of nanoparticles provides unique binding sites that promote efficient substrate conversion.

 DOI: 10.1201/9781003725930-3

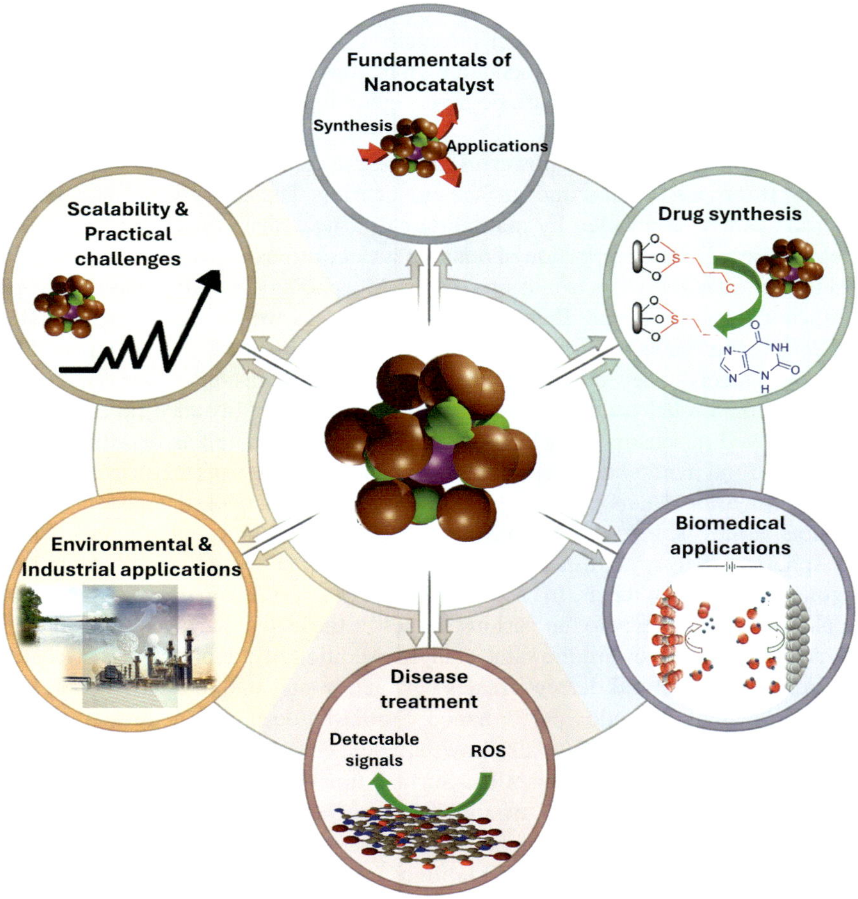

FIGURE 3.1 Schematic illustration of the applications of nanocatalysts in different fields such as drug synthesis, biomedical engineering, disease treatment, and environmental remediation.

3.1.2 Classes of Nanocatalysts

A wide range of nanomaterials have been investigated for catalytic applications in biomedical applications. Nanoparticles of transition metal oxides such as cerium oxide, manganese dioxide, and iron oxide are particularly attractive due to their redox flexibility, biocompatibility, and ability to mimic enzymes such as superoxide dismutase (SOD), catalase, or peroxidase. Noble metal nanoparticles, especially gold, platinum, and palladium, are prized for their superior catalytic activity and tunable electronic states, enabling applications in biosensing, imaging, and therapeutic interventions. Carbon-based nanomaterials, including graphene, carbon nanotubes, and fullerenes, offer high conductivity, stability, and ease of functionalization, which make them excellent support or co-catalysts in biomedical systems. Increasingly, hybrid systems that combine two or more classes of nanomaterials, such as metal–organic frameworks (MOFs) embedded with nanoparticles or carbon-based supports decorated with metal clusters, are being designed to harness synergistic effects and expand catalytic functionality.

Nanocatalysts evolves as a powerful tool for their ability to fine-tune the catalytic behavior through structural and surface engineering. The catalytic activity of nanomaterials can be controlled by manipulating particle size, since smaller nanoparticles expose a greater proportion of reactive surface atoms and may display quantum effects that alter their electronic properties. Morphology and dimension also play significant roles in varying their catalytic activity, as well as toxicological effects on humans and the environment, because nanocubes, rods, or sheets expose different crystal facets. They can be categorized as one-dimensional, two-dimensional, or three-dimensional according to their dimensions. For instance, thin-film coatings employed in sensors and electrical devices are designated as one-dimensional, whereas carbon nanotubes, wires, threads, and analogous structures are categorized as two-dimensional nanoparticles. Three-dimensional nanoparticles include quantum dots, hollow spheres, and dendrimers. According to morphology, they can display spherical, flat, crystalline, cubic, and various other shapes, occurring in either singular or composite forms. In case of gold (Au) or silver nanoparticle (AgNP), there are plenty of reports where the various shapes of these nanoparticles showed different catalytic activity toward the same analyte. Additionally, doping with heteroatoms or introducing structural defects creates new active sites and alters charge distribution, often enhancing redox performance. Similarly, designing heterostructures by combining different nanomaterials allows efficient charge separation at the interface, improving reaction rates and stability. Surface functionalization with biomolecules such as peptides, nucleic acids, or antibodies further enables selective interactions with biological targets, enhancing both biocompatibility and specificity.

Taken together, these principles highlight why nanocatalysis has become indispensable in modern biomedical research. The ability to design and control catalytic processes at the nanoscale has opened avenues ranging from biosensing and diagnostic imaging to therapeutic interventions. By uniting high catalytic efficiency with robust stability and engineerability, nanocatalysts stand at the interface of chemistry, biology, and medicine, laying the foundation for transformative advances in healthcare and beyond.

3.2 NANOCATALYSTS FOR DRUG SYNTHESIS AND BIOMOLECULAR APPLICATIONS

Nanocatalysts are increasingly recognized as transformative tools in pharmaceutical science and biomolecular engineering, offering unprecedented opportunities for selective synthesis, molecular modification, and controlled therapeutic activation. Unlike conventional catalytic systems, which often demand harsh reaction conditions and produce significant chemical waste, nanocatalysts function under milder environments, reduce activation barriers, and improve overall yields. Their tunable structural, electronic, and surface properties provide a versatile platform for designing reactions that are more sustainable, efficient, and adaptable to the growing complexity of drug molecules. Recent advancements have expanded this utility through the development of multicomponent designer nanoreactors (NRs), which are engineered to perform bioorthogonal catalysis, a "new-to-nature" reaction inside living systems without interfering with native biochemical pathways [3]. As illustrated in Figure 3.2a, these NRs often utilize porous, hollow, or open-mouth silica-based housings to compartmentalize and protect catalytic sites (such as metal nanocrystals) from the hostile biological environment. This compartmentalization allows for sophisticated spatiotemporal control over abiotic chemical synthesis, including the in cellulo generation of active drugs and bioimaging probes. Furthermore, these architectures can be integrated with plasmonic (gold) or magnetic components to harvest external energy sources, such as NIR light or alternating magnetic fields. This integration enables the selective activation of catalytic reactions via localized photothermal heating or magnetic stimuli, ensuring that high-energy chemical transformations occur precisely where needed without adversely affecting cell viability. In general, the roles of the nanocatalysts in drug synthesis and biomolecular applications are mainly responsible for the catalysis of organic reactions such as Knoevenagel condensation, coupling reaction, and sulfonamide synthesis. They are crucial in improving yield and the recovery via accelerating key organic transformations for drug intermediates. They also serve as antimicrobial and photocatalytic agents. Otherwise, the nanocatalysts act as carrier or prodrugs through bioorthogonal chemistry for in vivo drug activation and imaging, enabling targeted therapy and controlled drug release.

3.2.1 Nanocatalysts in Drug Synthesis and Green Chemistry

The pharmaceutical industry has long relied on catalytic strategies such as C–C bond formation, hydrogenation, and oxidation in the synthesis of small-molecule drugs. Nanocatalysts, particularly noble metal nanoparticles such as palladium, platinum, and gold, have significantly advanced these processes by offering higher surface reactivity, tunable electronic properties, and improved selectivity compared to bulk catalysts. Their large surface area-to-volume ratio allows for efficient substrate interaction, reducing reaction time and lowering energy requirements, which are essential for cost-effective and environmentally friendly drug production [4]. Palladium nanoparticles supported on carbon, alumina, or metal oxides are extensively employed in Suzuki–Miyaura and Heck coupling reactions, indispensable for constructing biaryl and vinyl-aryl frameworks [5]. These scaffolds form the backbone of numerous pharmaceutical reagents. Compared to conventional homogeneous palladium catalysts, nanoscale palladium offers the advantage of efficient recovery and reusability, minimizing residual metal contamination in the final drug product, a critical factor in meeting regulatory standards.

Gold nanoparticles have also emerged as highly effective nanocatalysts for redox transformations and selective oxidations under mild conditions. Supported on titania or ceria, they catalyze the oxidation of alcohols to aldehydes or ketones without the use of toxic oxidizing agents [6]. Such reactions are vital for preparing intermediates of drugs such as fluoxetine, an antidepressant, and atorvastatin, a cholesterol-lowering agent. The ability to operate under benign conditions not only minimizes hazardous

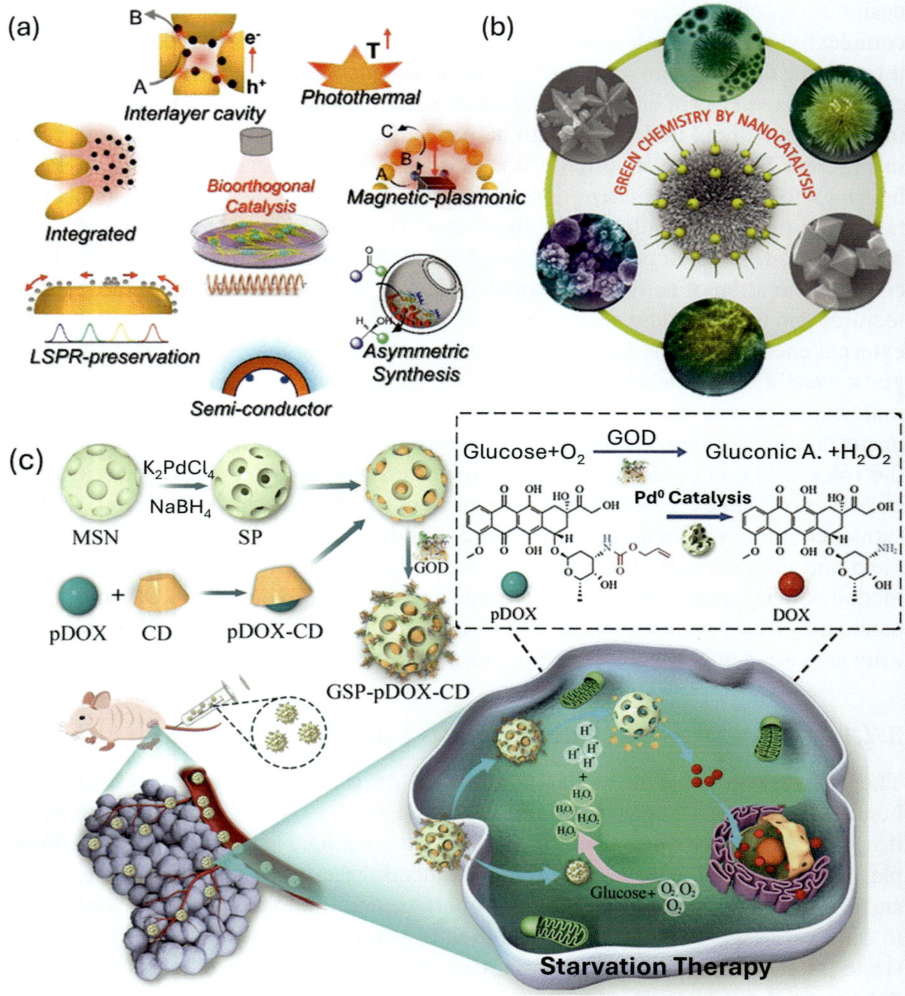

FIGURE 3.2 Advanced engineering and therapeutic applications of multifunctional nanocatalysts. (a) Strategies for bioorthogonal catalysis using engineered nanoreactors with various control mechanisms. (Adapted from Ref. [3] with permission from American Chemical Society.) (b) Diverse nanoparticle morphologies utilized in green chemistry applications and (c) mechanism of a prodrug-based nanoreactor (GSP-pDOX-CD) enabling synergistic cancer treatment by combining Pd-catalyzed prodrug activation (chemotherapy) with enzymatic glucose oxidation. (Adapted from Ref. [13] with permission from American Chemical Society.)

waste but also aligns strongly with the principles of green chemistry. Similarly, platinum nanoparticles have found wide application in hydrogenation reactions involving olefins, nitro compounds, and carbonyl groups [7]. These transformations are central to the synthesis of antibiotics such as chloramphenicol derivatives and anticancer agents, including platinum-based analogues. At the nanoscale, platinum catalysts can be engineered to achieve controlled selectivity, ensuring preferential hydrogenation of targeted functional groups while protecting sensitive moieties within complex drug molecules. Beyond noble metals, transitional metal nanocatalysts such as nickel, cobalt, and copper are increasingly being explored as sustainable low-cost alternatives. Copper nanocatalysts, for example, have been successfully applied in "click chemistry" reactions, particularly the copper-catalyzed azide-alkyne cycloaddition, which generates triazole-containing compounds with potent antiviral and anticancer activities. Cobalt- and iron-based nanocatalysts are also being developed for selective C–H activation, enabling late-stage functionalization of drug molecules and avoiding multiple protection and deprotection steps, thereby streamlining synthetic routes.

Another emerging area involves nanostructured frameworks such as MOFs and covalent organic frameworks (COFs), which provide ordered porous architectures and tunable active sites for confined catalysis [8,9]. These frameworks often mimic enzyme-like microenvironments, offering both selectivity and efficiency. For example, palladium-loaded MOFs have been reported to catalyze Suzuki couplings effectively in aqueous media, eliminating the need for toxic organic solvents, while COF-supported photocatalysts have been applied in visible light–driven oxidation reactions, offering renewable energy–based pathways to important drug intermediates. The integration of nanocatalysts into pharmaceutical manufacturing thus brings clear benefits by minimizing hazardous reagents, reducing energy consumption, enhancing atom economy, and enabling catalyst recyclability, all of which directly support the principles of green chemistry (Figure 3.2b). Furthermore, the use of bio-derived or biodegradable stabilizing agents, such as chitosan for metal nanoparticles, provides an additional layer of environmental compatibility, reinforcing the potential of nanocatalysts as a foundation for sustainable drug synthesis.

3.2.2 Nanocatalytic Platforms for Biomolecule Detection

Nanozymes like iron oxide nanoparticles with intrinsic peroxidase-like activity provide a prominent example of catalytic DNA, RNA, or protein detection. They have been successfully incorporated into nucleic acid detection assays, where they catalyze colorimetric or electrochemical reactions in response to hybridization events. For instance, in DNA biosensors, the hybridization of a target sequence triggers the catalytic breakdown of hydrogen peroxide by iron oxide nanozymes, generating a measurable color change or current signal. Such approaches have been applied to detect disease-associated genes, viral RNA, and microRNAs, offering platforms that are simpler, cheaper, and more stable than conventional enzyme-based assays that rely on horseradish peroxidase or other fragile biomolecules [10]. Nanocatalysts are also increasingly being harnessed to mediate site-specific modifications of proteins. Gold nanoparticles, for example, can catalyze selective bond formation between amino acid residues, enabling the construction of artificial protein conjugates or the attachment of therapeutic molecules. This has important implications for drug delivery, as proteins modified with nanocatalysts can be conjugated to drugs, fluorescent tags, or targeting ligands in a controlled manner. In some cases, nanocatalysts even facilitate post-translational modifications such as phosphorylation or glycosylation under biomimetic conditions, thereby expanding the chemical diversity of proteins beyond what natural biosynthetic pathways can achieve. Certain cerium oxide and manganese oxide nanoparticles display phosphatase- and nuclease-like activities, which can be exploited for controlled cleavage or remodeling of nucleic acids. Such properties have been applied in gene editing approaches, antisense oligonucleotide processing, and even in RNA interference pathways, where nanozyme activity enables precise and controllable manipulation of nucleic acid strands. By integrating nanocatalysts into these processes, researchers can bypass the instability and cost limitations of natural enzymes, paving the way for scalable molecular engineering techniques [11].

In diagnostics, they serve as catalytic amplifiers that translate biomolecular recognition events into detectable signals, allowing sensitive detection of nucleic acids, proteins, or metabolites. Specifically, nanocatalysts promote generation of ROS, radicals, or intermediates that enhance electrochemical or luminescent signals. For example, Pt nanoparticles catalyze H_2O_2 decomposition into superoxide radicals, boosting luminol ECL emission. Otherwise, structural confinement in nanocatalyst also crucial in increase active sites and improve sensitivity or selectivity. The enhanced stability of sensor is fulfilled via prevention of species aggregation and leaching issues in sensing performance. In therapeutics, they enable chemical transformations that attach drugs or functional groups to biomolecules in ways that were previously inaccessible, bridging the gap between synthetic chemistry and molecular biology. The convergence of nanocatalysis with biomolecular engineering thus promises a new era of hybrid technologies that combine the precision of biological systems with the robustness of inorganic catalysts.

3.2.3 Nanocatalysts for Prodrug Activation and Targeted Therapy

One of the most exciting biomedical applications of nanocatalysts lies in their ability to activate prodrugs directly at the site of disease. Traditional chemotherapy is often plagued by systemic toxicity, since active drugs circulate throughout the body and indiscriminately damage both malignant and healthy tissues. Prodrugs, which are chemically modified inactive or less toxic forms of therapeutics, were developed to address this problem, but their activation typically relies on physiological processes that lack spatial precision. Nanocatalysts introduce a transformative solution by enabling localized, controllable conversion of prodrugs into their active forms within diseased tissues, thereby enhancing efficacy while minimizing collateral damage. Platinum-based nanocatalysts show several examples of this strategy [12]. When accumulated in the tumor microenvironment (TME), they can catalyze the reduction or oxidation of prodrugs into cytotoxic species in situ. Platinum nanozymes have been shown to activate alkylating agents and Pt(IV) prodrugs into active Pt(II) complexes that bind DNA and induce apoptosis, while sparing healthy tissues from systemic exposure. This localized conversion is particularly advantageous in solid tumors, where nanoparticle accumulation is facilitated by the enhanced permeability and retention effect. Gold and palladium nanocatalysts have also been investigated for bioorthogonal catalysis, a concept in which catalytic reactions proceed selectively in biological environments without interfering with native biochemical pathways. Palladium nanoparticles, for instance, can mediate deprotection reactions that liberate active drug molecules from caged prodrugs once they reach the tumor.

A recent example of this advanced capability is the development of prodrug-based NRs for multisynergistic cancer therapy, as illustrated in Figure 3.2c [13]. In this platform, palladium (Pd^0) nanoparticles are synthesized in situ within the pores of mesoporous silica to serve as catalytic centers for the specific activation of a doxorubicin prodrug (pDOX) into its active cytotoxic form. To further enhance therapeutic efficacy, glucose oxidase (GOD) is integrated into the system to catalyze the oxidation of intratumoral glucose into gluconic acid and hydrogen peroxide (H_2O_2). This dual-catalytic approach achieves a three-pronged attack: Pd-mediated chemotherapy, GOD-driven starvation therapy (via glucose consumption), and oxidation therapy (via H_2O_2 generation), resulting in the effective suppression of tumor growth. Similarly, gold nanocatalysts can also exploit redox gradients in the TME to activate thiol- or disulfide-based prodrugs, achieving a degree of spatiotemporal precision that conventional pharmacology cannot provide.

This catalytic control shows wide applications beyond oncology. For example, enzyme-mimicking nanocatalysts have been applied in antimicrobial therapy, where they convert prodrugs into bactericidal species at the site of infection, minimizing systemic side effects. Iron oxide nanozymes, with peroxidase-like activity, can generate ROS in situ from benign precursors, effectively creating a localized oxidative stress environment lethal to pathogens but tolerable to surrounding tissues. The principle of using nanocatalysts for prodrug activation thus aligns with the broader goals of precision medicine. This approach not only reduces off-target toxicity but also opens the possibility of combining therapeutic action with diagnostic capability, as the same nanocatalyst can be engineered to serve as an imaging probe. Such dual-function systems exemplify the concept of "theranostics," where therapy and diagnostics converge into a single nanoplatform.

3.2.4 Microfluidic and On-Demand Nanocatalytic Drug Production

Another promising frontier in biomedical nanotechnology is the integration of nanocatalysts into microfluidic systems for on-demand drug production [14]. Microreactors that incorporate catalytic nanoparticles can execute multistep chemical reactions within confined, precisely controlled volumes, offering unique advantages such as rapid reaction kinetics, reduced reagent consumption, and exceptional reproducibility. These platforms mimic the concept of "chemical factories on a chip," where complex synthetic pathways are miniaturized and automated, enabling both fundamental research and translational applications in medicine. In personalized medicine, this technology is particularly transformative. For example, catalytic nanoparticles can mediate selective coupling or activation reactions to generate customized small molecules or biomolecule conjugates on demand, ensuring that the therapy precisely matches the patient's disease state. This not only reduces reliance on centralized manufacturing but also allows for dynamic adjustments in treatment regimens as the patient's condition evolves.

Microfluidic-nanocatalyst systems also show immense promise in outbreak and emergency scenarios, where the ability to rapidly synthesize antiviral or antimicrobial agents can have life-saving consequences. During viral epidemics, for instance, nanocatalyst-driven microreactors can be programmed to quickly assemble nucleoside analogues or small-molecule inhibitors, bypassing lengthy industrial-scale synthesis pipelines. The confined volumes of microfluidics enhance safety by limiting exposure to hazardous intermediates, while the precision of nanocatalytic reactions ensures consistent product quality, even under urgent conditions. Metal nanoparticles such as palladium, platinum, or copper can catalyze bond-forming reactions, while enzyme-mimicking nanozymes can mediate selective transformations that require biomimetic conditions. The result is a compact and versatile platform capable of synthesizing a wide variety of therapeutics in a continuous-flow manner. Recent innovations have advanced this concept further through AI-assisted autonomous manufacturing of tailored drug-loaded nanoparticles [15]. By leveraging a multi-objective Bayesian optimization algorithm, researchers have developed a multistep continuous-flow platform that seamlessly integrates combinatorial synthesis, ultrafast flow dialysis for purification, and real-time characterization. This autonomous system was able to screen multistep parameters and swiftly manufacture doxorubicin (DOX)-loaded liposomes and polymeric nanoparticles, precisely customized in terms of size and drug loading efficiency, within just 6h. Such AI-driven platforms demonstrate the potential to accelerate the development timeline for bespoke drug delivery systems, addressing diverse therapeutic needs with unprecedented speed and precision. By combining the catalytic efficiency of nanomaterials with the precision of microfluidics, researchers are advancing toward a future where medicines can be designed, produced, and delivered on demand, revolutionizing how healthcare systems respond to both individual needs and global crises.

3.3 BIOMIMETIC NANOCATALYSTS IN DISEASE TREATMENT

A particularly exciting frontier in nanocatalysis is the development of biomimetic nanocatalysts that replicate the catalytic functions of natural enzymes while maintaining stability under harsh physiological conditions. These nanozymes are engineered to catalyze key biological reactions involved in both normal physiology and disease progression. Unlike natural enzymes, which often suffer from high production costs, limited stability, and sensitivity to pH or temperature fluctuations, nanozymes can be rationally designed with tunable properties such as size, morphology, charge, and surface chemistry. Nanocatalysts represent a versatile and powerful platform for disease treatment, especially in oncology and infectious diseases. First, they enable precise activation of therapeutics inside target cells or tissues. Several biomimetic nanocatalysts, which mimic enzyme-like catalytic activities such as catalase, oxidase, and peroxidase, can efficiently generate cytotoxic ROS to overcome tumor or biofilm microenvironment challenges and help modulate immune responses and cell death pathways (e.g., ferroptosis and cuproptosis). Enhanced targeting and reduced systemic toxicity during disease have been improved through rational design of catalytic centers, nanoscaffolds, and surface functionalities, combined with stimuli-responsive behavior.

3.3.1 Cancer Therapy Applications

In cancer therapy, nanozymes have been particularly impactful. The TME is characterized by specific conditions such as hypoxia, acidic pH, and elevated concentrations of hydrogen peroxide (H_2O_2). Nanocatalysts such as manganese dioxide (MnO_2) and iron oxide (Fe_3O_4) nanoparticles exploit these conditions by catalyzing the decomposition of H_2O_2 into highly reactive hydroxyl radicals (OH) through Fenton-like reactions. This strategy, termed chemodynamic therapy (CDT), has attracted considerable attention as a minimally invasive cancer treatment. Furthermore, CDT is often combined with photothermal therapy or photodynamic therapy, where external heat or light enhances tumor destruction. Such multifunctional nanoplatforms not only maximize therapeutic efficacy but also allow simultaneous imaging, creating theranostic systems that integrate diagnosis and treatment into a single nanoscale construct. Besides, tumor and bacterial microenvironments often have high GSH, which neutralizes ROS. Nanocatalysts deplete GSH to enhance oxidative stress and therapeutic efficacy [16]. Thus, there is case of using Cu–Au doped polypyrrole nanocatalysts that consume GSH and catalyze ROS generation with the NIR II laser in cancer therapy.

3.3.2 Antimicrobial Therapy Using Nanozymes

Biomimetic nanocatalysts are also emerging as powerful tools in combating infectious diseases, especially against multidrug-resistant bacteria. Nanozymes with oxidase or peroxidase-like activities generate ROS that disrupt bacterial membranes, inactivate enzymes, and interfere with metabolic pathways. A notable example is cerium oxide (CeO_2) nanoparticles, which display a unique dual redox behavior. In healthy cellular environment, they act as antioxidants by scavenging harmful ROS, whereas in infected or inflamed environments, they switch to pro-oxidant activity, producing ROS that kill pathogens. This selective catalytic modulation provides a highly effective means of treating infections while minimizing collateral damage to host tissues. The therapeutic potential of nanozymes is not limited to oncology and infectious diseases.

3.3.3 Neuroprotective Applications in Neurodegenerative Disorders

In neurodegenerative disorders such as Parkinson's and Alzheimer's diseases, oxidative stress plays a central role in neuronal injury and disease progression. Excessive accumulation of ROS damages proteins, lipids, and nucleic acids in neural tissues, accelerating cognitive and motor decline. Nanozymes such as platinum nanoparticles and CeO_2-based materials mimic the activity of antioxidant enzymes including SOD and catalase, neutralizing ROS and restoring redox balance in neurons. By alleviating oxidative stress, these materials have shown promise in protecting neuronal cells, preserving synaptic function, and potentially slowing disease progression. Their stability, controllable activity, and long-term persistence in vivo make them particularly suitable for chronic neurological conditions, where natural enzymes would degrade rapidly [17].

The diverse applications of biomimetic nanocatalysts in cancer therapy, antimicrobial treatment, and neuroprotection highlight their remarkable versatility in addressing complex disease pathologies. As research progresses toward translational and clinical applications, nanozymes hold immense promise for reshaping the future of disease treatment, offering more effective, safer, and personalized therapeutic options.

3.4 ENVIRONMENTAL APPLICATIONS AND INDUSTRIAL USE

Beyond their direct impact in medicine, nanocatalysts play a pivotal role in addressing environmental and industrial challenges that ultimately shape human health and well-being. Many pollutants and byproducts of modern industry including pesticides, organic dyes, heavy metals, and pharmaceutical residues express significant risks to ecosystems and public health through water and food contamination. Nanocatalysis offers powerful solutions for these problems by enabling efficient degradation, detoxification, and recycling processes under environmentally friendly conditions. Nanocatalysts with tailored composition, structure, and surface chemistry play pivotal roles in industrial processes via mechanisms that often involve radical generation, enhanced electron transfer, and adsorption facilitation. At the same time, nanocatalysts have been adopted in industrial settings to promote sustainable production, reduce energy consumption, and advance the principles of green chemistry. Magnetic nanocatalysts and green synthesis approaches improve catalyst recovery, reusability, and environmental sustainability. Composite and doped nanomaterials show superior catalytic performance due to synergistic effects. Their dual relevance to environmental protection and industrial innovation makes them a cornerstone technology with wide-ranging biomedical implications.

3.4.1 Environmental Remediation and Water Purification

One of the most established applications of nanocatalysts is in environmental remediation, with water purification being a primary focus. Semiconductor nanomaterials such as titanium dioxide (TiO_2) and zinc oxide (ZnO) are extensively studied for their photocatalytic activity under ultraviolet (UV) and visible light. Upon irradiation, these materials generate ROS capable of degrading a wide range of contaminants, including synthetic dyes, pesticides, and pharmaceutical residues, into harmless end products such as water and carbon dioxide. This process not only detoxifies contaminated water but also prevents the accumulation of persistent organic pollutants that might otherwise enter the food chain and pose long-term health risks. For example, TiO_2-based nanocatalysts have been employed to degrade methylene blue and Rhodamine B, two dyes commonly used to simulate industrial wastewater treatment, while ZnO nanoparticles have demonstrated high efficiency in breaking down organophosphorus pesticides.

Recent advances in doping and surface engineering of TiO_2 and ZnO have further enhanced their photocatalytic efficiency by extending light absorption into the visible spectrum, making them more practical for solar-driven purification systems. Nitrogen-doped TiO_2, for instance, exhibits superior activity under natural sunlight, while silver-decorated ZnO nanoparticles show improved charge separation and stability during prolonged photocatalysis. Beyond laboratory studies, TiO_2-coated membranes and ZnO-based nanocomposites are being developed for large-scale water treatment plants, where they combine filtration with catalytic degradation of pollutants, offering dual functionality in a single platform. Nanocatalysts are also proving effective in tackling heavy metal contamination, another major threat to water safety. Iron oxide nanoparticles, for instance, have been explored for their ability to reduce toxic hexavalent chromium (Cr^{6+}) to the less harmful trivalent form (Cr^{3+}), while bimetallic nanocatalysts such as palladium–copper systems have been employed to degrade chlorinated solvents in groundwater. Such multifunctional nanocatalysts not only detoxify water but also contribute to restoring ecological balance in contaminated aquatic environments.

Beyond water purification, nanocatalysts play a growing role in air quality improvement. Photocatalytic coatings of TiO_2 are increasingly applied to building surfaces, self-cleaning windows, and air filters, where they degrade volatile organic compounds, formaldehyde, and nitrogen oxides released from vehicles and industrial processes. Pilot studies in urban environments have shown that TiO_2-treated road surfaces can reduce concentrations of nitrogen oxides in the surrounding air, highlighting their potential in mitigating air pollution at a city-wide scale. Similarly, nanocatalyst-enabled catalytic converters are being optimized for vehicle exhaust treatment, offering improved removal of carbon monoxide and unburnt hydrocarbons compared to traditional systems.

3.4.2 Nanocatalysts for Biomedical Energy and Gas Modulation

Hydrogen, traditionally regarded as a clean energy carrier, has recently attracted attention in medicine due to its ability to act as a selective antioxidant. Unlike conventional antioxidants, molecular hydrogen can neutralize highly reactive hydroxyl radicals (OH) without interfering with beneficial ROS that are essential for normal cellular signaling. Nanocatalysts such as platinum nanoparticles, molybdenum sulfide (MoS_2) nanosheets, and nickel-based hybrids have been engineered to catalyze the in situ production of hydrogen in biological environments. For example, injectable MoS_2 nanosheets under mild conditions can release therapeutic levels of hydrogen, offering potential for treating oxidative stress-related diseases, including neurodegenerative disorders and even cancer. In parallel, oxygen modulation via nanocatalysis plays a critical role in overcoming hypoxia within diseased tissues, particularly solid tumors. Nanocatalysts that facilitate oxygen generation or controlled oxygen reduction have been developed to address this challenge. For instance, manganese dioxide (MnO_2) and platinum-based nanocatalysts can decompose endogenous hydrogen peroxide into molecular oxygen, relieving tumor hypoxia and thereby enhancing the efficacy of oxygen-dependent therapies. Similarly, nanocatalysts mimicking ORR pathways are being integrated into implantable devices and biosensors, where they function to manage local oxygen concentrations or generate power from biofluids.

The biomedical integration of HER and ORR catalysis extends further into self-powered biosensing systems and implantable energy devices. Micro- and nanoscale fuel cells that exploit nanocatalysts for ORR are being designed as sustainable power sources for pacemakers, glucose monitors, and neurostimulators. These devices harness endogenous fuels such as glucose and oxygen from body fluids, eliminating the need for frequent battery replacements and offering continuous operation in vivo. Together, these emerging applications demonstrate how nanocatalysts originally developed for energy research are now crossing into the biomedical domain.

3.4.3 Industrial Synthesis and Green Chemistry

In the industrial sector, nanocatalysts are transforming chemical manufacturing by enhancing efficiency, selectivity, and sustainability. Traditional synthetic routes in pharmaceutical and fine chemical production often rely on energy-intensive processes, excessive solvent usage, and hazardous reagents, leading to significant environmental burdens. Nanocatalysis provides a powerful alternative by lowering activation energies, enabling reactions under milder conditions, and improving atom economy, all of which align with the principles of green chemistry.

Porous nanostructured materials such as MOFs and COFs emerging as versatile catalytic platforms. Their tunable pore size, high surface area, and capacity to host active sites make them ideal for multistep transformations. For instance, MOF-based catalysts have been employed in the sustainable synthesis of amino acids and peptide derivatives, while COFs incorporating metal nanoparticles have shown promise in large-scale vitamin and antibiotic production. These frameworks can also integrate enzymatic components, creating hybrid biocatalytic systems that couple the selectivity of enzymes with the robustness of nanomaterials, as schematically presented in Figure 3.3. Green chemistry applications extend further into polymer and fine chemical manufacturing. Nanocatalysts such as nickel, cobalt, and iron nanoparticles are increasingly used in polymerization reactions, replacing toxic organometallic catalysts and enabling recyclable, energy-efficient processes. In the agrochemical sector, nanocatalysts accelerate the synthesis of herbicides and insecticides with reduced byproduct formation, lowering the environmental impact of large-scale agriculture.

Importantly, these innovations not only improve process sustainability but also enhance economic viability by lowering raw material usage, energy costs, and waste management requirements. For instance, continuous-flow reactors incorporating nanocatalysts are being adopted in pharmaceutical plants, offering superior scalability and reproducibility compared to conventional batch processes. This integration of nanocatalysis with flow chemistry is paving the way toward decentralized, on-demand drug manufacturing facilities that align with the future of precision medicine.

3.4.4 Biomedical Device Coatings and Antifouling Applications

Beyond chemical synthesis, nanocatalysts are increasingly finding practical applications in the biomedical device industry, where long-term functionality and sterility are critical. A persistent challenge with medical devices such as catheters, stents, orthopedic implants, and prosthetics is biofouling, the unwanted accumulation of proteins, microbial cells, and biofilms on surfaces. Biofouling not only compromises device performance but also creates reservoirs for infection, leading to complications that often necessitate device removal or replacement. Nanocatalyst-enabled surface coatings offer a promising strategy to mitigate these problems by combining antimicrobial activity with self-cleaning properties.

One approach is the incorporation of silver-based nanocatalysts into device coatings. Silver nanoparticles release Ag^+ ions with well-documented antimicrobial effects, while also catalyzing redox reactions that generate ROS capable of disrupting

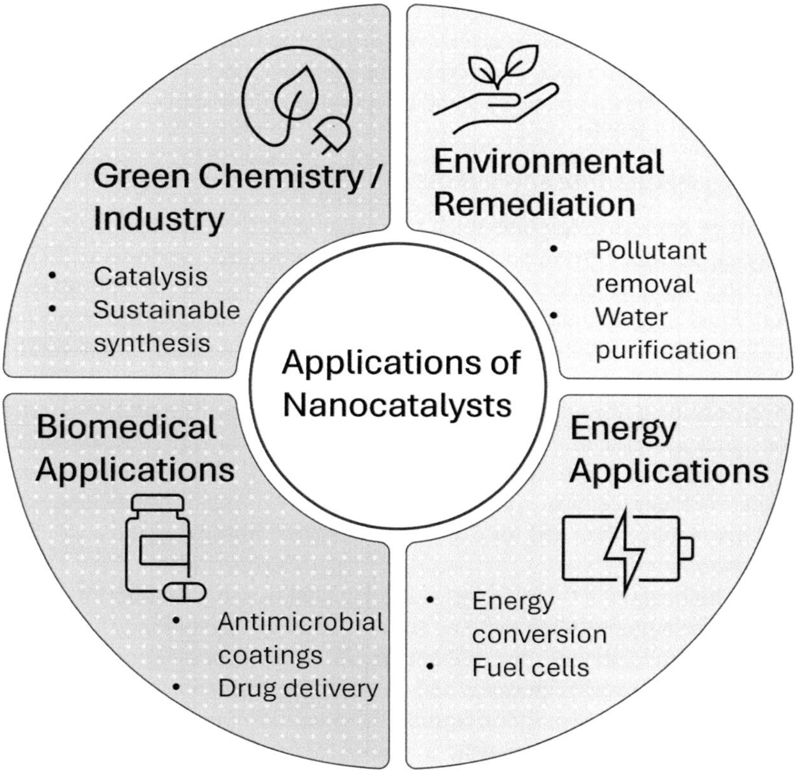

FIGURE 3.3 Schematic overview of the diverse environmental and industrial applications of nanocatalysts.

microbial membranes and metabolic pathways. This dual action prevents colonization at the early stages and minimizes the risk of biofilm maturation. Silver–titania composites have been employed in catheter and wound dressing coatings, where their catalytic activity maintains a sterile surface over extended periods.

Another well-studied system involves titanium dioxide (TiO_2) coatings, which exhibit photocatalytic properties under UV or visible light. Upon activation, TiO_2 generates hydroxyl radicals and superoxide anions that degrade organic deposits and kill surface-adhered microbes. This photocatalytic self-sterilization makes TiO_2 particularly attractive for coatings on orthopedic implants, surgical tools, and dental devices, where surface cleanliness is critical for patient safety. Recent engineering strategies, such as doping TiO_2 with nitrogen or silver, have extended its photocatalytic activity into the visible light range, enabling activation under indoor lighting rather than requiring UV irradiation. Beyond silver and titanium dioxide, enzyme-mimicking nanocatalysts (nanozymes) are being explored for antifouling applications. Iron oxide and cerium oxide nanozymes exhibit peroxidase- or oxidase-like activities, producing ROS in situ when exposed to physiological levels of hydrogen peroxide. These catalytic coatings not only disrupt microbial growth but also break down bioorganic layers, preserving the functional integrity of device surfaces. For example, Fe_3O_4 nanozyme coatings have been investigated for use in vascular stents to prevent restenosis and infection simultaneously.

3.4.5 Large-Scale Industrial Bioreactors and Sustainable Biotechnology

Nanocatalysts are also being integrated into large-scale industrial bioreactors, where they play an increasingly important role in the controlled synthesis of high-value biomolecules for pharmaceutical, nutraceutical, and bio-based industries. Their reusability and long operational lifespans make them particularly attractive for continuous-flow and large-volume reactor systems, where efficiency and durability are critical. For example, iron oxide (Fe_3O_4) nanoparticles with peroxidase-like activity have been explored for scalable biotransformation processes, catalyzing oxidative reactions that are essential in pharmaceutical intermediate production. Similarly, cerium oxide (CeO_2) nanozymes are used in antioxidant-related pathways to support the synthesis of nutraceutical compounds. These systems not only accelerate reaction rates but also reduce the need for expensive cofactors, improving the cost-efficiency of bioproduction.

A major innovation in this area is the development of hybrid nanocatalyst–enzyme systems, where nanoparticles serve as support or co-catalysts for natural enzymes. By stabilizing the enzyme and enhancing substrate accessibility, these hybrids achieve higher turnover frequencies and extended operational stability compared to free enzymes. For instance, lipase immobilized on mesoporous silica nanoparticles have been applied in the sustainable synthesis of biodiesel and therapeutic lipids, demonstrating improved yield and reusability. In another example, GOD integrated with gold nanoparticles has been utilized in bioreactors for controlled synthesis of gluconic acid, a key industrial metabolite.

The advantages extend to amino acid and vitamin production, where nanocatalyst-augmented systems are streamlining synthesis pathways. Cobalt- and nickel-based nanocatalysts have been employed in reductive amination and hydrogenation reactions, enabling efficient production of amino acid derivatives for pharmaceuticals. Similarly, MOF- and COF-supported nanocatalysts are being tested in the green synthesis of vitamins such as riboflavin (B_2) and cobalamin (B_{12}), where their porous frameworks provide confined catalytic spaces that mimic enzyme active sites while offering recyclability. Importantly, the adoption of nanocatalysts in bioreactors aligns with the principles of sustainable biotechnology. By enabling higher reaction efficiency, lowering energy demands, and reducing waste generation, these systems contribute to greener manufacturing pipelines. For instance, continuous bioreactors equipped with nanocatalyst-immobilized membranes allow for simultaneous reaction and product separation, minimizing downstream purification steps and water consumption. This integration of catalysis and process intensification is paving the way for decentralized, modular biomanufacturing facilities capable of producing therapeutics and nutraceuticals locally, reducing reliance on centralized plants. Collectively, these advances highlight the transformative potential of nanocatalysts in industrial biotechnology. From amino acid synthesis to vitamin production and enzyme stabilization, they are redefining the efficiency, cost-effectiveness, and ecological footprint of large-scale bioprocesses. As research continues to refine hybrid catalytic systems and scalable nanomaterial designs, nanocatalyst-enabled bioreactors are set to become cornerstones of a sustainable and resilient bioeconomy.

3.5 CHALLENGES IN SCALABILITY AND COMMERCIALIZATION

While nanocatalysts have demonstrated extraordinary potential in biomedical, environmental, and industrial applications, their transition from laboratory-scale research to large-scale manufacturing and commercialization remains challenging. Unlike conventional catalysts, they demand precise control over particle size, shape, surface chemistry, and distribution to maintain catalytic activity and reproducibility, and achieving such precision on an industrial scale is a difficult task. Questions regarding cost-effectiveness, safety, regulatory approval, and long-term environmental implications further complicate their path toward widespread adoption.

One of the foremost hurdles is the scalability of synthesis. Producing nanocatalysts in bulk with consistent properties is difficult, as many laboratory methods such as hydrothermal treatment, sol–gel processing, or chemical vapor deposition, are not easily scalable due to their complexity and dependence on specialized conditions. Batch-to-batch variability remains a significant issue, since even small changes in reaction parameters can alter catalytic efficiency or introduce unwanted side effects. Without robust and reproducible synthesis approaches, nanocatalysts risk remaining confined to proof-of-concept demonstrations. Stability and storage further limit the commercialization of these methodologies. Many nanomaterials are prone to agglomeration, oxidation, or structural degradation, leading to a loss of activity over time. Surface modifications such as coatings with polymers, surfactants, or biomolecules can improve stability, but not up to the mark yet. Economic considerations also weigh heavily on the viability of nanocatalyst commercialization. Precious metals like platinum, gold, and palladium exhibit outstanding catalytic efficiency but are expensive and limited in availability, restricting large-scale adoption in industries such as pharmaceuticals or water purification. Recycling and recovery strategies may reduce the costs, but efficient separation technologies are still under development. Alternatives based on earth-abundant metals such as iron, manganese, or cobalt, as well as hybrid nanocatalysts that combine low-cost supports with highly active sites, are being actively explored to strike a balance between affordability and performance.

Safety and regulatory concerns represent another major barrier. In biomedical applications, nanocatalysts may accumulate in organs, cross biological barriers, or generate ROS in unintended contexts, raising serious questions about toxicity and long-term biocompatibility. Comprehensive testing, including cytotoxicity, immunogenicity, and environmental impact studies, is essential before approval can be granted. Yet the absence of standardized international guidelines for evaluating nanomaterial safety complicates regulatory pathways and slows down translation. Environmental release of nanocatalysts during manufacturing or disposal adds another layer of risk, demanding rigorous assessment. Without harmonized frameworks, industrial stakeholders may remain hesitant to invest heavily in commercialization. With sustained innovation and regulatory harmonization, nanocatalysts have the potential to move beyond niche, high-value markets and become mainstream tools in biomedical, environmental, and industrial applications. Until these obstacles are addressed, however, their impact will remain significant but limited in scope.

3.6 CONCLUSION

Nanocatalysis has rapidly emerged as a transformative field at the interface of nanotechnology, chemistry, and biomedical science, enabling precise manipulation of chemical reactions with high efficiency. Their nanoscale features, high surface area-to-volume ratios, tunable electronic structures, and abundant active sites provide superior catalytic performance compared to bulk materials. These unique properties have been harnessed in drug synthesis and biomolecular engineering, where nanocatalysts accelerate complex reactions under mild conditions, improve yields, and enable site-specific drug activation. The rise of biomimetic nanocatalysts, or nanozymes, adds further momentum by replicating enzymatic functions even under harsh physiological environments. Such systems hold promises for disease treatment, including cancer, microbial infections, and neurodegenerative disorders, where they selectively regulate oxidative stress or disrupt pathological microenvironments. At the same time, their applications extend beyond biomedicine into environmental remediation, green chemistry, and antifouling coatings for biomedical devices, underscoring their versatility in protecting both human health and ecosystems. Yet, the translation of these advances into industrial and clinical practice faces challenges. Reproducibility in large-scale synthesis, long-term stability, high material costs, and concerns regarding safety and regulatory approval remain major barriers. Overcoming these limitations, it is required to innovate in green and scalable fabrication methods, the design of cost-effective alternatives to precious metals, and the establishment of harmonized safety frameworks. In essence, nanocatalysts embody a unifying platform that bridges biomedical, environmental, and industrial domains. Their unique precision and adaptability position them as catalysts not only of chemical transformations but also of next-generation technologies. With continued interdisciplinary collaboration and attention to scalability and safety, nanocatalysts are poised to move from proof-of-concept innovations to real-world solutions with direct impact on health, sustainability, and industry.

REFERENCES

1. R. Zhang, X. Yan, L. Gao, and K. Fan, “Nanozymes expanding the boundaries of biocatalysis,” *Nature Communications,* vol. 16, no. 1, p. 6817, 2025.
2. B. Zhao et al., “Photocatalysis-mediated drug-free sustainable cancer therapy using nanocatalyst,” *Nature Communications,* vol. 12, no. 1, p. 1345, 2021.
3. A. Kumar and I. S. Lee, “Designer nanoreactors for bioorthogonal catalysis,” *Accounts of Chemical Research,* vol. 57, no. 3, pp. 413–427, 2024.
4. V. Polshettiwar, J. M. Basset, and D. Astruc, “Nanoscience makes catalysis greener,” *ChemSusChem*, vol. 5, no. 1, pp. 6–8, 2012.

5. M. Díaz-Sánchez, D. Díaz-García, S. Prashar, and S. Gómez-Ruiz, "Palladium nanoparticles supported on silica, alumina or titania: Greener alternatives for Suzuki–Miyaura and other C–C coupling reactions," *Environmental Chemistry Letters,* vol. 17, no. 4, pp. 1585–1602, 2019.
6. A. Corma and H. Garcia, "Supported gold nanoparticles as oxidation catalysts," *Nanoparticles and Catalysis,* D. Astruc (ed.), Wiley, pp. 389–426, 2008.
7. G. Vilé, N. Almora-Barrios, N. r. López, and J. Pérez-Ramírez, "Structure and reactivity of supported hybrid platinum nanoparticles for the flow hydrogenation of functionalized nitroaromatics," *ACS Catalysis,* vol. 5, no. 6, pp. 3767–3778, 2015.
8. J. Yang and Y. W. Yang, "Metal–organic frameworks for biomedical applications," *Small,* vol. 16, no. 10, p. 1906846, 2020.
9. X. Wang et al., "Covalent organic frameworks as a biomacromolecule immobilization platform for biomedical and related applications," *Advanced Therapeutics,* vol. 5, no. 10, p. 2200053, 2022.
10. A. A. Mansur, H. S. Mansur, and S. M. Carvalho, "Engineered hybrid nanozyme catalyst cascade based on polysaccharide-enzyme-magnetic iron oxide nanostructures for potential application in cancer therapy," *Catalysis Today,* vol. 388, pp. 187–198, 2022.
11. R. Zhang, B. Jiang, K. Fan, L. Gao, and X. Yan, "Designing nanozymes for in vivo applications," *Nature Reviews Bioengineering,* vol. 2, no. 10, pp. 849–868, 2024.
12. J. I. Garcia-Peiro, J. Bonet-Aleta, J. Santamaria, and J. L. Hueso, "Platinum nanoplatforms: classic catalysts claiming a prominent role in cancer therapy," *Chemical Society Reviews,* vol. 51, no. 17, pp. 7662–7681, 2022.
13. C. Ren et al., "Prodrug-based nanoreactors with tumor-specific in situ activation for multisynergistic cancer therapy," *ACS Applied Materials & Interfaces,* vol. 12, no. 31, pp. 34667–34677, 2020.
14. V. Sebastian, "Toward continuous production of high-quality nanomaterials using microfluidics: nanoengineering the shape, structure and chemical composition," *Nanoscale,* vol. 14, no. 12, pp. 4411–4447, 2022.
15. A. Mottafegh, J.-U. Joo, G.-S. Na, V. Sharma, and D.-P. Kim, "AI-assisted autonomous manufacturing of tailored drug-loaded nanoparticles by multi-step continuous-flow platform," *Chemical Engineering Journal,* vol. 500, p. 157454, 2024.
16. B. Niu et al., "Application of glutathione depletion in cancer therapy: enhanced ROS-based therapy, ferroptosis, and chemotherapy," *Biomaterials,* vol. 277, p. 121110, 2021.
17. Y. Cai et al., "Cerium oxide nanozymes: exploring synthesis, catalytic activity, and biomedical potential," *Small,* vol. 31, no. 34, p. 2504436, 2025.

4 Radioactive Applications Using Nanomaterials

Avik Chakraborty

4.1 INTRODUCTION

The integration of nanotechnology with radiochemistry has opened a new paradigm in nuclear medicine, radiological diagnostics, and targeted radionuclide therapy (TRT). Nanomaterials, owing to their tunable size, shape, surface chemistry, and high surface area-to-volume ratio, offer improved stability, enhanced payload capacity, and selective organ or tumor targeting compared to conventional radiopharmaceuticals, as schematically presented in Figure 4.1. Radiolabeled nanoparticles have demonstrated significant advantages in both imaging and therapy, enabling multimodal diagnostics positron emission tomography/magnetic resonance imaging/computed tomography–positron emission tomography (PET/MRI/CT-PET) and image-guided drug delivery. Their ability to carry β, γ, or α emitters within tumor microenvironments provides better biodistribution, deeper tissue penetration, and reduced off-target radiation exposure.

This chapter discusses the fundamental principles of radioisotope selection, radiolabeling strategies, nano–bio interactions, and the rationale for nano-radiomedicine in cancer theranostics. Beyond healthcare, the role of nanomaterials in environmental radiotracing, industrial monitoring, food sterilization, and nuclear waste remediation is explored with relevant case studies. Key translational barriers, including pharmacokinetics, regulatory governance, radiotoxicity, and good manufacturing practice (GMP) manufacturing challenges, are critically examined. The chapter concludes with future perspectives underscoring the convergence of artificial intelligence (AI), personalized radiopharmacy, and nanotheranostics for next-generation precision medicine.

4.2 OVERVIEW OF RADIOLABELED NANOMATERIALS

4.2.1 Introduction to Radiolabeled Nanomaterials

The convergence of nanotechnology with nuclear medicine has led to the development of radiolabeled nanomaterials, an emerging class of engineered platforms that combine the physicochemical benefits of nanoscale systems with the functional capabilities of diagnostic and therapeutic radioisotopes. Conventional radiopharmaceuticals, though widely used for PET and single-photon emission computed tomography (SPECT) imaging, often suffer from rapid systemic clearance, poor tumor retention, and limited payload capacity. In contrast, radiolabeled nanoparticles enable enhanced

 DOI: 10.1201/9781003725930-4

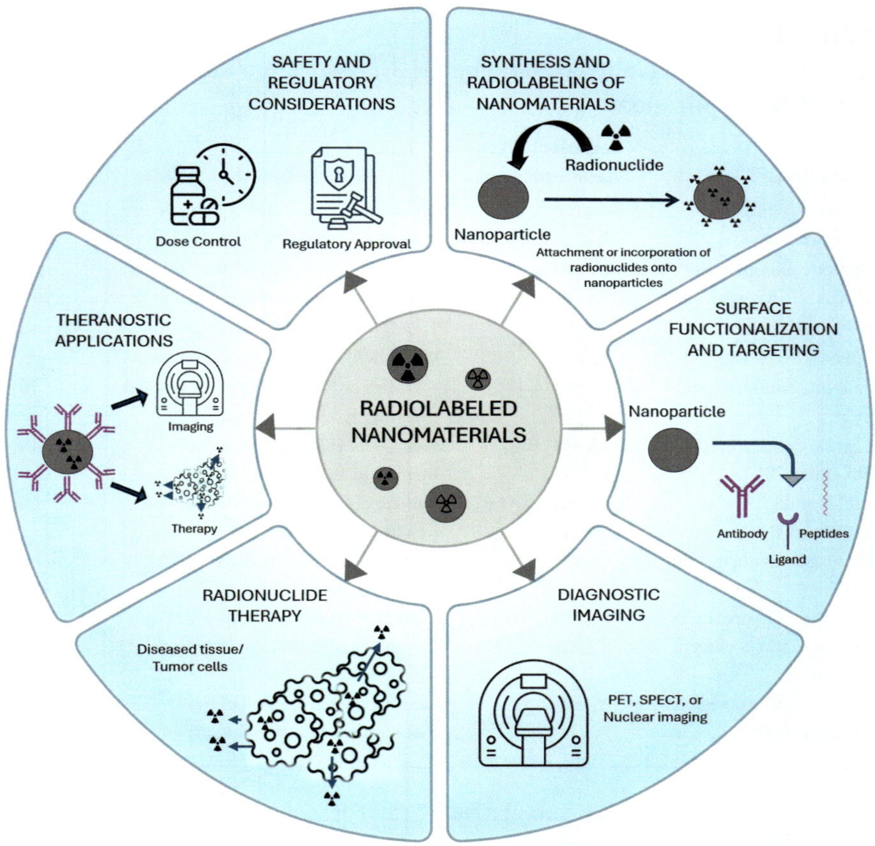

FIGURE 4.1 Schematic representation of radiolabeled nanomaterials for diagnostic and therapeutic applications. Nanoparticles of varying composition (lipid-based, polymeric, metallic, and hybrid systems) are functionalized with targeting ligands and radiolabeled with diagnostic (PET/SPECT) or therapeutic (β-, α-, Auger-emitting) radioisotopes.

pharmacokinetics, improved biological specificity, and multifunctional integration for theranostic applications [1]. A list of applications of radiolabeled nanomaterials and their associated radioisotopes is presented in Table 4.1.

Nanomaterials can be precisely engineered in terms of size, composition, surface charge, and ligand presentation. Their nanoscale dimensions (typically 10–150 nm) allow prolonged circulation and preferential accumulation at pathological sites through the enhanced permeability and retention (EPR) effect. Additionally, surface functionalization with antibodies, peptides, aptamers, and small-molecule ligands enables active targeting of overexpressed receptors in cancer, inflammation, or other disease microenvironments. The large surface area of nanocarriers supports high radiolabel loading and enables co-delivery of drugs, photosensitizers, or immunomodulators, establishing them as powerful platforms for personalized medicine.

TABLE 4.1
Representative Radiolabeled Nanomaterials, Associated Radioisotopes, and Biomedical Applications

Nanomaterial Class	Representative Radioisotopes	Primary Application(s)	Refs.
Liposomes/lipid nanoparticles	^{99m}Tc, ^{64}Cu, ^{111}In, ^{177}Lu	Tumor imaging, sentinel lymph node mapping, targeted radionuclide therapy	[5]
Polymeric nanoparticles (PLGA-, PEG-based)	^{64}Cu, ^{68}Ga, ^{89}Zr, ^{177}Lu	PET/SPECT imaging, theranostics, controlled radionuclide delivery	[6,7]
Gold nanoparticles (spheres, rods, shells)	^{64}Cu, ^{125}I, ^{131}I, ^{177}Lu	PET/CT imaging, radiosensitization, photothermal–radio combination therapy	[8]
Iron oxide nanoparticles	^{64}Cu, ^{68}Ga, ^{111}In	PET/MRI or SPECT/MRI multimodal imaging, lymph node mapping	[6]
Quantum dots/carbon nanodots	^{64}Cu, ^{18}F, ^{111}In	Multimodal PET–optical imaging, image-guided surgery	[9]
Metal–organic frameworks	^{64}Cu, ^{89}Zr, ^{177}Lu	High-capacity radionuclide loading, imaging-guided therapy	[6]
Silica-based nanoparticles	^{64}Cu,^{99m}Tc, ^{131}I	Drug–radionuclide co-delivery, PET/SPECT imaging	[10]
Biomimetic nanoparticles (cell membrane–coated, exosomes)	^{64}Cu, ^{68}Ga, ^{177}Lu	Immune evasion, personalized theranostics, metastatic targeting	[11,12]
Microspheres/nanospheres (intra-arterial)	^{90}Y, ^{166}Ho	Selective internal radiotherapy, locoregional tumor treatment	[13]

Radiolabeling strategies are broadly categorized into chelator-based and chelator-free approaches. Chelator-based systems employ macrocyclic ligands such as DOTA, NOTA, and HYNIC to form stable coordination complexes with radioisotopes. Chelator-free methods, more recent and increasingly attractive, rely on inherent affinity between the metallic or semiconductive nanomaterial surface and the isotope, resulting in improved labeling stability and minimal structural alteration. This versatility enables integration of a wide range of isotopes, including γ emitters for SPECT (e.g., ^{99m}Tc, ^{111}In), positron emitters for PET (e.g., ^{64}Cu, ^{68}Ga, ^{89}Zr), and β or α emitters for TRT (e.g., ^{177}Lu, ^{225}Ac) [2]. Applications of radiolabeled nanomaterials extend far beyond conventional oncology imaging. In cancer, they enhance tumor delineation, allow monitoring of therapeutic response, and enable targeted radionuclide delivery. In cardiovascular medicine, they assist in imaging atherosclerotic plaques and ischemic injury [3]. In neurology, radiolabeled nanosystems are being developed for tracking neuroinflammation and blood–brain barrier permeability. Their multimodal capacity allows integration of PET/SPECT with MRI, computed tomography (CT), or optical modalities, improving anatomical and molecular co-localization [4].

Beyond clinical contexts, nanotechnology-enabled radiotracers are gaining traction in environmental monitoring, oil and gas pipeline diagnostics, wastewater mapping, and nuclear waste tracking, owing to their high stability and detection sensitivity. Despite their promise, translational adoption faces several challenges. Pharmacokinetic unpredictability, opsonization by serum proteins, and reticuloendothelial system (RES) clearance can alter biodistribution. Long-term safety and biodegradability remain active research areas, particularly for inorganic nanocarriers. Regulatory frameworks for nano-radiopharmaceuticals are still evolving, requiring harmonization between nuclear regulatory standards and nanomedicine guidelines.

4.2.2 Historical Context and Evolution

The clinical use of radiopharmaceuticals began in the mid-20th century, when radioisotopes such as ^{131}I and ^{99m}Tc were integrated into small molecules and antibodies for diagnostic imaging and targeted radiotherapy. These early agents significantly improved clinical detection of thyroid disorders, bone metastasis, and organ physiology mapping [14]. However, their utility was constrained by rapid systemic clearance, limited tumor penetration, off-target toxicity, and low payload capacity. Antibody-based radiotracers improved specificity but suffered from slow pharmacokinetics and immunogenicity, limiting their widespread application. The emergence of nanotechnology in the late 20th and early 21st centuries created a paradigm shift in radiopharmaceutical design. Nanomaterials provided new opportunities to overcome biological and physicochemical limitations inherent to small-molecule tracers. Their tunable size enabled longer circulation times and preferential tumor accumulation via EPR effect, while surface modification with ligands introduced active targeting strategies toward cancer biomarkers, inflamed tissues, or ischemic microenvironments. Additionally, nanoplatforms offered modularity for multimodal payload delivery, combining therapeutic radionuclides, imaging isotopes, chemotherapeutic drugs, or photosensitizers on a single carrier.

Early milestones in the field included radiolabeled liposomes for extended drug delivery, followed by gold nanoparticles conjugated with γ- or PET-emitting isotopes for high-contrast tumor visualization and radiosensitization. Iron oxide nanoparticles later gained prominence due to their dual role as MRI contrast enhancers and radionuclide carriers, facilitating hybrid PET/MRI and SPECT/MRI imaging. The introduction of chelator-free radiolabeling techniques, particularly for metallic nanostructures and quantum dots, marked a breakthrough by enhancing label stability and simplifying radiochemical synthesis.

This historical trajectory reflects a steady transition from "radiation delivery through molecules" to "biologically intelligent nanosystems with integrated radiochemical function." Today, radiolabeled nanomaterials occupy a unique translational niche bridging molecular imaging, image-guided therapy, and theranostics. Their evolution has been driven not only by advances in material science and radiochemistry but also by an improved understanding of tumor biology, immune microenvironments, and biodistribution dynamics.

4.2.3 Classes of Radiolabeled Nanomaterials

Radiolabeled nanomaterials can be broadly classified according to their chemical composition, structural architecture, and radiolabeling strategy. Classification of radiolabeled nanomaterials based on chemical composition and structural architecture is presented in Figure 4.2. Among the most established systems are lipid-based nanocarriers, such as liposomes, solid lipid nanoparticles, and polymeric micelles, which are widely used owing to their biocompatibility, ease of surface modification, and ability to encapsulate both hydrophilic and hydrophobic agents. These platforms can be either surface-labeled or radionuclide-encapsulated, providing controlled biodistribution and stimuli-responsive release.

Metallic nanoparticles, particularly those derived from noble metals such as gold and platinum, serve as robust radiolabel carriers with inherent photothermal or radiosensitizing properties. Their high atomic number improves radiation dose deposition, making them suitable for combined imaging and radiotherapy. Similarly, metal oxide nanoparticles, such as iron oxide or manganese oxide, integrate diagnostic capabilities, for example, MRI contrast enhancement with nuclear imaging when conjugated with PET or SPECT isotopes, enabling effective multimodal theranostics.

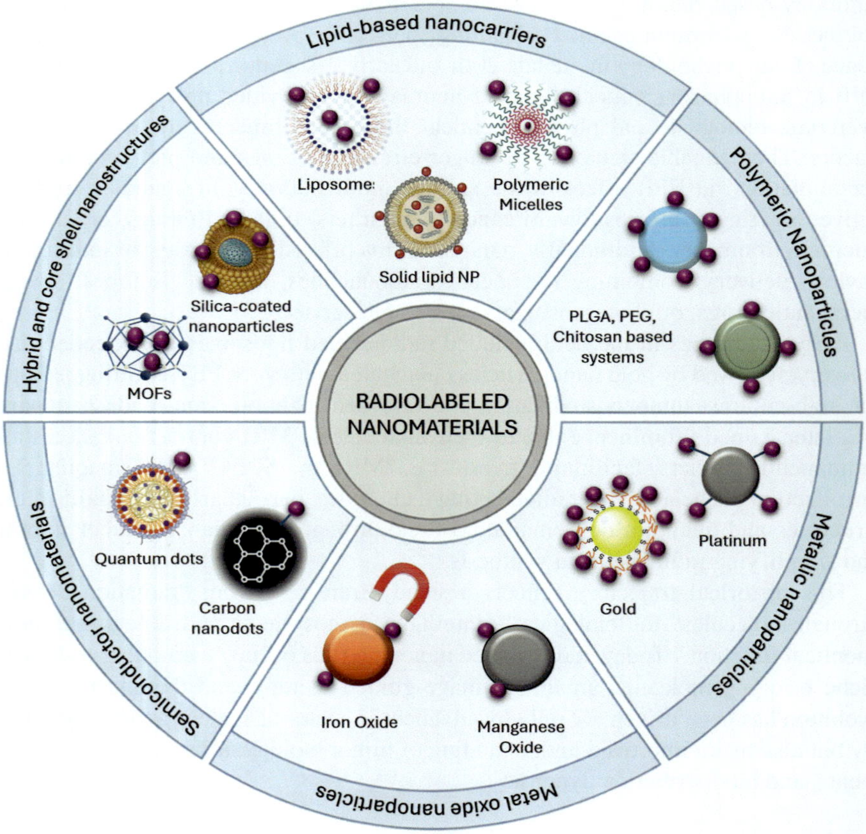

FIGURE 4.2 Classification of radiolabeled nanomaterials based on chemical composition and structural architecture. The schematic highlights diverse platforms from organic lipid-based vesicles to inorganic metallic clusters and hybrid frameworks.

Polymeric nanoparticles, fabricated from biodegradable materials like poly(lactic-co-glycolic acid) (PLGA), polyethylene glycol (PEG), or chitosan, offer tunable pharmacokinetics and controlled degradation profiles. Their surface can be engineered with chelators, peptides, or antibodies to facilitate targeted radionuclide delivery. Quantum dots and carbon nanodots represent semiconductor-based nanosystems that exhibit photoluminescence, enabling optical imaging in conjunction with radioisotopic tracking, although concerns regarding long-term toxicity have limited their clinical translation. More recently, hybrid and core–shell nanostructures have emerged as multifunctional platforms that unify diagnostic, therapeutic, and targeting features within a single architecture. These include metal–organic frameworks, silica-coated nanoparticles, and biomimetic cell membrane–coated nanocarriers, which provide enhanced stability and improved tumor microenvironment interaction.

4.2.4 Advantages of Nanoparticles in Radiopharmaceuticals

Nanoparticles offer distinct advantages over conventional small-molecule radiopharmaceuticals by improving targeting efficiency, circulation behavior, and therapeutic precision [15]. Their nanoscale dimensions facilitate passive tumor accumulation via the EPR effect, which arises from leaky tumor vasculature and impaired lymphatic drainage. In addition to passive targeting, nanoparticles also support multivalency, allowing simultaneous conjugation of multiple ligands, such as antibodies, peptides, or aptamers, thereby enhancing binding avidity and molecular selectivity toward diseased tissues. The larger surface area and protective coating strategies confer superior pharmacokinetics, including prolonged blood circulation and reduced rapid renal clearance, which is a major limitation of traditional radiotracers. A key advantage of nanoparticle-based radiopharmaceuticals is their inherent multimodality, enabling the co-integration of radionuclides with MRI, CT, or optical imaging agents, as well as chemotherapeutic or radiosensitizing payloads within a single platform. This multifunctionality forms the basis for modern nano-radiotheranostics, allowing simultaneous disease detection, monitoring, and treatment. Furthermore, many nanosystems can be engineered for controlled or stimuli-responsive release, activating payload delivery preferentially within the tumor microenvironment through pH, enzyme, or redox triggers. These properties collectively contribute to reduced off-target toxicity, as radionuclides and therapeutics are concentrated at the target site rather than distributed systemically, thereby improving the therapeutic index, and minimizing radiation-induced side effects.

4.2.5 Challenges and Considerations

Despite their advantages, the clinical translation of radiolabeled nanomaterials is constrained by several critical challenges. One major concern is the incomplete understanding of their long-term biodistribution and biological fate. Unlike small-molecule tracers that clear rapidly through renal excretion, nanoparticles can persist in the RES, accumulating primarily in the liver and spleen, which increases the risk of chronic retention or delayed toxicity. Another important limitation arises from nontarget organ uptake and immune sequestration, particularly by macrophages. This can reduce effective tumor delivery and compromise imaging sensitivity or therapeutic efficacy. Additionally, radiolysis-induced instability poses a technical barrier; exposure to ionizing radiation can degrade nanoparticle coatings or alter surface chemistry, leading to premature release of the radionuclide and loss of targeting ability.

Radiolabeling itself can be complex, often requiring stringent conditions to ensure radiochemical purity and in vivo stability, especially for chelator-based systems. From a translational standpoint, scaling up nanoparticle production under GMP-compliant conditions remains difficult, as precise control over particle size, ligand density, and labeling efficiency is essential for regulatory approval. Furthermore, nano-radiopharmaceuticals fall at the regulatory intersection of drug, device, and radioactive material frameworks, complicating approval pathways and safety evaluation. Toxicity assessments must account for both radiation dose and nanoparticle composition, including biodegradability and potential immunogenicity. Together, these considerations highlight the need for harmonized radiopharmacy protocols, improved material design, and coordinated regulatory guidance to facilitate clinical adoption. With these design principles and challenges in mind, the following section focuses on the synthesis, isotope integration, and characterization strategies that govern the performance of radiolabeled nanomaterials.

4.3 DESIGN, SYNTHESIS, AND CHARACTERIZATION OF RADIOLABELED NANOMATERIALS

4.3.1 Radioisotope Selection Criteria for Nanomaterials

The selection of an appropriate radioisotope is a critical determinant of the success of radiolabeled nanomaterials in both diagnostic and therapeutic applications. Unlike conventional small-molecule radiopharmaceuticals, nanoparticle-based systems exhibit prolonged circulation times, complex biodistribution patterns, and multistep biological interactions. Consequently, isotope choice must be carefully matched to nanoparticle pharmacokinetics, biological targeting strategy, and intended clinical application.

A primary consideration is physical half-life, which must be compatible with the in vivo residence time of the nanocarrier. Short-lived isotopes such as ^{68}Ga ($t_{1/2} \approx 68$ min) are suitable for rapidly distributing nanoparticles or local delivery systems, whereas longer-lived isotopes such as ^{64}Cu ($t_{1/2} \approx 12.7$ h) and ^{89}Zr ($t_{1/2} \approx 78.4$ h) are preferred for slow-clearing nanoparticles that require extended imaging windows [16]. For therapeutic applications, isotopes such as ^{177}Lu and ^{225}Ac are selected to align with prolonged tumor retention and sustained radiation delivery.

The type and energy of emitted radiation further influence isotope selection. Positron emitters are chosen for PET imaging based on positron range and image resolution, while γ emitters are optimized for SPECT detection efficiency. For therapy, β emitters provide crossfire effects suitable for heterogeneous tumors, whereas α emitters deliver high-linear energy transfer (LET) radiation with subcellular precision, making them ideal for micrometastatic disease.

Radiochemical compatibility with the nanomaterial is another key factor. Metallic radioisotopes such as ^{64}Cu, ^{68}Ga, and ^{177}Lu readily coordinate with chelators (e.g., DOTA, NOTA), while certain nanomaterials enable chelator-free labeling through intrinsic surface affinity. Isotope stability under physiological and radiolytic conditions is essential to prevent premature dissociation and off-target irradiation.

Finally, availability, production route, and regulatory acceptance influence translational feasibility. Generator-produced isotopes (e.g., ^{99m}Tc, ^{68}Ga) offer logistical advantages, whereas cyclotron-produced isotopes may require centralized manufacturing and distribution. Together, these criteria underscore the importance of integrating radiochemistry, material science, and biological considerations in the rational design of radiolabeled nanomaterials.

4.3.2 Nanoparticle Synthesis Methods

The synthesis pathway selected for a nanoparticle plays a decisive role not only in determining its morphology and surface chemistry but also in governing radiolabeling efficiency and in vivo performance. Unlike conventional nanomedicines, radiolabeled nanoparticles must be synthesized under constraints related to isotope half-life, radiation handling safety, and GMP scalability. Therefore, synthesis methods that are both reproducible and radionuclide-compatible are preferred.

Chemical co-precipitation is one of the most widely used methods for iron oxide nanoparticles and offers fine control over particle size by modulating pH, temperature, salt concentration, and reductive environment. Because the process can incorporate radioisotopes such as ^{59}Fe directly during precipitation, it aligns well with direct radiolabeling strategies. Moreover, the mild aqueous reaction conditions support further surface functionalization with chelators or targeting ligands without requiring extensive purification steps.

Seed-mediated growth, frequently utilized in the synthesis of gold nanoparticles and nanorods, enables exquisite control over particle geometry. The optical and pharmacokinetic properties of gold nanostructures vary considerably with shape and aspect ratio, making this method highly relevant for radiotheranostics in which photothermal transduction or radiosensitization accompany imaging. Radiolabeling can occur post-synthetically via thiol–gold affinity or silane functionalization followed by chelation. Due to the chemical inertness of gold, isotopic stability is typically high once labeling is completed.

Emulsion polymerization is particularly advantageous for generating polymeric nanocarriers such as PLGA, PEG-polylactic acid, or chitosan-based nanoparticles. These systems are well suited for radiometal chelation, as chelators may be introduced either pre- or post-polymerization. Their biodegradability and modularity make them attractive for clinical translation; for example, ^{64}Cu- or ^{177}Lu-labeled polymeric nanosystems have been investigated for combined imaging and TRT.

Emerging technologies now favor microfluidic synthesis, which provides unprecedented control over nanoparticle uniformity, reaction conditions, and reproducibility. Microfluidic reactors are particularly attractive from a radiopharmacy standpoint, because they reduce operator exposure, minimize reagent consumption, and are compatible with automated GMP production. Furthermore, microfluidic platforms facilitate rapid "just-in-time" synthesis, an essential advantage when working with short-lived PET isotopes such as ^{68}Ga and ^{64}Cu. The combination of microfluidics and radiochemistry is increasingly being viewed as the future of decentralized radiolabeled nanoparticle manufacturing.

4.3.3 In Vitro and In Vivo Characterization

Following physicochemical confirmation, biological evaluation ensures that nanoparticle architecture translates into functional activity. In vitro assays typically include cellular uptake, conducted using cancer or immune cell lines expressing target receptors, and cytotoxicity assays, which establish safe dose windows prior to animal studies. Confocal microscopy or radiometric quantification is used to track internalization efficiency and receptor-mediated targeting. In vivo characterization begins with preliminary pharmacokinetic assessment using small-animal PET or SPECT imaging to determine circulation half-life, tumor accumulation, and organ distribution. These datasets are often corroborated through biodistribution studies, in which excised organs are gamma-counted to yield quantitative uptake values (e.g., %ID/g). A critical translational element is dosimetry, which estimates absorbed radiation dose to both tumor and healthy tissues. By integrating time–activity curves derived from PET/SPECT imaging with biological clearance models, dosimetric estimates guide therapeutic index optimization and ensure safety prior to clinical translation. This step is especially crucial for therapeutic isotopes such as ^{177}Lu,^{225}Ac, or ^{131}I, where off-target deposition may induce organ-specific toxicity [17,18].

4.4 APPLICATIONS FOR CANCER DIAGNOSIS AND THERAPY

Radiolabeled nanomaterials have emerged as a transformative class of agents in oncology due to their ability to combine molecular imaging with targeted radionuclide delivery [18]. Unlike conventional radiotracers, which predominantly rely on passive biodistribution and rapid clearance, nanoparticles offer prolonged circulation, tumor-selective accumulation, and the capacity to integrate multimodal functions such as imaging, radiosensitization, and drug co-delivery. These features enable earlier detection of malignancies, improved staging accuracy, and enhanced therapeutic index in radionuclide-based interventions.

4.4.1 Radiolabeled Nanomaterials in Cancer Imaging

The oncological utility of radiolabeled nanoparticles in imaging arises from their capacity to accumulate preferentially in tumors through both passive (EPR) and ligand-mediated targeting, enabling visualization at superior contrast and persistence compared to small molecules, as presented in Figure 4.3.

4.4.1.1 PET and SPECT Imaging

Nanoparticles labeled with positron emitters (^{64}Cu, ^{89}Zr, ^{68}Ga) or γ emitters (^{99m}Tc, ^{111}In) serve as high-sensitivity imaging agents in PET and SPECT, respectively. Gold nanoparticles have been widely explored in PET/CT hybrid imaging platforms,

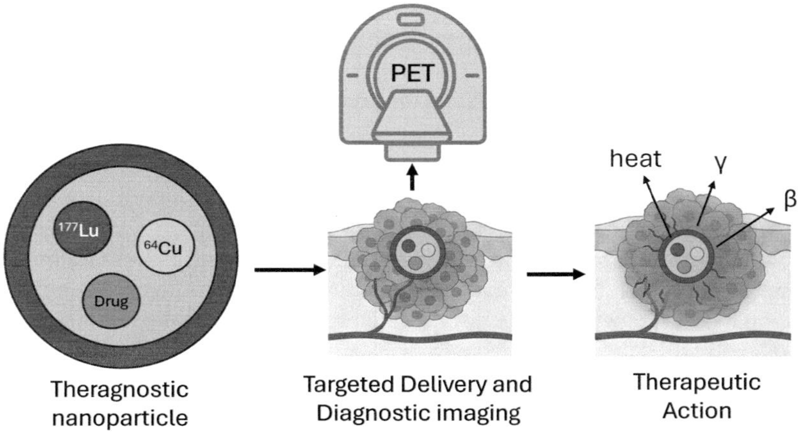

FIGURE 4.3 Radiolabeled nanotheranostic platform integrating PET-based diagnosis, personalized dose planning, and targeted radionuclide therapy with real-time response monitoring.

where their high electron density simultaneously enhances CT contrast. Similarly, ^{99m}Tc- or ^{111}In-labeled liposomes and micelles have been used to track tumor uptake and vascular permeability in solid tumors.

Magnetic and metallic nanoplatforms provide unique multimodal advantages. Radiolabeled iron oxide nanoparticles, for instance, enable concurrent PET/MRI visualization, combining anatomical soft-tissue detail with molecular signal tracking. This dual functionality offers more accurate tumor margin assessment and treatment planning than PET alone, particularly in brain tumors, prostate cancer, and metastatic lesions where microenvironmental heterogeneity limits small-molecule tracer performance [18,19].

4.4.1.2 Multimodality Imaging

A major advancement introduced by nanoparticle-based radiotracers is their ability to integrate nuclear, optical, and magnetic imaging modalities. Quantum dots or carbon nanodots radiolabeled with PET emitters provide simultaneous fluorescence and nuclear detection, facilitating intraoperative surgical navigation following preoperative PET-based mapping. Likewise, gold nanoparticles allow PET/CT/photothermal hybrid detection, while silica- or polymer-based nanosystems can co-encapsulate radiolabels and near-infrared dyes to support real-time image-guided interventions. These platforms enable longitudinal tumor monitoring, early assessment of therapeutic response, and improved surgical precision [20].

4.4.2 Targeted Radionuclide Therapy with Nanoparticles

Beyond imaging, nanoparticles can be engineered as carriers for therapeutic radionuclides, enabling controlled delivery of cytotoxic radiation to the tumor site while minimizing off-target exposure. By shielding healthy tissues and prolonging tumor residence time, nanocarrier-based TRT significantly improves therapeutic index [18].

4.4.2.1 Beta-Particle Emitting Nanotherapeutics

β emitters such as ^{177}Lu, ^{131}I, and ^{90}Y are widely used in nanocarrier-based therapies due to their intermediate tissue penetration range, which is suitable for solid tumors. Polymeric nanoparticles functionalized with targeting ligands (e.g., antibodies, arginine–glycine–aspartic acid peptides, or folate receptors) selectively deliver these isotopes to malignant cells while sparing surrounding tissues. Radiolabeled liposomes loaded with ^{177}Lu have demonstrated durable tumor control in preclinical breast and ovarian cancer models by enabling prolonged internal irradiation [18].

4.4.2.2 Alpha Particle Therapy

α-emitting isotopes, including ^{225}Ac and ^{211}At, represent a next-generation paradigm in targeted therapy due to their high LET and extremely localized cytotoxicity. When conjugated to nanoparticles, these isotopes achieve higher stability and reduced systemic dissemination compared to small chelate complexes alone. Nanocarriers also protect alpha daughters (decay products) from diffusing away from the tumor, a key translational challenge in alpha therapy. This approach is particularly promising for micrometastatic disease and minimal residual disease, where high-intensity localized irradiation may eradicate tumor cells resistant to conventional therapies [21].

4.4.2.3 Auger Electron Emitters

Auger emitters, such as ^{125}I and ^{111}In, release very short-range electrons capable of inducing lethal DNA damage when delivered intracellularly. Nanoparticles enable efficient intracellular localization, particularly nuclear-targeted or mitochondria-targeted nanosystems, enhancing therapeutic potency. These agents hold promise for precision oncology applications where subcellular targeting is essential to efficacy [22].

4.4.3 Theranostic Applications

The convergence of diagnosis and therapy within the same nanosystem termed "nanotheranostics" is one of the most clinically relevant advances of radiolabeled nanomaterials. By carrying both diagnostic and therapeutic radioisotopes, or combining radioisotopes with chemotherapeutics or radiosensitizers, theranostic nanoplatforms enable patient stratification, personalized dose planning, and real-time monitoring of therapeutic efficacy. Dual-labeled nanosystems such as ^{64}Cu/^{177}Lu-polymeric nanoparticles exemplify this integration: the PET isotope (^{64}Cu) is first used to visualize tumor uptake and determine suitability for treatment, followed by ^{177}Lu-mediated therapy using the same nanocarrier [23]. Similarly, gold nanoparticles co-loaded with radiolabels and photothermal sensitizers support synergistic radio-thermal ablation.

4.4.4 Challenges in Cancer Applications

Despite their promise, several factors limit the universal effectiveness of radiolabeled nanomaterials in oncology. Tumor heterogeneity and dense stromal barriers can hinder nanoparticle penetration, reducing therapeutic payload delivery in hypoxic or fibrotic tumor regions. Accelerated uptake by the RES reduces systemic bioavailability, necessitating surface modifications such as PEGylation or biomimetic cloaking. Furthermore, isotope half-life must be carefully matched to nanoparticle pharmacokinetics: slow-clearing nanocarriers paired with short-lived isotopes risk suboptimal dose delivery, while long-lived isotopes may increase radiation burden if clearance is incomplete [24].

4.5 NANOMATERIALS IN NUCLEAR MEDICINE

The integration of nanotechnology with nuclear medicine represents a major transition from conventional molecular radiotracers toward multifunctional nanoscale platforms that enable improved detection sensitivity, theranostic precision, and multimodal imaging (Figure 4.4). Beyond oncology, radiolabeled nanoparticles are expanding applications in cardiovascular disease, inflammation, infection imaging, and regenerative medicine. Their versatility lies in their tunable biodistribution, prolonged circulation, and capacity to internalize multiple functional payloads including imaging isotopes, therapeutic radionuclides, and contrast agents [25].

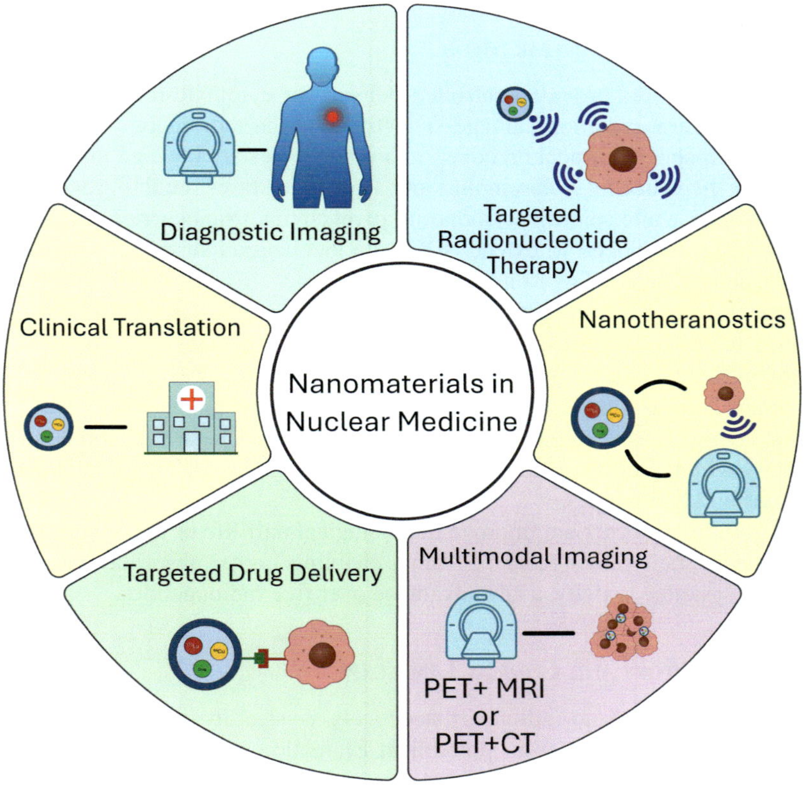

FIGURE 4.4 Nanomaterials in nuclear medicine: broad applications of nanotechnology in nuclear medicine, spanning diagnostic imaging, targeted therapeutic interventions, and the path toward clinical translation.

4.5.1 Diagnostic Nuclear Medicine

In diagnostic imaging, radiolabeled nanomaterials improve lesion visualization by enhancing tumor retention and reducing background signal. Their multivalent surfaces facilitate the attachment of receptor-targeting ligands, outperforming monoclonal antibodies and peptides in terms of stability and circulation time. For example, radiolabeled iron oxide nanoparticles have demonstrated success in PET/MRI fusion imaging for glioma and lymph node mapping, providing superior anatomical resolution alongside molecular specificity. Similarly, ^{99m}Tc-labeled polymeric micelles have shown utility in sentinel lymph node imaging and vascular permeability assessment. An emerging area in diagnostic nuclear medicine is image-guided intervention, where radiolabeled nanoparticles provide intraoperative surgical navigation by delineating tumor margins more effectively than conventional dyes or free radionuclides. Dual radiolabel–fluorescent nanoplatforms assist surgeons in real-time lesion localization, especially in oncologic resections requiring high precision (e.g., head and neck tumors, hepatobiliary lesions). Additionally, nanoparticle-based tracers enable earlier detection of micro-lesions that fall below the sensitivity threshold of conventional radiotracers, improving staging accuracy [26].

4.5.2 Therapeutic Nuclear Medicine

In TRT, nanocarriers provide controlled delivery of cytotoxic radioisotopes while reducing collateral radiation damage. Selective internal radiotherapy (SIRT) exemplifies this concept in clinical practice. ^{90}Y microspheres are injected intra-arterially for treating hepatocellular carcinoma and liver metastases, enabling locoregional dose escalation while sparing surrounding parenchyma. Nanocarrier-based systems are now being developed to extend SIRT-like localization strategies to other solid tumors using ^{177}Lu or ^{131}I as β emitters [27].

Nanoplatforms also support site-specific therapeutic targeting for metastatic and disseminated disease. Bone-seeking radiolabeled nanoparticles are under investigation for skeletal metastases, while membrane-coated nanocarriers functionalized with tumor-homing ligands enable enhanced selectivity for hematological malignancies. Hybrid constructs, such as radioimmunonano conjugates, combine immune specificity with radiotherapeutic delivery, representing a next-generation strategy for leukemias and lymphomas.

Importantly, nanocarriers improve the biological half-life of therapeutic isotopes and modulate their tumor residence time, enabling higher absorbed dose without increasing systemic toxicity, a key advantage over free radionuclides.

4.5.3 Regulatory and Clinical Landscape

Clinical interest in nano-radiopharmaceuticals is steadily increasing, with several candidates advancing from preclinical evaluation into regulatory review and early-phase human trials. ^{64}Cu-labeled liposomal formulations, ^{89}Zr-labeled iron oxide PET/MRI agents, and ^{177}Lu-bearing polymeric nanocarriers represent notable examples demonstrating translational feasibility. Regulatory agencies now encourage more robust nanoparticle characterization, harmonized dosimetry protocols, and long-term biodistribution studies to ensure safety. The convergence of nanotechnology and radiopharmaceutical regulations has prompted the adoption of hybrid approval pathways that account for both nanomedicine and nuclear medicine oversight. This dual-governance framework emphasizes reproducibility, GMP-compliant manufacturing, and traceability of the radionuclide synthesis chain. The growing emphasis on precision medicine and image-guided therapy further strengthens the role of radiolabeled nanoparticles in future nuclear medicine practice. Their capacity to unify diagnosis and therapy within a single platform aligns with modern theranostic paradigms and facilitates treatment personalization based on real-time biological response [28].

4.6 SAFETY CONSIDERATIONS AND REGULATORY FRAMEWORK

The translation of radiolabeled nanomaterials from laboratory platforms to clinical application requires rigorous safety evaluation that encompasses both radiopharmaceutical and nanomedicine risk profiles. Safety considerations extend beyond radionuclide toxicity to include nanocarrier biodegradability, long-term biodistribution, and immunological compatibility. Because these systems introduce a hybrid therapeutic modality, regulatory assessment must simultaneously address radiation protection, pharmacology, and material science criteria, necessitating multidisciplinary oversight [29].

4.6.1 Toxicity and Biocompatibility

Nanoparticles interact with biological systems in ways that differ from conventional drugs. Their nanoscale size facilitates cellular uptake but also increases the likelihood of RES sequestration in the liver, spleen, and lymphatic tissues. Persistent accumulation can pose risks of chronic inflammation or oxidative stress if materials are not biodegradable. Therefore, the choice between organic (polymeric, lipid-based) and inorganic (metallic, metal oxide) systems has significant safety implications. Toxicity assessment begins with in vitro cytotoxicity assays followed by in vivo evaluation of acute and chronic toxicity across major organs. Beyond general toxicity, the biocorona effect, adsorption of biomolecules onto nanoparticle surfaces in circulation can modify biodistribution and immunogenicity. For clinical translation, nanocarriers must demonstrate predictable metabolism or safe excretion pathways, without unexpected long-term retention. Radiation-related toxicity also requires careful evaluation. Although targeted delivery minimizes systemic exposure, residual activity in nontarget organs must be quantified. The therapeutic window depends on optimizing absorbed dose to tumors while maintaining acceptable thresholds for healthy tissues [30].

4.6.2 Radiation Safety

Because these systems contain radioisotopes, radiological safety extends to manufacturing, storage, administration, and waste disposal. The incorporation of nanoparticles does not diminish the need for radiation protection; in fact, prolonged handling during synthesis can increase occupational exposure if not automated. Safe formulation requires secure radiolabel attachment to prevent leaching and off-target irradiation. For α emitters, daughter nuclide recoil is an additional concern; nanoparticle-based internal shielding is often required to prevent diffusion of radioactive progeny into healthy tissues.

4.6.3 Regulatory Guidelines

Radiolabeled nanomaterials occupy a dual-regulatory space, falling under both nanomedicine and radiopharmaceutical governance. Agencies such as the Food and Drug Administration, European Medicines Agency, and International Atomic Energy Agency mandate extensive preclinical characterization including pharmacokinetics, dosimetry, immunogenicity, and stability. GMP guidelines require reproducibility of nanoparticle size, surface chemistry, ligand density, and radiochemical purity. Because radionuclides may alter degradation profiles or induce structural instability, regulators increasingly require in vivo radiostability data and post-radiosynthesis quality control beyond conventional nanoparticle assays. Furthermore, labeling efficiency must exceed minimum thresholds (typically >95%) to prevent free isotope accumulation. The approval pathway often follows a hybrid model: radionuclide-specific evaluation under radiopharmaceutical frameworks merged with nanocarrier assessment under advanced therapy medicinal product or drug–device combination regulations.

4.6.4 Ethical and Environmental Considerations

Ethical oversight includes ensuring informed consent, particularly for first-in-human studies where long-term clearance remains uncertain. Patients must be made aware of both radiological and nanoparticle-related risks. Accessibility is an additional ethical issue, as high production costs may limit widespread availability unless standardized manufacturing platforms evolve. Environmentally, disposal of radioactive nanoparticle waste requires stricter containment compared to conventional radiopharmaceuticals, as the persistence of nanomaterials can prolong decay storage requirements. Prevention of inadvertent environmental exposure is critical, particularly for long-lived isotopes or nonbiodegradable nanocarriers.

4.7 FUTURE DIRECTIONS AND PERSPECTIVES

The field of radiolabeled nanomaterials is rapidly evolving toward smarter, more biologically responsive, and clinically adaptable platforms. The next generation of nano-radiopharmaceuticals is expected to go beyond passive tumor targeting and incorporate real-time biological feedback, adaptive dose modulation, and precision delivery tailored to individual patient profiles. Three key technological shifts are shaping this trajectory: smart activatable nanoplatforms, AI-enabled design and dosimetry, and the development of novel radionuclide–nanocarrier combinations [31].

4.7.1 Development of Smart Radiolabeled Nanomaterials

A major future direction centers on stimuli-responsive and intelligent nanoparticles capable of releasing radionuclides or therapeutic payloads selectively within pathological microenvironments. These systems leverage endogenous stimuli such as pH, enzymes, hypoxia, or redox gradients to trigger activation only at the tumor site, thereby minimizing systemic exposure. For example, pH-sensitive polymer–lipid hybrids can retain radiolabels in circulation but release co-loaded chemotherapeutics intracellularly, supporting synergistic radio-chemo effects. DNA-responsive nanosystems are also emerging as a platform for controlled nuclear delivery of Auger emitters, enabling subcellular precision therapy. As tumor biology becomes increasingly understood through imaging genomics and metabolomics, these "smart" nanoplatforms will allow more dynamic response-driven theranostics [31].

4.7.2 Artificial Intelligence in Design and Dosimetry

The integration of AI and machine learning (ML) into nano-radiopharmaceutical design is poised to accelerate optimization pipelines. Data-driven modeling can predict nanoparticle biodistribution, ligand density thresholds for targeting, and radionuclide retention stability before synthesis, reducing empirical trial-and-error [32]. In dosimetry, ML-assisted reconstruction of PET/SPECT signals enables individualized radiation dose mapping based on patient-specific tumor perfusion and clearance kinetics. This paves the way for adaptive radiotheranostics, where nanoparticle-mediated therapy is recalibrated based on real-time imaging feedback [33].

4.7.3 Emerging Radionuclides and Nanocarriers

The discovery of novel radioisotopes with favorable half-lives and decay signatures is expanding the radiotheranostic landscape. Isotopes such as ^{67}Cu, ^{47}Sc, and ^{161}Tb offer balanced imaging–therapy properties that match nanoparticle circulation times more effectively than conventional radiotracers [34]. Parallel advances in biomimetic and biodegradable nanocarriers, including exosome-derived vesicles, cell membrane–coated nanoparticles, and protein-based scaffolds, are expected to improve immune evasion, enhance tumor penetration, and reduce long-term organ retention. An additional frontier is the convergence of immunotherapy and radiotheranostics, where nanoparticles not only deliver radionuclides but also modulate the tumor immune microenvironment. By combining targeted radiation with immune-stimulating payloads or checkpoint inhibitors, nanoplatforms may overcome immune resistance and enable synergistic treatment outcomes [33,35].

4.8 CONCLUSION

Radiolabeled nanomaterials represent a paradigm shift at the intersection of nanotechnology and nuclear medicine, offering solutions to several long-standing limitations of conventional radiopharmaceuticals. Their unique physicochemical properties, high surface area, tunable size, and the ability to co-deliver imaging and therapeutic payloads enable superior targeting, prolonged circulation, and enhanced signal retention in malignant tissue. By integrating diagnostic and therapeutic capabilities within a single nanosystem, they embody the principle of theranostics and support precision oncology through real-time monitoring of treatment response. The versatility of nanoparticle platforms accommodates a wide spectrum of radionuclides, ranging from PET and SPECT isotopes for improved lesion visualization to high-LET α emitters for targeted cytotoxicity in micrometastatic disease. Moreover, hybrid and multimodal nanoplatforms extend the role of nuclear medicine beyond imaging toward image-guided interventions and adaptive therapy planning. These advantages collectively position radiolabeled nanomaterials as next-generation radiotheranostics with strong translational potential. However, successful clinical integration requires careful navigation of safety, biodistribution, and radiochemical stability challenges. Regulatory approval pathways remain complex due to the dual nature of these constructs as both nanomedicines and radiopharmaceuticals. Harmonized GMP manufacturing and predictive dosimetry models will be essential for widespread clinical adoption. Looking forward, advances in smart stimuli-responsive designs, biomimetic nanocarriers, and AI-enabled dosimetric modeling are anticipated to elevate radiolabeled nanoparticles from experimental platforms to routine clinical tools. With continued multidisciplinary collaboration among chemists, radiopharmacists, material scientists, and clinicians, these technologies have the potential to significantly expand the therapeutic reach of nuclear medicine and deliver truly personalized cancer care.

REFERENCES

1. G. Tiwari, V. Shirsat, P. Desale, S. Karale, Critical perspectives on nanoparticle-enabled radiopharmaceuticals: integrating molecular imaging, targeted therapy, and theranostic translation, *Current Radiopharmaceuticals*, 19(2026) 100018.
2. S. Patra, S. Ghosh, K. Singh, B. Dutta, A. Chakraborty, N. Gamre, et al., Accelerator production, radiochemical separation and nanoradiopharmaceutical formulation using 69Ge: a next generation PET probe, *Journal of Drug Delivery Science and Technology*, 91(2024) 105204.
3. A. Maier, A.J. Teunissen, S.A. Nauta, E. Lutgens, Z.A. Fayad, M.M. van Leent, Uncovering atherosclerotic cardiovascular disease by PET imaging, *Nature Reviews Cardiology*, 21(2024) 632–51.
4. K.C. Black, W.J. Akers, G. Sudlow, B. Xu, R. Laforest, S. Achilefu, Dual-radiolabeled nanoparticle SPECT probes for bioimaging, *Nanoscale*, 7(2015) 440–4.
5. H. Lee, D. Gaddy, M. Ventura, N. Bernards, R. de Souza, D. Kirpotin, et al., Companion diagnostic 64Cu-liposome positron emission tomography enables characterization of drug delivery to tumors and predicts response to cancer nanomedicines, *Theranostics*, 8(2018) 2300.
6. M.S.O. Pijeira, H. Viltres, J. Kozempel, M. Sakmár, M. Vlk, D. İlem-Özdemir, et al., Radiolabeled nanomaterials for biomedical applications: radiopharmacy in the era of nanotechnology, *EJNMMI Radiopharmacy and Chemistry*, 7(2022) 8.
7. J. Fu, L. Chen, J. Hu, C. Yu, J. Yin, Radiolabelled nanomaterials for diagnostic and therapeutic applications in hepatocellular carcinoma and other liver diseases, *Precision Medicine and Engineering*, 2(2025) 100018.
8. X.-D. Zhang, D. Wu, X. Shen, J. Chen, Y.-M. Sun, P.-X. Liu, et al., Size-dependent radiosensitization of PEG-coated gold nanoparticles for cancer radiation therapy, *Biomaterials*, 33(2012) 6408–19.

9. J.T. Robinson, K. Welsher, S.M. Tabakman, S.P. Sherlock, H. Wang, R. Luong, et al., High performance in vivo near-IR (>1 μm) imaging and photothermal cancer therapy with carbon nanotubes, *Nano Research*, 3(2010) 779–93.
10. M. Martínez-Carmona, D. Lozano, M. Colilla, M. Vallet-Regí, Lectin-conjugated pH-responsive mesoporous silica nanoparticles for targeted bone cancer treatment, *Acta Biomaterialia*, 65(2018) 393–404.
11. A. Najdian, D. Beiki, M. Abbasi, A. Gholamrezanezhad, H. Ahmadzadehfar, A.M. Amani, et al., Exploring innovative strides in radiolabeled nanoparticle progress for multimodality cancer imaging and theranostic applications, *Cancer Imaging*, 24(2024) 127.
12. S. Zhang, A. Zhang, X. Qi, Z. Han, L. Song, J. Zhou, et al., Radionuclide-labeled biomaterials: a novel strategy for tumor-targeted therapy, *Biomimetics*, 10(2025) 394.
13. P. Sólymos, M. Rédei, C. Turan, B. Szabó, A. Ádám, Z. Molnár, et al., Holmium-166 radioembolization is a safe and effective locoregional treatment for primary and secondary liver tumors: a systematic review and meta-analysis, *Cancers*, 17(2025) 1841.
14. D.V. Becker, C.T. Sawin, Radioiodine and thyroid disease: the beginning, *Seminars in Nuclear Medicine*, 26 (1996) 155–64.
15. S.F. Mirshojaei, A. Ahmadi, E. Morales-Avila, M. Ortiz-Reynoso, H. Reyes-Perez, Radiolabelled nanoparticles: novel classification of radiopharmaceuticals for molecular imaging of cancer, *Journal of Drug Targeting*, 24(2016) 91–101.
16. D. Chen, D. Yang, C.A. Dougherty, W. Lu, H. Wu, X. He, et al., In vivo targeting and positron emission tomography imaging of tumor with intrinsically radioactive metal–organic frameworks nanomaterials, *ACS Nano*, 11(2017) 4315–27.
17. S. Kunjachan, J. Ehling, G. Storm, F. Kiessling, T. Lammers, Noninvasive imaging of nanomedicines and nanotheranostics: principles, progress, and prospects, *Chemical Reviews*, 115(2015) 10907–37.
18. J. Pellico, P.J. Gawne, R.T. de Rosales, Radiolabelling of nanomaterials for medical imaging and therapy, *Chemical Society Reviews*, 50(2021) 3355–423.
19. B.R. Jarrett, B. Gustafsson, D.L. Kukis, A.Y. Louie, Synthesis of 64Cu-labeled magnetic nanoparticles for multimodal imaging, *Bioconjugate Chemistry*, 19(2008) 1496–504.
20. F. Chen, P.A. Ellison, C.M. Lewis, H. Hong, Y. Zhang, S. Shi, et al., Chelator-free synthesis of a dual-modality PET/MRI agent, *Angewandte Chemie (International ed in English)*, 52(2013) 13319–23. doi: 10.1002/anie.201306306.
21. M.R. McDevitt, D. Ma, L.T. Lai, J. Simon, P. Borchardt, R.K. Frank, et al., Tumor therapy with targeted atomic nanogenerators, *Science*, 294(2001) 1537–40.
22. F. Buchegger, F. Perillo-Adamer, Y.M. Dupertuis, A. Bischof Delaloye, Auger radiation targeted into DNA: a therapy perspective, *European Journal of Nuclear Medicine and Molecular Imaging*, 33(2006) 1352–63.
23. E.B. Ehlerding, S. Goel, W. Cai, Cancer theranostics with 64Cu/177Lu-loaded liposomes, *European Journal of Nuclear Medicine and Molecular Imaging*, 43(2016) 938–40.
24. R.H. Fang, A.V. Kroll, W. Gao, L. Zhang, Cell membrane coating nanotechnology, *Advanced Materials*, 30(2018) 1706759.
25. M.J. Salgueiro, M. Zubillaga, Theranostic nanoplatforms in nuclear medicine: Current advances, emerging trends, and perspectives for personalized oncology, *Journal of Nanotheranostics*, 6(2025) 27.
26. R. Madru, P. Kjellman, F. Olsson, K. Wingårdh, C. Ingvar, F. Ståhlberg, et al., 99mTc-labeled superparamagnetic iron oxide nanoparticles for multimodality SPECT/MRI of sentinel lymph nodes, *Journal of Nuclear Medicine*, 53(2012) 459–63.
27. A.B. Satterlee, H. Yuan, L. Huang, A radio-theranostic nanoparticle with high specific drug loading for cancer therapy and imaging, *Journal of Controlled Release*, 217(2015) 170–82.
28. F. Chen, H. Hong, S. Goel, S.A. Graves, H. Orbay, E.B. Ehlerding, et al., In vivo tumor vasculature targeting of CuS@ MSN based theranostic nanomedicine, *ACS Nano*, 9(2015) 3926–34.

29. M.P. Monopoli, C. Aberg, A. Salvati, K.A. Dawson, Biomolecular coronas provide the biological identity of nanosized materials, *Nano-Enabled Medical Applications*, L.P. Balogh (ed.), Routledge (2020) 205–29.
30. G. Sgouros, Dosimetry of internal emitters, *Journal of Nuclear Medicine*, 46(2005) 18S–27S.
31. B.K. Kashyap, V.V. Singh, M.K. Solanki, A. Kumar, J. Ruokolainen, K.K. Kesari, Smart nanomaterials in cancer theranostics: challenges and opportunities, *ACS Omega*, 8(2023) 14290–320.
32. J. Tao, L. Liang, S. Hao, Y. Chen, Z. Yang, Y. Cai, et al., Artificial intelligence for radiopharmaceutical and molecular imaging, *Acta Pharmaceutica Sinica B*, 15(2025) 6199–21.
33. R. Seifert, M. Weber, E. Kocakavuk, C. Rischpler, D. Kersting, Artificial intelligence and machine learning in nuclear medicine: future perspectives, *Seminars in Nuclear Medicine*, 51(2021), 170–7.
34. C. Champion, M.A. Quinto, C. Morgat, P. Zanotti-Fregonara, E. Hindié, Comparison between three promising ß-emitting radionuclides, 67Cu, 47Sc and 161Tb, with emphasis on doses delivered to minimal residual disease, *Theranostics*, 6(2016) 1611.
35. J. Shi, P.W. Kantoff, R. Wooster, O.C. Farokhzad, Cancer nanomedicine: progress, challenges and opportunities, *Nature Reviews Cancer*, 17(2017) 20–37.

5 Progress in Food Technology by Nanocomposites

Jasmina Vidic, Petar Todorovic, and Petar Ristivojevic

5.1 INTRODUCTION

Food waste and spoilage have become pressing challenges for global food systems, affecting food security, straining economies, and worsening environmental damage. The Food and Agriculture Organization estimates that nearly one-third of all food produced worldwide, about 1.3 billion tons annually is lost or wasted, with associated economic costs exceeding 940 billion USD. Beyond financial losses, this waste misuses precious natural resources such as land and water, while decomposing organic matter in landfills accounts for an estimated 8%–10% of global greenhouse gas emissions, largely in the form of methane. The paradox of food abundance alongside widespread hunger is particularly visible in third world countries where nearly several million tons of food are wasted each year, despite persistent malnutrition and micronutrient deficiencies [1]. Much of this loss occurs before consumption, with up to 40% of perishable fruits and vegetables spoiled due to inadequate refrigeration and storage infrastructure. Developed regions face similar inefficiencies: the United States discards nearly 119 billion pounds of food annually, amounting to 40% of its total production, while Europe wastes around 88 million tons at an estimated cost of €143 billion.

Nanotechnology offers powerful avenues to overcome these interconnected challenges by enhancing food preservation, improving safety monitoring, and enriching nutritional quality. As presented in Figure 5.1, the food sector can develop packaging with superior barrier and antimicrobial properties, nanosensors capable of real-time contamination detection, and nano-encapsulation systems that protect and deliver sensitive nutrients [2]. Practical demonstrations already highlight this promise: antimicrobial nanocomposite packaging has reduced microbial contamination in meat by up to 90% in experimental studies, while nano-silicon additives in dairy products have improved shelf-life and reduced spoilage. By integrating these nano-enabled innovations into the food supply chain, it is possible to not only reduce economic losses and environmental impact but also move closer to achieving global food security and sustainability targets.

DOI: 10.1201/9781003725930-5

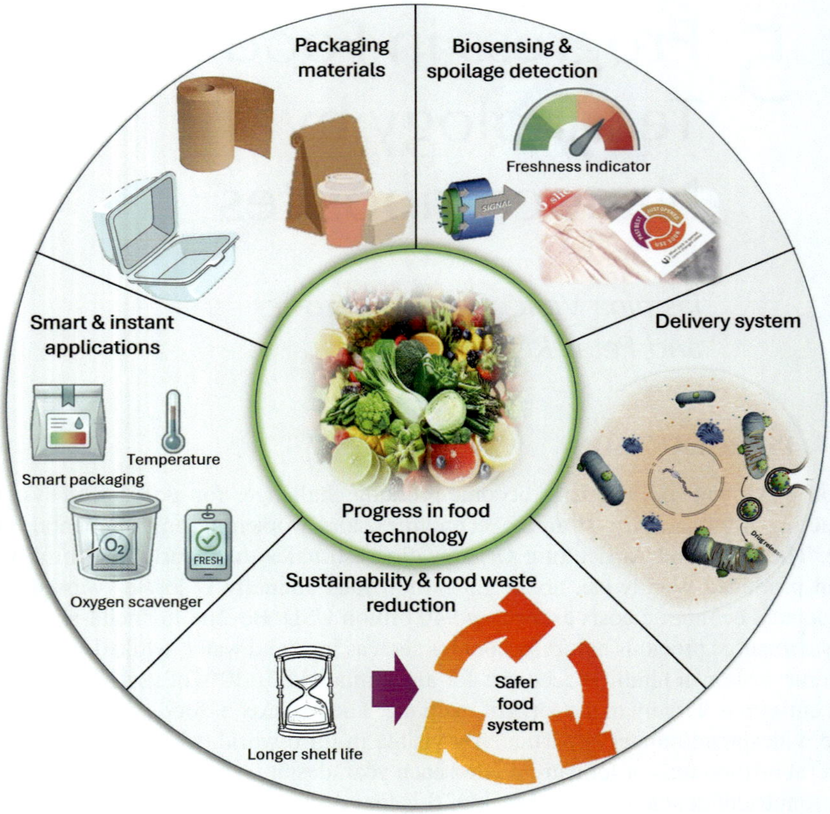

FIGURE 5.1 General schematic overview of food waste and how nanotechnology addresses it (packaging, biosensing, nutrient enrichment, and smart applications).

5.2 NANOMATERIALS FOR FOOD PACKAGING AND PRESERVATION

Packaging is a vital component of the food supply chain, serving not only to contain and transport food but also to protect it from physical damage, microbial contamination, moisture loss, and oxidative degradation. Conventional packaging materials such as plastics, glass, and aluminum have provided basic functionality for decades, but they often lack active protective properties, contribute to environmental waste, and fail to ensure extended shelf-life in modern distribution networks. Nanotechnology introduces nanomaterials and nanocomposites with enhanced functionalities into food packaging, leading to improved shelf-life, safety, and sustainability. Incorporating nanoparticles into polymeric matrices or designing hybrid nanocomposites enables properties such as antimicrobial activity, oxygen and moisture barrier enhancement, UV protection, and even "intelligent" sensing of food quality [2–4]. These nano-enabled packaging systems represent a major step toward active, intelligent, and sustainable food packaging solutions.

5.2.1 Silver Nanoparticles: The Antimicrobial Powerhouse

Silver nanoparticles (AgNPs) are among the most widely explored nanomaterials in food packaging due to their broad-spectrum antimicrobial activity against bacteria, fungi, and even some viruses [5,6]. The antimicrobial mechanism of AgNPs involves the release of silver ions (Ag^+), which disrupt microbial cell membranes, interact with thiol groups of enzymes, generate reactive oxygen species, and interfere with DNA replication. This multi-targeted mode of action makes microbial resistance less likely compared to conventional chemical preservatives.

AgNPs are frequently embedded into polymer matrices such as polyethylene (PE), polypropylene, and polyvinyl alcohol to create antimicrobial films. These films actively inhibit microbial growth on food surfaces. For instance, PE films with dispersed AgNPs were shown to extend the shelf-life of packaged bread by preventing mold growth. Biopolymer-based edible coatings (e.g., chitosan or starch) incorporated with AgNPs have been developed for perishable fruits such as strawberries and apples. The coatings suppress fungal growth, delay ripening, and maintain firmness. Studies have demonstrated that AgNP-embedded films effectively reduce bacterial contamination in raw chicken, fish fillets, and cheese, thus extending shelf-life by several days under refrigeration. AgNPs presents several advantages when incorporated into food packaging systems. Their most notable strength is their potent antimicrobial activity at relatively low concentrations, which ensures effectiveness against a broad spectrum of bacteria, fungi, and even some viruses. Moreover, AgNPs are highly versatile and can be readily integrated into a variety of polymeric and biopolymeric matrices, allowing for applications in both conventional plastic films and biodegradable alternatives. Another advantage lies in their compatibility with edible coatings, particularly when combined with natural polymers such as chitosan or starch, which makes them attractive for fresh fruit and vegetable preservation. This multifunctionality positions AgNPs as one of the most reliable nanomaterials for extending food shelf-life.

However, the limitations of AgNPs stem largely from safety and regulatory concerns [2,7]. The potential migration of silver ions or nanoparticles from packaging materials into food has raised questions about long-term health effects, particularly regarding cytotoxicity and bioaccumulation in human tissues. The extent of migration is influenced by particle size, polymer composition, food type, and storage conditions, making it difficult to establish universal safety thresholds. Regulatory authorities such as the U.S. Food and Drug Administration and European Food Safety Authority have therefore imposed strict guidelines, limiting the commercial use of AgNPs in direct food-contact applications. Furthermore, the high cost of large-scale AgNP synthesis compared to more conventional antimicrobials can hinder widespread adoption [3]. To address these issues, current research is directed toward hybrid packaging systems that combine AgNPs with natural antimicrobials, which can reduce the required silver dosage while maintaining antimicrobial efficiency and consumer safety.

5.2.2 Clay-Based Nanocomposites: Enhancing Mechanical Integrity and Barrier Properties

Layered silicate clays, such as montmorillonite (MMT) and halloysite nanotubes, are widely used in nanocomposite packaging materials due to their ability to reinforce polymers and create indirect paths for gas and vapor diffusion [8]. When exfoliated or intercalated into polymer matrices, clay nanoparticles significantly improve mechanical strength, thermal stability, and barrier properties against oxygen, carbon dioxide, ethylene, and moisture, critical factors for food preservation.

Incorporating MMT nanoclay into polylactic acid or polyethylene terephthalate (PET) reduces oxygen permeability by up to 50%–80%. This makes nanoclay composites highly suitable for packaging oxygen-sensitive foods such as nuts, coffee, and dairy products. Clay-polymer nanocomposites have been used to package cereals and bakery products, preventing moisture-induced spoilage while maintaining texture and crispness. Adding nanoclays into PET enhances its thermal resistance, making it viable for hot-fill beverage bottles and microwaveable food trays. Recent research has combined clays with antimicrobial nanoparticles (e.g., Ag, ZnO) or biopolymers to create multifunctional films that both block gases and inhibit microbial growth. This property makes them ideal for protecting oxygen-sensitive foods, moisture-prone bakery products, and beverages. In addition to barrier improvements, their low cost, natural abundance, and compatibility with biodegradable polymers also align with global demands for sustainable packaging materials.

Despite these advantages, clay-based nanocomposites face limitations that must be addressed before widespread commercialization. One of the primary challenges is achieving uniform dispersion of clay particles within the polymer matrix, as agglomeration reduces both barrier performance and mechanical reinforcement. The processing techniques required to achieve exfoliation or intercalation of clay layers can also be complex and costly at an industrial scale. Furthermore, although clays are generally regarded as safe, the possibility of nanoparticle migration into food, particularly under acidic or high moisture conditions, requires thorough toxicological assessment. These concerns have slowed regulatory approval and raised questions about consumer acceptance. Future research is therefore focusing on green fabrication methods, layer-by-layer nanostructuring, and the use of biopolymers to develop next-generation clay nanocomposites that balance performance, safety, and sustainability.

5.3 DETECTION OF FOODBORNE PATHOGENS USING NANOTECHNOLOGY

Foodborne illnesses remain one of the most persistent threats to global health and food security. Each year, contaminated food leads to millions of illnesses and significant economic losses, with bacterial pathogens such as *Salmonella*, *Escherichia coli O157:H7*, *Listeria monocytogenes*, and *Campylobacter jejuni* among the most notorious culprits [7,9–12]. Traditional methods of pathogen detection such as culture plating, enzyme-linked immunosorbent assay (ELISA), and polymerase chain reaction (PCR) though reliable, are often time-consuming, labor-intensive, and require well-equipped laboratories. These limitations hinder their application in rapid screening at food production and distribution points, where early detection is most critical. Nanotechnology provides transformative solutions for pathogen detection by enabling rapid, sensitive, and specific sensing at the point of need. Nanomaterials such as metal nanoparticles, quantum dots (QDs), carbon nanostructures, and hybrid nanocomposites offer unique physicochemical properties, including high surface area, tunable optical and electronic characteristics, and compatibility with biomolecular functionalization. These properties allow nanosensors to transduce pathogen recognition events whether through antibody–antigen binding, deoxyribonucleic acid (DNA) hybridization, or aptamer interactions into measurable optical, electrical, or mechanical signals.

5.3.1 Surface-Enhanced Raman Spectroscopy Nanosensors

Surface-enhanced Raman spectroscopy (SERS) has emerged as one of the most powerful nanotechnology-enabled techniques for pathogen detection [13]. Conventional Raman spectroscopy provides rich molecular "fingerprint" spectra, but its weak scattering intensity limits sensitivity. By placing analyte molecules near metallic nanostructures, typically gold (Au) or silver (Ag) nanoparticles or nanostructured substrates, the local electromagnetic field is enormously amplified, enhancing Raman signals by factors of 10^6–10^{14}. This dramatic signal enhancement enables detection of even single bacterial cells or trace biomolecules, making SERS a prime candidate for foodborne pathogen diagnostics. SERS nanosensors are typically constructed using roughened metallic substrates, nanoparticle aggregates, or engineered nanogap structures. When bacterial cells or pathogen-associated biomolecules (proteins, DNA, or cell wall components) come into close contact with these plasmonic "hot spots," their Raman scattering signals are amplified [13]. Functionalization of nanoparticles with recognition elements such as antibodies, aptamers, or lectins improves specificity, allowing targeted detection of pathogens even in complex food matrices.

Direct pathogen identification using SERS has demonstrated remarkable promise in distinguishing foodborne bacteria based on their intrinsic vibrational signatures. Each bacterial species produces a unique Raman fingerprint arising from its cell wall components, nucleic acids, and proteins. For example, *E. coli*, *Salmonella enterica*, and *L. monocytogenes* were successfully discriminated using AgNP-decorated nanostructured substrates, which provided strong electromagnetic enhancement of Raman scattering. In one study, contaminated milk samples were directly analyzed without the need for lengthy culture, achieving accurate species-level identification within 30 min. Such rapid discrimination is particularly valuable in perishable food systems where early intervention can prevent outbreaks.

Immuno-SERS assays further improve specificity by integrating antibody recognition with plasmonic enhancement. Antibody-functionalized gold nanoparticles (AuNPs) can selectively bind to target pathogens, while Raman reporter molecules attached to the AuNPs provide distinct spectral signatures. For instance, an immuno-SERS platform developed for *Salmonella Typhimurium* in chicken meat achieved detection limits as low as 10^2 CFU/mL, a sensitivity far superior to conventional culture-based techniques that require 24–72 h. Similar antibody–nanoparticle conjugates have been designed for *E. coli O157:H7* and *C. jejuni*, illustrating the adaptability of this method to diverse pathogens of concern in food safety.

Label-free SERS detection of viruses and toxins highlights the versatility of this technique beyond bacteria. Viral pathogens such as noroviruses, which are notoriously difficult to culture, have been directly identified using SERS through their capsid protein spectral features. Staphylococcal enterotoxin B, a potent foodborne toxin, has also been detected using label-free SERS with spectral shifts corresponding to its peptide backbone and aromatic amino acid residues. These studies illustrate how SERS can be applied not only for bacterial pathogens but also for viral and toxin detection, providing a comprehensive tool for food safety monitoring.

Portable SERS devices are combined with various SERS sensors bringing this technology closer to real-world application. Handheld Raman spectrometers integrated with nanostructured SERS substrates enable rapid, on-site analysis without the need for laboratory infrastructure. A notable example involved a portable SERS chip coated with AuNP arrays, which successfully detected *L. monocytogenes* under 1 h. Other field-deployable SERS platforms have been demonstrated for detecting pesticide residues and adulterants alongside pathogens, underscoring the multifunctionality of portable systems. The combination of portability, speed, and molecular specificity positions SERS as a transformative technology for food inspection and public health surveillance.

SERS offers unparalleled sensitivity and molecular specificity, enabling detection at very low pathogen concentrations. The ability to obtain fingerprint spectrum provides not only presence/absence information but also species-level discrimination. However, challenges remain in substrate reproducibility, signal variation due to matrix effects (e.g., fats, proteins in food samples), and the high cost of fabricating nanostructured substrates.

5.3.2 Quantum Dot–Based Fluorescent Biosensors

QDs are semiconductor nanocrystals with exceptional optical properties, including size-tunable fluorescence, high brightness, narrow emission spectra, and resistance to photobleaching. These features make them ideal for biosensing applications that require sensitive and stable fluorescence signals. In pathogen detection, QDs are often conjugated with antibodies, aptamers, or nucleic acid probes, enabling specific binding to bacterial or viral targets while providing strong optical readouts. When QDs are excited by a light source, they emit fluorescence at specific wavelengths determined by their size and composition. By conjugating QDs with pathogen-specific biomolecules, the binding of a target pathogen can modulate the fluorescence signal through mechanisms such as fluorescence resonance energy transfer, quenching, or signal amplification [7]. This allows for quantitative detection of pathogens with high sensitivity.

In multiplex detection, several pathogens are simultaneously identified within a single sample. Unlike organic dyes, which require multiple excitation sources for different colors, QDs of varying sizes can all be excited by the same light source but emit at distinct, narrow wavelengths. This advantage has been exploited in QD-based immunoassays for the simultaneous detection of multiple foodborne pathogens. In one study, three differently sized CdSe/ZnS QDs were conjugated with pathogen-specific antibodies and used to detect *S. enterica*, *E. coli O157:H7*, and *L. monocytogenes*

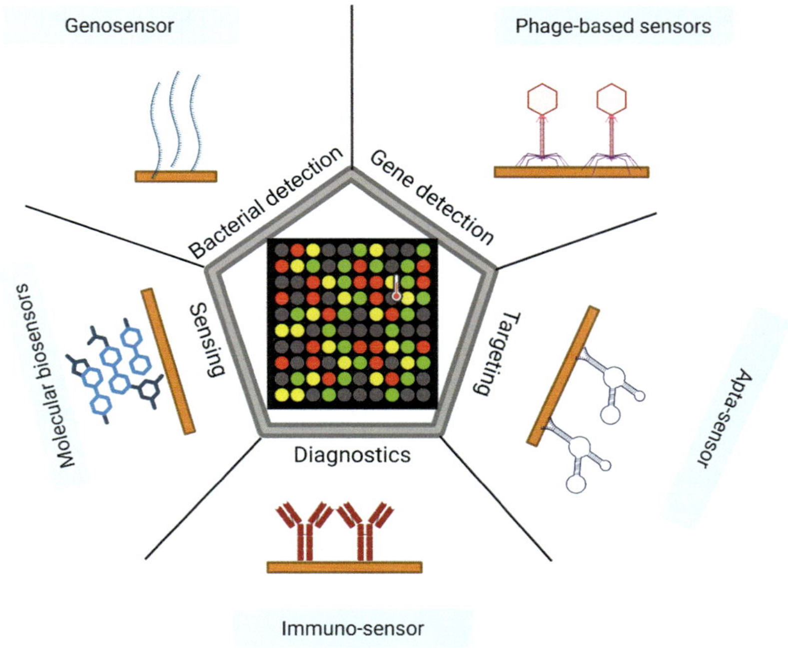

FIGURE 5.2 Schematic illustration summarizing examples of the more commonly used recognition elements in different types of biosensors.

in contaminated milk. The assay produced distinct fluorescent signals for each pathogen, enabling multiplexed analysis with high sensitivity and minimal cross-reactivity, a capability particularly valuable in complex food safety monitoring.

Beyond immunoassays, QDs have also been conjugated with DNA and aptamer probes to detect pathogen-specific genetic sequences (Figure 5.2). The combination of nucleic acid recognition and QD fluorescence enables sensitive and specific detection without the need for thermal cycling, as required in PCR. For instance, CdSe/ZnS QDs functionalized with complementary DNA probes successfully identified *Salmonella* DNA sequences in under 1 h. This approach not only reduced assay time but also eliminated the requirement for bulky instrumentation, offering a practical alternative to PCR for rapid on-site testing. Aptamer-functionalized QDs further extend this approach, as aptamers can selectively bind to whole cells or toxins, allowing for flexible and cost-effective pathogen recognition platforms [14].

The versatility of QDs is also reflected in their integration with lateral flow assays (LFAs), which are widely used for field-deployable diagnostics due to their simplicity and low cost. Traditional LFAs employing AuNPs provide colorimetric signals visible to the naked eye but often lack sufficient sensitivity for trace-level detection. Incorporating QDs into the test line addresses this limitation by producing highly sensitive fluorescence readouts. In one notable example, a QD-LFA designed for *L. monocytogenes* achieved a detection limit as low as 10 CFU/mL, with the results clearly visible under a handheld ultraviolet (UV) lamp. Such improvements significantly expand the utility of LFAs for point-of-care and on-site food inspection.

Importantly, QD-based sensors have demonstrated strong robustness in real food matrices, an essential step toward practical deployment [15–17]. Studies have shown successful detection of *E. coli* in apple juice and *Salmonella* in poultry meat, where the fluorescence signal remained stable despite the complex background of organic matter, proteins, and other interfering molecules. These results confirm that QDs maintain their sensitivity and specificity even in challenging environments, making them promising candidates for integration into routine food safety testing and portable diagnostic devices.

QDs offer high sensitivity, stability, and multiplexing capacity, surpassing traditional fluorophores. Their ability to resist photobleaching is particularly advantageous for long-term monitoring and repeated measurements. However, toxicity concerns, especially with cadmium-based QDs, limit their direct application in food systems and pose regulatory challenges. The development of heavy metal–free alternatives, such as carbon dots and indium phosphide QDs, is helping to address these safety concerns; however, graphene quantum dots (GQDs) or carbon quantum dots (CQDs) are not as efficient as inorganic QDs.

5.3.3 Other Biosensors

In addition to SERS and QD-based platforms, a wide range of nanotechnology-enabled biosensors are being developed to provide rapid, sensitive, and cost-effective detection of foodborne pathogens. These include electrochemical sensors [5,18,19], magnetic nanoparticle (MNP)-based assays, and nano-enabled colorimetric tests, as well as integrated nanosensing platforms designed to combine multiple detection strategies [20].

Electrochemical biosensors show the superior sensitivity and tunable surface chemistry of nanomaterials such as graphene, carbon nanotubes (CNTs), transition metal carbides, nitrides, or carbonitrides (MXenes), and conducting polymers to transduce pathogen recognition into electrical signals [21]. A notable example is a graphene oxide–modified electrode functionalized with *Salmonella*-specific aptamers, which enabled rapid, label-free detection of the bacteria in chicken broth with detection limits as low as 10 CFU/mL. Techniques such as electrochemical impedance spectroscopy and voltammetry are widely employed in these systems to achieve high sensitivity and reproducibility. Beyond bacterial detection, electrochemical nanosensors have also been adapted for viral diagnostics, such as norovirus detection in leafy greens using CNT-modified electrodes. Their main strengths are portability, low cost, and compatibility with smartphone-based or wearable electronics, making them suitable for decentralized monitoring along the food supply chain.

MNP-based biosensors are particularly effective for pathogen enrichment and separation from complex food matrices, thereby improving both sensitivity and specificity. Functionalized with antibodies, aptamers, or even phage proteins, MNPs selectively capture target organisms and allow for rapid magnetic isolation. For instance, antibody-coated iron oxide nanoparticles were used to isolate *L. monocytogenes* from milk, followed by detection using a portable magneto-resistive sensor. This integrated approach reduced total assay time from several hours to less than

45 min. MNPs can also be coupled with PCR or isothermal nucleic acid amplification to further enhance sensitivity, enabling near single-cell detection in contaminated samples. Such strategies have already been validated for pathogens like *Salmonella* in poultry rinses and *E. coli O157:H7* in ground beef.

Nano-enabled colorimetric assays exploit the localized surface plasmon resonance properties of AuNPs, which produce visible color changes upon aggregation. These systems are extremely simple, requiring no advanced instrumentation, and are especially valuable in resource-limited settings [7,17]. An example is an AuNP-based colorimetric test for *E. coli* in fruit juice, where a clear red-to-blue color change appeared within 15 min, indicating the presence of the pathogen. While colorimetric sensors generally lack the ultra-sensitivity of SERS or QD-based methods, coupling with amplification strategies (e.g., rolling circle amplification, clustered regularly interspaced short palindromic repeats-based readouts) or digital quantification using smartphone cameras has significantly improved their performance.

Integrated nanosensing platforms represent the next generation of food safety tools by combining multiple nanotechnologies into single hybrid devices [22]. For example, microfluidic chips integrating MNP enrichment with electrochemical sensing have been developed for multiplexed detection of *E. coli*, *Salmonella*, and *Listeria* in fresh produce wash water [23]. Another approach couples plasmonic AuNPs with carbon nanomaterials to produce dual-mode electrochemical and optical signals, increasing both reliability and sensitivity. Such platforms demonstrate the versatility of nanosensors when engineered for real-world applications where food samples are often complex and variable.

Beyond pathogen detection, nanomaterial-based biosensors are also finding applications in monitoring food freshness markers such as ethylene, a natural plant hormone that regulates ripening in fruits and vegetables [24–26]. Ethylene is released at trace levels (ppm to ppb) during postharvest storage, and its accumulation accelerates spoilage. Nanomaterial-enabled ethylene sensors provide a powerful way to monitor ripening in real time. SnO_2 and ZnO nanowire-based chemiresistive sensors have shown high sensitivity to ethylene at sub-ppm levels, making them suitable for smart packaging applications. More advanced designs incorporate Pd- or Pt-decorated nanostructures to lower detection limits and reduce cross-sensitivity to interfering gases. Recently, graphene–metal oxide hybrid sensors have been demonstrated for detecting ethylene released from bananas and mangoes, enabling early intervention to extend shelf-life. These advances highlight how nanosensors can expand beyond pathogen detection to encompass comprehensive food quality monitoring, integrating microbial safety with freshness and spoilage indicators.

For real-world applications, the requirement for efficient sample preparation, and ensuring reproducibility across diverse food types is still the big challenge including interference (fat, proteins, sugars). Furthermore, achieving regulatory approval and consumer trust remains essential for large-scale deployment. While challenges remain in standardization, reproducibility, and translation to field settings, the integration of nanosensors into portable, multiplexed, and digitally connected devices points to a future where foodborne pathogen detection and freshness monitoring are proactive, continuous, and highly reliable, ultimately ensuring safer food and healthier populations worldwide.

5.4 NUTRIENTS ENRICHMENT

Nutrient enrichment is a vital strategy to address global malnutrition and improve public health. Micronutrient deficiencies, often referred to as "hidden hunger," affect billions of people worldwide, with iron, vitamin A, vitamin D, and zinc deficiencies being among the most prevalent. Traditional supplementation and fortification strategies, while valuable, face limitations such as poor stability during food processing, low bioavailability in the gastrointestinal tract, and undesirable changes in food products. Nanotechnology offers innovative solutions to these challenges by improving nutrient protection, enhancing absorption, and enabling targeted release within the digestive system. Through nano-encapsulation, lipid-based carriers, polymeric systems, and nanocomposite films, essential vitamins, minerals, and functional bioactives can be incorporated into food matrices without compromising sensory qualities, as presented in Figure 5.3 [2]. These approaches not only improve the nutritional value of foods but also open pathways toward personalized nutrition, where specific dietary needs are met with precision.

5.4.1 Nano-Encapsulation of Nutrients

Nano-encapsulation is a widely adopted strategy for enhancing stability, bioavailability, and controlled release of sensitive nutrients. Encapsulation within lipid nanoparticles, polymeric nanocapsules, or protein-based nanocarriers provides a protective barrier against environmental factors such as light, oxygen, and heat, which otherwise degrade vulnerable compounds. Lipid-based carriers, such as solid lipid nanoparticles (SLNs) and nanostructured lipid carriers (NLCs), are particularly effective for fat-soluble nutrients like vitamins A, D, E, and K, as well as omega-3 fatty acids. These nanocarriers not only protect the encapsulated compounds but

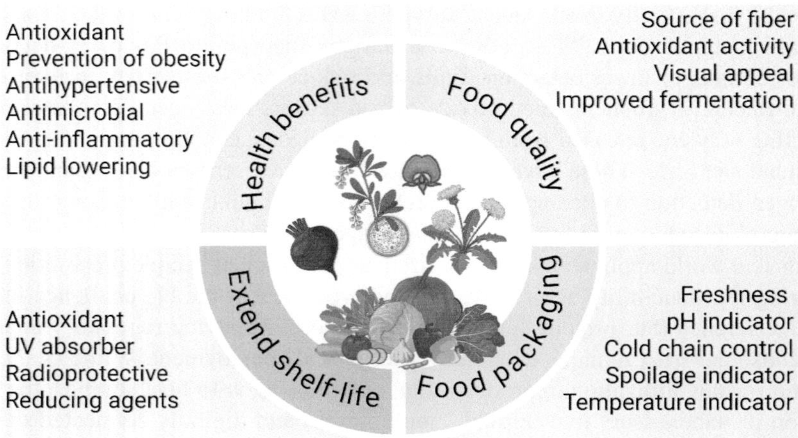

FIGURE 5.3 Health benefits and solutions that can be obtained by encapsulation of nutrients.

also improve solubility in aqueous food systems [27]. For example, vitamin A encapsulated in SLNs demonstrated significantly higher stability in dairy products compared to free vitamin A, with minimal losses during pasteurization and storage. Polymeric nanocapsules, often made from biocompatible materials such as PLGA (poly(lactic-co-glycolic acid)) or chitosan, are also widely studied for encapsulating polyphenols and flavonoids, which are otherwise prone to rapid degradation.

In one study, curcumin encapsulated in chitosan nanoparticles exhibited a three-fold increase in bioavailability compared to free curcumin, while retaining its anti-oxidant activity in functional beverages. Protein-based nanocarriers, such as casein micelles or zein nanoparticles, offer natural, food-grade encapsulation systems. Casein micelles have been shown to effectively entrap hydrophobic bioactives such as quercetin and resveratrol, improving their solubility and intestinal uptake. These protein nanocarriers also align well with clean-label consumer preferences, as they rely on naturally occurring food proteins.

5.4.2 Fortification of Iron to Combat Anemia

Iron deficiency anemia remains one of the most widespread nutritional disorders globally, excessively affecting women and children in developing countries. Conventional iron fortification methods, such as adding ferrous sulfate to flour or salt, often suffer from poor absorption, metallic taste, and gastrointestinal side effects. Nanotechnology has introduced iron oxide nanoparticles encapsulated in biocompatible polymers to improve both bioavailability and stability. The encapsulation minimized the metallic taste, reduced reactivity with other food components, and ensured gradual release of iron in the intestine. Similar strategies have been extended to rice fortification, where iron nanoparticles are incorporated into rice kernels through extrusion. These fortified grains retain their sensory qualities while delivering enhanced bioavailable iron, presenting scalable solutions for staple food fortification in low-resource regions [28–30].

5.4.3 Nanostructured Lipid Carriers for Fat-Soluble Vitamins

Fat-soluble vitamins such as D3 and E are particularly susceptible to degradation during food processing and storage. NLCs provide a robust solution by embedding these vitamins within a lipid matrix that shields them from oxidation and thermal breakdown. For instance, commercial dairy products in Europe supplemented with vitamin D-loaded NLCs retained up to 95% of vitamin content after pasteurization, compared to less than 60% in conventional fortification systems. Similarly, vitamin E encapsulated in NLCs demonstrated enhanced stability in fruit juices, with minimal loss during high-pressure processing. NLCs not only improve stability but also enable controlled release in the gastrointestinal tract, thereby enhancing absorption efficiency. This feature is especially important for populations in northern regions with limited sun exposure, where vitamin D deficiency is highly prevalent. The incorporation of NLCs into widely consumed products such as milk, yogurt, and fortified juices offers a practical and consumer-friendly strategy to combat micronutrient deficiencies.

5.4.4 Protein and Peptide Delivery

Proteins and bioactive peptides are increasingly recognized for their therapeutic and functional benefits, ranging from muscle repair and satiety regulation to immune enhancement. However, their oral delivery is often compromised by enzymatic degradation in the gastrointestinal tract [31]. Nanotechnology addresses this issue through protective encapsulation. Studies have shown that nanoencapsulated peptides reach the bloodstream in bioactive form, enhancing their physiological effects. For example, collagen peptides encapsulated in zein nanoparticles demonstrated superior bioavailability in human trials, leading to improved muscle recovery after exercise compared to non-encapsulated formulations. Similarly, nano-encapsulation of lactoferrin, a milk protein with immune-boosting properties, ensured intact delivery to the intestine, enhancing its antimicrobial activity and supporting gut health. The application of nano-encapsulation in protein delivery represents an important advance for functional foods targeting specific health outcomes, such as sports nutrition, aging-related muscle loss, and immune system support.

5.4.5 Edible Nanoclay and Chitosan Films

Beyond encapsulation, nutrient enrichment can also be achieved through active food-contact surfaces. Edible nanocomposite films made from nanoclays, chitosan, or starch are increasingly being developed to release essential micronutrients directly onto food surfaces during storage. For instance, chitosan films embedded with zinc oxide nanoparticles not only acted as antimicrobial agents but also gradually released zinc ions, enriching fresh produce and enhancing its nutritional value. Similarly, selenium-loaded nanoclay films have been applied to fruits and vegetables, delivering trace nutrients while also providing antioxidant protection against spoilage. Such films are particularly relevant in low-resource regions, where nutrient deficiencies are widespread and access to fortified processed foods may be limited. By packaging fresh produce in nutrient-releasing films, it becomes possible to improve both food safety and micronutrient intake simultaneously.

5.4.6 Commercial and Consumer Products

The food industry has rapidly recognized the potential of nanotechnology for nutrient delivery, with several products already reaching the market. Leading companies such as Danone and Nestlé are actively investing in nano-encapsulation research to improve the stability and efficacy of probiotics, vitamins, and micronutrients in functional foods and beverages. Commercially available examples include functional beverages containing nano-curcumin for anti-inflammatory benefits and nano-coenzyme Q10 for cardiovascular health, which are particularly popular in Asian markets. These formulations not only improve bioavailability but also enable lower dosages, reducing potential side effects while maintaining efficacy. In addition, probiotic encapsulation using nanocarriers has been explored to improve the survival of beneficial bacteria through gastric conditions, ensuring effective colonization in the intestine. Such advances are paving the way toward personalized nutrition, where nanoformulations can be tailored to deliver specific nutrient combinations based on individual dietary needs and genetic profiles.

5.5 FUTURE APPLICATIONS AND PROSPECTS OF NANOTECHNOLOGY IN FOOD

The integration of nanotechnology into the food sector is still in its early stages; however, the progress is shaping the future of food production, preservation, and consumption. Beyond current applications in packaging, pathogen detection, and nutrient enrichment, emerging nanotechnologies are composed to enable smart packaging, personalized nutrition, sustainable materials, and even adaptive food manufacturing. These innovations align with global goals of food safety, sustainability, and improved public health, while also responding to growing consumer demand for transparency, functionality, and personalization.

5.5.1 Smart Packaging and Real-Time Monitoring

Smart packaging systems enhanced with nanotechnology will provide more than passive protection; they will actively monitor, communicate, and even respond to changes in food quality. Embedded nanosensors based on graphene oxide, CNTs, or metal oxide nanostructures can detect spoilage gases (such as ammonia or hydrogen sulfide), microbial metabolites, or chemical contaminants, providing real-time indicators of freshness and safety. A notable example comes from researchers at Amity University, who developed a nanosensor system that changes resistance under UV exposure when meat spoilage gases are detected. Such signals allow consumers or transporters to instantly assess product freshness. Similarly, nanomaterial-based colorimetric indicators have been integrated into packaging films, changing color when oxygen permeability increases, or microbial contamination occurs. Nanocellulose, extracted from plant fibers, is one of the most promising candidates for biodegradable packaging materials. Its high mechanical strength, transparency, and barrier properties make it suitable for replacing petroleum-based plastics [1,2]. Studies demonstrated that nanocellulose films could double the shelf-life of bakery products without the need for chemical preservatives, underscoring both sustainability and functionality. Similarly, plant-derived nanoparticles and starch-based nanocomposites have been explored to produce edible coatings that can degrade naturally without harming the environment.

The adoption of smart nanosensors promises to significantly reduce food waste at retail and household levels by providing accurate indicators of spoilage. However, scalability, cost, and regulatory approval remain barriers to widespread commercial deployment. Future systems are expected to integrate these nanosensors with Internet of Things (IoT) platforms, allowing real-time data transmission to consumers, retailers, and regulatory authorities. This connected framework will not only reduce waste but also improve food traceability and outbreak management.

5.5.2 Personalized Nutrition and Nano-Delivery Systems

The convergence of nanotechnology with nutrigenomics and digital health platforms will drive the next revolution in personalized nutrition. Advances in genomic and metabolic profiling enable precise identification of an individual's nutritional requirements, while nanocarriers provide targeted delivery of specific nutrients at optimal doses. For example, functional foods could be customized by analyzing saliva or gut microbiome samples, with results processed by artificial intelligence (AI)-driven nutrient planning systems. Based on this profile, nanoformulated nutrient supplements such as lipid nanoparticles encapsulating vitamin D for individuals with deficiency, or nano-iron formulations for those prone to anemia, can be tailored to the consumer. Prototype systems under development involve integrating nanoparticle-based nutrient delivery with wearable health monitoring devices, creating a closed-loop feedback system for diet optimization. This personalized approach is particularly relevant for managing chronic diseases such as diabetes, cardiovascular disorders, and obesity, where precise nutritional interventions are essential. While the potential is vast, challenges include consumer acceptance of ingestible nanomaterials, regulatory oversight of personalized functional foods, and ensuring equitable access to these advanced nutrition technologies [32]. Nevertheless, the combination of nanotechnology, genomics, and AI is expected to redefine dietary practices in the coming decades.

5.6 CONCLUSION

Nanotechnology has emerged as a transformative force in food technology, offering solutions that address some of the most pressing global challenges of food waste, safety, and malnutrition. By exploring the unique physicochemical properties of nanomaterials, researchers have developed innovative packaging systems with superior barrier and antimicrobial performance. Additionally, the development of nanosensors capable of detecting pathogens and spoilage markers in real time, and nanoformulations that protect and enhance the bioavailability of essential nutrients are also emerging in research. Practical demonstrations such as AgNP-embedded antimicrobial films extending the shelf-life of bread and meat, QD-based multiplex biosensors detecting pathogens in milk, and nanostructured lipid carriers safeguarding vitamins through pasteurization highlight how nano-enabled strategies are steadily moving from laboratory research toward commercial reality. At the same time, advances in ethylene nanosensors and smart packaging signal the rise of integrated systems that not only protect food but also actively monitor and communicate its quality to consumers. Challenges remain, including regulatory approval, standardization, toxicity concerns, and consumer acceptance; however, ongoing research into biocompatible nanomaterials, green synthesis, and hybrid systems is steadily addressing these issues. Looking ahead, the convergence of nanotechnology with digital health, IoT, and personalized nutrition platforms will redefine food systems, making them safer, more sustainable, and more responsive to individual and societal needs.

ACKNOWLEDGMENT

This work was supported by the European Union under grants MOBILES HORIZON-CL6-2023-ZEROPOLLUTION-01, No. 101135402 and PURE-WAY HORIZON-MSCA-2024-SE-01-01, No. 101236277.

REFERENCES

1. N. Omerović, M. Djisalov, K. Živojević, M. Mladenović, J. Vunduk, I. Milenković, et al., Antimicrobial nanoparticles and biodegradable polymer composites for active food packaging applications, *Comprehensive Reviews in Food Science and Food Safety*, 20(2021) 2428–54.
2. M.V. Nikolic, Z.Z. Vasiljevic, S. Auger, J. Vidic, Metal oxide nanoparticles for safe active and intelligent food packaging, *Trends in Food Science & Technology*, 116(2021) 655–68.
3. S. Stankic, S. Suman, F. Haque, J. Vidic, Pure and multi metal oxide nanoparticles: synthesis, antibacterial and cytotoxic properties, *Journal of Nanobiotechnology*, 14(2016) 73.
4. J. Vidic, S. Stankic, F. Haque, D. Ciric, R. Le Goffic, A. Vidy, et al., Selective antibacterial effects of mixed ZnMgO nanoparticles, *Journal of Nanoparticle Research*, 15(2013) 1595.
5. I. Bobrinetskiy, M. Radovic, F. Rizzotto, P. Vizzini, S. Jaric, Z. Pavlovic, et al., Advances in nanomaterials-based electrochemical biosensors for foodborne pathogen detection, *Nanomaterials*, 11(2021) 2700.
6. R. Mukherjee, K. Gunjan, K. Himanshu, J. Vidic, R.P. Pandey, C.-M. Chang, Advancing influenza prevention through a one health approach: a comprehensive analysis, *Journal of Hazardous Materials Advances*, 14(2024) 100419.
7. M. Marin, M.V. Nikolic, J. Vidic, Rapid point-of-need detection of bacteria and their toxins in food using gold nanoparticles, *Comprehensive Reviews in Food Science and Food Safety*, 20(2021) 5880–900.
8. S.P. Bangar, W.S. Whiteside, V. Chaudhary, P.P. Akhila, K.V. Sunooj, Recent functionality developments in Montmorillonite as a nanofiller in food packaging, *Trends in Food Science & Technology*, 140(2023) 104148.
9. J. Malet-Villemagne, F. Rizzotto, V. Léguillier, J. Vidic, V. Escobar, Y. Hou, et al., Advances in rapid detection of zoonotic pathogens in poultry production and processing environments, *Improving Poultry Meat Safety and Sustainability*, S.C. Ricke, N. Corcionivoschi, J. Hite, T. Callaway, N. Jaffrezic-Renault, D. Biswas, et al. (eds.), Springer (2025) 81–108.
10. F. Zhao, Y. Wang, H. An, Y. Hao, X. Hu, X. Liao, New insights into the formation of viable but nonculturable *Escherichia coli* O157: H7 induced by high-pressure CO_2, *MBio*, 7(2016) 10.1128/mbio.00961-16.
11. Z. Kotsiri, A. Vantarakis, F. Rizzotto, D. Kavanaugh, N. Ramarao, J. Vidic, Sensitive detection of *E. coli* in artificial seawater by aptamer-coated magnetic beads and direct PCR, *Applied Sciences*, 9(2019) 5392.
12. F. Rizzotto, M. Khalife, Y. Hou, C. Chaix, F. Lagarde, N. Scaramozzino, et al., Recent advances in electrochemical biosensors for food control, *Micromachines*, 14(2023) 1412.
13. S. Balbinot, A.M. Srivastav, J. Vidic, I. Abdulhalim, M. Manzano, Plasmonic biosensors for food control, *Trends in Food Science & Technology*, 111(2021) 128–40.
14. V. Léguillier, B. Heddi, J. Vidic, Recent advances in aptamer-based biosensors for bacterial detection, *Biosensors*, 14(2024) 210.
15. J. Vidic, M. Manzano, C.-M. Chang, N. Jaffrezic-Renault, Advanced biosensors for detection of pathogens related to livestock and poultry, *Veterinary research*, 48(2017) 11.
16. M. Manceau, C. Farre, F. Lagarde, R. Mathey, A. Buhot, J. Vidic, et al., Investigation of the affinity of aptamers for bacteria by surface plasmon resonance imaging using nanosomes, *ACS Applied Materials & Interfaces*, 16(2024) 29645–56.
17. M. Marin, F. Rizzotto, V. Léguillier, C. Péchoux, E. Borezee-Durant, J. Vidic, Naked-eye detection of *Staphylococcus aureus* in powdered milk and infant formula using gold nanoparticles, *Journal of Microbiological Methods*, 201(2022) 106578.

18. Z. Novakovic, M. Khalife, V. Costache, M.J. Camacho, S. Cardoso, V. Martins, et al., Rapid detection and identification of vancomycin-sensitive bacteria using an electrochemical apta-sensor, *ACS Omega*, 9(2024) 2841–9.
19. J. Vidic, M. Manzano, Electrochemical biosensors for rapid pathogen detection, *Current Opinion in Electrochemistry*, 29(2021) 100750.
20. M. Ghosh, K. Isago, U. Dasgupta, H. Shimizu, T. Suzuki, J. Vidic, et al., Duplex-specific nuclease assisted magnetic nanoprobe for cyclic amplified RNA detection, *Sensors and Actuators B: Chemical*, 399(2024) 134833.
21. J. Vidic, C. Chaix, M. Manzano, M. Heyndrickx, Food sensing: detection of *Bacillus cereus* spores in dairy products, *Biosensors*, 10(2020) 15.
22. S. Auger, C. Henry, C. Péchoux, S. Suman, N. Lejal, N. Bertho, et al., Exploring multiple effects of $Zn_{0.15}Mg_{0.85}O$ nanoparticles on *Bacillus subtilis* and macrophages, *Scientific reports*, 8(2018) 12276.
23. V. Escobar, N. Scaramozzino, J. Vidic, A. Buhot, R. Mathey, C. Chaix, et al., Recent advances on peptide-based biosensors and electronic noses for foodborne pathogen detection, *Biosensors*, 13(2023) 258.
24. Z.Z. Vasiljevic, J. Vunduk, M.P. Dojcinovic, G. Miskovic, N.B. Tadic, J. Vidic, et al., ZnO and Fe_2TiO_5 nanoparticles obtained by green synthesis as active components of alginate food packaging films, *Food Packaging and Shelf Life*, 43(2024) 101280.
25. F. Rizzotto, Z.Z. Vasiljevic, G. Stanojevic, M.P. Dojcinovic, I. Jankovic-Castvan, J.D. Vujancevic, et al., Antioxidant and cell-friendly Fe_2TiO_5 nanoparticles for food packaging application, *Food Chemistry*, 390(2022) 133198.
26. P. Vizzini, E. Beltrame, V. Zanet, J. Vidic, M. Manzano, Development and evaluation of qPCR detection method and Zn-MgO/alginate active packaging for controlling *Listeria monocytogenes* contamination in cold-smoked salmon, *Foods*, 9(2020) 1353.
27. Y. Dutt, R.P. Pandey, M. Dutt, A. Gupta, A. Vibhuti, J. Vidic, et al., Therapeutic applications of nanobiotechnology, *Journal of Nanobiotechnology*, 21(2023) 148.
28. P. Ristivojević, J. Trifković, F. Andrić, D. Milojković-Opsenica, Poplar-type propolis: chemical composition, botanical origin and biological activity, *Natural Product Communications*, 10(2015) 1934578X1501001117.
29. I. Dimkić, S. Stanković, M. Nišavić, M. Petković, P. Ristivojević, D. Fira, et al., The profile and antimicrobial activity of Bacillus lipopeptide extracts of five potential biocontrol strains, *Frontiers in Microbiology*, 8(2017) 925.
30. P. Ristivojević, I. Dimkić, J. Trifković, T. Berić, I. Vovk, D. Milojković-Opsenica, et al., Antimicrobial activity of Serbian propolis evaluated by means of MIC, HPTLC, bioautography and chemometrics, *PLoS one*, 11(2016) e0157097.
31. R.P. Pandey, J. Vidic, R. Mukherjee, C.-M. Chang, Experimental methods for the biological evaluation of nanoparticle-based drug delivery risks, *Pharmaceutics*, 15(2023) 612.
32. V. Zanet, J. Vidic, S. Auger, P. Vizzini, G. Lippe, L. Iacumin, et al., Activity evaluation of pure and doped zinc oxide nanoparticles against bacterial pathogens and *Saccharomyces cerevisiae*, *Journal of Applied Microbiology*, 127(2019) 1391–402.

6 Biosensors

Akhilesh Babu Ganganboina

6.1 INTRODUCTION

Biosensors are analytical devices designed to translate a specific biological interaction into a measurable, quantifiable, and processable signal. Over the past several decades, they have fundamentally transformed the landscape of diagnostics by enabling rapid, sensitive, and highly specific detection of a broad range of biological targets. At a fundamental level, a biosensor consists of three tightly integrated components: a biorecognition element that provides molecular specificity through selective interaction with the target analyte, commonly employing enzymes, antibodies, antigens, nucleic acids, aptamers, receptors, or even living cells; a transducer that converts this biorecognition event into a physicochemical signal, which may be electrical, electrochemical, optical, mechanical, or thermal in nature; and a signal processing and display unit that amplifies, filters, and interprets the generated signal to yield a quantitative and user-readable output. The performance of a biosensor is governed by a set of essential static and dynamic characteristics that collectively determine its efficiency, reliability, and suitability for practical and commercial applications [1]. Selectivity refers to the ability of a biosensor to specifically recognize its target analyte in complex samples with minimal interference. Sensitivity defines the lowest detectable analyte concentration, enabling trace-level detection. Linearity describes the proportional relationship between analyte concentration and sensor response, ensuring accurate quantification. Response time indicates how quickly the sensor reaches a stable signal after exposure. Reproducibility reflects consistent and accurate performance across repeated measurements, while stability denotes the sensor's ability to maintain reliable functionality over time under varying conditions. The conceptual foundation of biosensors dates to the 1960s, with the development of enzyme-based electrochemical sensors such as the glucose biosensor, which marked a pivotal shift toward real-time biochemical analysis [2]. Since then, advances in materials science, micro- and nanofabrication, surface functionalization, and microelectronics have transformed biosensors from bulky laboratory instruments into compact, portable, and point-of-care platforms. These innovations have broadened biosensor applications across clinical diagnostics and therapeutic monitoring, environmental and pathogen surveillance, food safety assessment, and biodefense and biosecurity. The growing global demand for rapid, accurate, and decentralized diagnostic tools became particularly evident during health emergencies such as the COVID-19 pandemic [3]. In this context, the integration of nanomaterials including metallic and semiconductor nanoparticles, carbon-based nanostructures, and two-dimensional (2D) materials has emerged as a transformative strategy, as their high surface-to-volume ratio, tunable electronic and optical properties, and enhanced

DOI: 10.1201/9781003725930-6

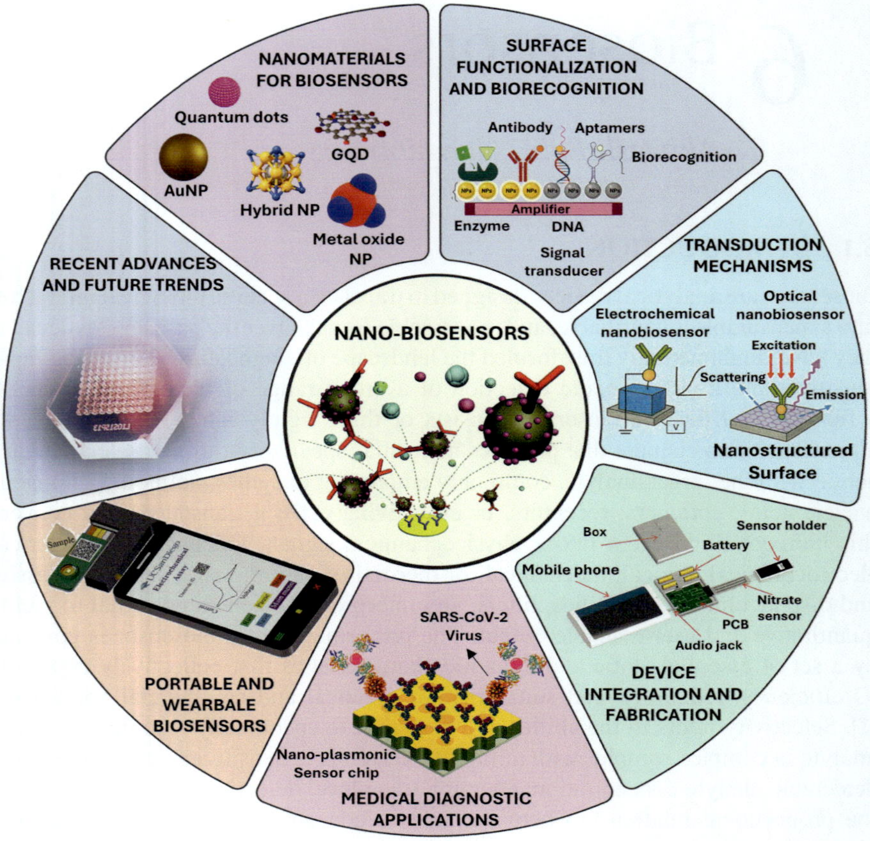

FIGURE 6.1 Overview of nano-biosensors for medical diagnostics.

bioconjugation capabilities significantly improve analyte capture efficiency, signal transduction, detection sensitivity, and overall biosensor performance (Figure 6.1).

6.2 TYPES OF BIOSENSORS

Biosensors are classified based on the nature of their biorecognition elements and the transduction mechanisms they employ.

6.2.1 Classification by Biorecognition Element

6.2.1.1 Enzymatic Biosensors

Enzymatic biosensors employ enzymes as biocatalysts to selectively recognize target substrates and generate detectable signals through enzyme-mediated reactions. The high specificity of enzymes toward their substrates enables accurate analyte detection. The primary limitation of these systems is their high cost, which arises from the use of enzymes [4]. For instance, glucose oxidase in combination with peroxidase is commonly employed to quantify hydrogen peroxide formation in serum or blood plasma for diagnostic purposes [5].

6.2.1.2 Immunosensors

Immunosensors utilize antibodies as recognition elements and operate on the principle of specific antigen–antibody interactions. Labeled immunosensors rely on signal-producing tags to enable analyte detection, including enzymes such as catalase and glucose oxidase, fluorescent molecules, and metal ions, as well as nanomaterial-based labels which enhance signal generation and detection sensitivity [6,7]. Owing to their exceptional selectivity, these biosensors are extensively applied in clinical diagnostics, particularly for the detection of infectious agents, disease biomarkers, and toxins.

6.2.1.3 Nucleic Acid Biosensors

Nucleic acid biosensors use single-stranded DNA or RNA probes that are complementary to target nucleic acid sequences. Target recognition occurs through hybridization, enabling highly specific detection of genetic material, which is essential for pathogen identification, mutation analysis, and molecular diagnostics. Key applications include rapid pathogen detection (e.g., COVID-19 using CRISPR-Cas), genetic screening, and environmental monitoring.

6.2.1.4 Cell-Based Biosensors

Cell-based biosensors incorporate whole living cells as sensing elements that respond to chemical or biological stimuli via measurable physiological, metabolic, or morphological changes. These biosensors are particularly valuable in environmental monitoring, toxicity testing, and metabolite sensing, as they provide information on the overall biological impact of analytes.

6.2.1.5 Aptasensors

Aptasensors employ aptamers, i.e., synthetic single-stranded DNA or RNA oligonucleotides selected for high affinity and specificity toward diverse targets. Compared to antibodies, aptamers offer advantages such as enhanced stability, ease of chemical synthesis and modification, reduced batch-to-batch variability, and greater design flexibility, making aptasensors a promising alternative in advanced biosensing applications.

6.2.2 Classification by Transduction Principle

6.2.2.1 Electrochemical Biosensors

They operate by measuring electrical parameters such as current, voltage, or impedance changes that arise from biochemical interactions at the electrode–electrolyte interface. These sensors typically rely on amperometric, potentiometric, or impedimetric detection modes, making them highly sensitive to redox reactions and charge-transfer processes. Their simple instrumentation, and compatibility with microfabrication techniques enable easy miniaturization and integration into portable devices. The operating principle of an electrochemical DNA biosensor is based on the interaction between the biorecognition element and the target nucleic acid, which leads to the generation or consumption of ions or electrons, thereby altering the current, potential, or other electrical characteristics of the sensing system [8].

6.2.2.2 Optical Biosensors

These detect analyte-induced variations in optical properties, including light absorption, fluorescence, luminescence, and refractive index changes, as well as surface plasmon resonance phenomena. An optical biosensor is a miniaturized analytical platform in which a biorecognition component is coupled with an optical transduction system to convert biological interactions into measurable optical signals [9]. These biosensors offer high sensitivity and the advantage of real-time, often label-free detection, allowing direct monitoring of biomolecular interactions without altering the target or recognition element.

6.2.2.3 Piezoelectric Biosensors

They function by converting mass changes on the sensor surface into measurable frequency shifts, typically using quartz crystal microbalance or similar devices. When biomolecules bind to the functionalized sensor surface, the resulting increase in mass alters the resonant frequency, enabling highly sensitive and label-free detection of biomolecular interactions. The piezoelectric immunosensors with immobilized antigen are a suitable tool for diagnosis of infectious diseases [10]. These sensors are especially useful for studying binding kinetics and affinity in real time.

6.2.2.4 Thermal Biosensors

They detect changes in temperature or heat flow generated during biochemical reactions, such as enzymatic catalysis or binding events. The sensing principle is based on measuring the enthalpy changes associated with these reactions. Although thermal biosensors offer universal detection capability, their broader application is limited by challenges related to sensitivity, thermal noise, and the requirement for precise temperature control.

6.2.2.5 Mechanical Biosensors

These employ micro- or nanoscale structures, such as microcantilevers and nanowires, to detect mechanical changes induced by biomolecular interactions. Binding events generate surface stress, deflection, or resonance frequency shifts in these structures, which are subsequently measured to infer analyte presence. Due to their high sensitivity and potential for label-free detection at very low analyte concentrations, mechanical biosensors are gaining increasing attention in advanced sensing and nanotechnology-based diagnostic applications.

6.2.3 Emerging Categories of FET-based Biosensors

6.2.3.1 Field-Effect Transistor (FET) Biosensors

They operate by transducing biological interactions into electrical signals through modulation of the electric field or charge distribution at the surface of a semiconductor channel (Figure 6.2). In these devices, the biorecognition element is immobilized near

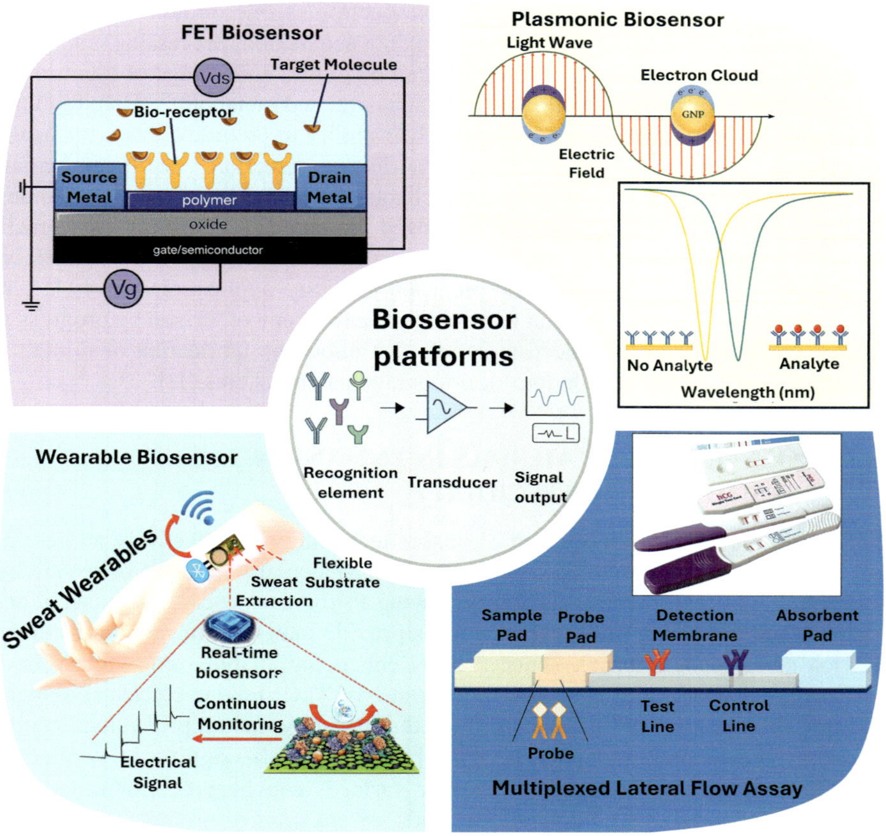

FIGURE 6.2 Schematic overview of emerging biosensor platforms and their signal transduction mechanisms.

or on the gate region, and binding of charged biomolecules induces changes in the surface potential, leading to measurable variations in channel conductivity. Owing to this direct charge-based sensing mechanism, FET biosensors offer exceptionally high sensitivity, often reaching femtomolar or even attomolar detection limits. Their ability to provide rapid, real-time, and label-free detection makes them particularly attractive for applications in clinical diagnostics, environmental monitoring, and early disease detection. Advances in nanomaterials, such as graphene, silicon nanowires, and transition metal dichalcogenides, have further enhanced the performance of FET biosensors by improving charge transport, surface functionalization, and signal-to-noise ratios, positioning them as next-generation sensing platforms.

6.2.3.2 Wearable Biosensors

These are designed for continuous and noninvasive monitoring of physiological and biochemical parameters by integrating biosensing elements into flexible and conformable substrates, such as textiles, wristbands, or skin-mounted patches. These systems combine biosensing technologies with flexible electronics, microfluidics, and wireless communication modules to enable real-time data acquisition, processing, and transmission (Figure 6.2). Wearable biosensors can monitor a wide range of biomarkers, including glucose, lactate, electrolytes, and stress-related metabolites, from biofluids such as sweat, interstitial fluid, or saliva. Their ability to provide continuous health data supports personalized healthcare, early disease detection, and remote patient monitoring. Recent developments in stretchable materials, low-power electronics, and data analytics have significantly improved the comfort, reliability, and practicality of wearable biosensors, making them an increasingly important component of next-generation digital health and precision medicine applications. Flexible sensors have emerged as a significant technological advancement, driven by progress in printed electronics and advanced materials that allow the fabrication of miniature sensors suitable for integration into skin-mounted patch systems [11].

6.3 ROLE OF NANOMATERIALS IN ENHANCING SENSITIVITY AND SPECIFICITY

Nanomaterials have revolutionized biosensor technology by effectively addressing key limitations of conventional sensing systems, particularly in terms of sensitivity, selectivity, and multiplexing capability. Owing to their nanoscale dimensions and high surface-to-volume ratio, nanomaterials provide many active sites for immobilization of biorecognition elements, thereby enhancing analyte–probe interactions and enabling detection at very low concentrations. Their unique electrical, optical, and magnetic properties further contribute to intrinsic signal amplification, leading to improved detection limits. Selectivity in biosensors is also significantly enhanced through nanomaterial integration, as their surfaces can be precisely functionalized with antibodies, aptamers, nucleic acids, or enzymes to promote specific target recognition while minimizing nonspecific binding. Additionally, nanostructured interfaces help preserve biomolecular activity and improve signal-to-noise ratios in complex biological samples. Importantly, nanomaterials facilitate multiplexed detection by offering tunable and distinct transduction signals, allowing simultaneous sensing of multiple analytes within a single platform. This capability is crucial for comprehensive disease diagnostics and biomarker profiling. Overall, the incorporation of nanomaterials has enabled the development of highly sensitive, selective, and multifunctional biosensors, expanding their applicability across clinical diagnostics, environmental monitoring, and point-of-care testing.

6.3.1 Unique Properties of Nanomaterials

Nanoscale materials play a transformative role in modern biosensor design due to their unique physicochemical properties that are unattainable in bulk materials. One of their most significant advantages is the exceptionally high surface-to-volume ratio, which provides abundant active sites for the immobilization of biorecognition elements such as antibodies, enzymes, aptamers, peptides, and nucleic acids. This dense and stable loading of bioreceptors increases the probability of target–probe interactions, improves analyte capture efficiency, and ultimately enhances the sensitivity and detection capability of biosensors. In addition, the nanoscale dimensions allow closer proximity between the target molecule and the transducer surface, reducing diffusion limitations and accelerating signal generation.

Beyond surface effects, nanomaterials exhibit distinctive size-dependent optical, electrical, and magnetic properties that are highly advantageous for signal transduction. Phenomena such as localized surface plasmon resonance (LSPR) in metallic nanoparticles, quantum confinement effects in semiconductor nanostructures, and superior charge transport in carbon-based nanomaterials enable subtle biorecognition events to be converted into strong and measurable optical or electrical signals. These properties allow biosensors to achieve ultralow detection limits and high signal-to-noise ratios, even in complex biological or environmental matrices.

Certain nanomaterials function as nanozymes, displaying intrinsic enzyme-like catalytic activity while overcoming many limitations associated with natural enzymes, such as poor stability, high cost, and sensitivity to environmental conditions. Nanozymes can catalyze signal-generating reactions efficiently over a wide range of pH and temperature, thereby enhancing sensor robustness, extending operational lifetimes, and enabling long-term or repeated use. Their catalytic activity can be finely tuned through material composition, size, and surface modification, offering additional control over sensor performance.

Surface functionalization is another key strength of nanomaterials. Well-established chemical modification strategies allow precise conjugation of biomolecules under mild conditions, ensuring correct orientation, preserved bioactivity, and strong attachment. This contributes to reproducible sensor fabrication and consistent analytical performance. Furthermore, nanostructured surfaces inherently amplify sensing signals by concentrating electromagnetic fields, increasing surface energy, or facilitating rapid electron transfer between redox-active biomolecules and electrode interfaces. Conductive nanomaterials, such as graphene, carbon nanotubes, and metallic nanostructures, significantly improve electrochemical signal resolution and reduce detection limits without the need for additional amplification steps.

Importantly, nanomaterials enable multifunctional biosensing platforms in which a single material can simultaneously perform target recognition, signal transduction, amplification, and even therapeutic delivery. This multifunctionality supports the development of compact, integrated, and intelligent biosensors capable of real-time, point-of-care, and multiplexed analysis. Collectively, these attributes position nanomaterials as essential components in the next generation of highly sensitive, reliable, and versatile biosensing technologies.

6.3.2 Commonly Used Nanomaterials

There are some commonly used nanomaterials for biosensing applications, presented in Figure 6.3.

Metallic Nanoparticles: Gold and silver nanoparticles are extensively employed due to their strong plasmonic properties, particularly LSPR, which enhances optical biosensing signals. Their excellent electrical conductivity also facilitates efficient electron transfer, making them highly suitable for electrochemical biosensing and signal amplification strategies.

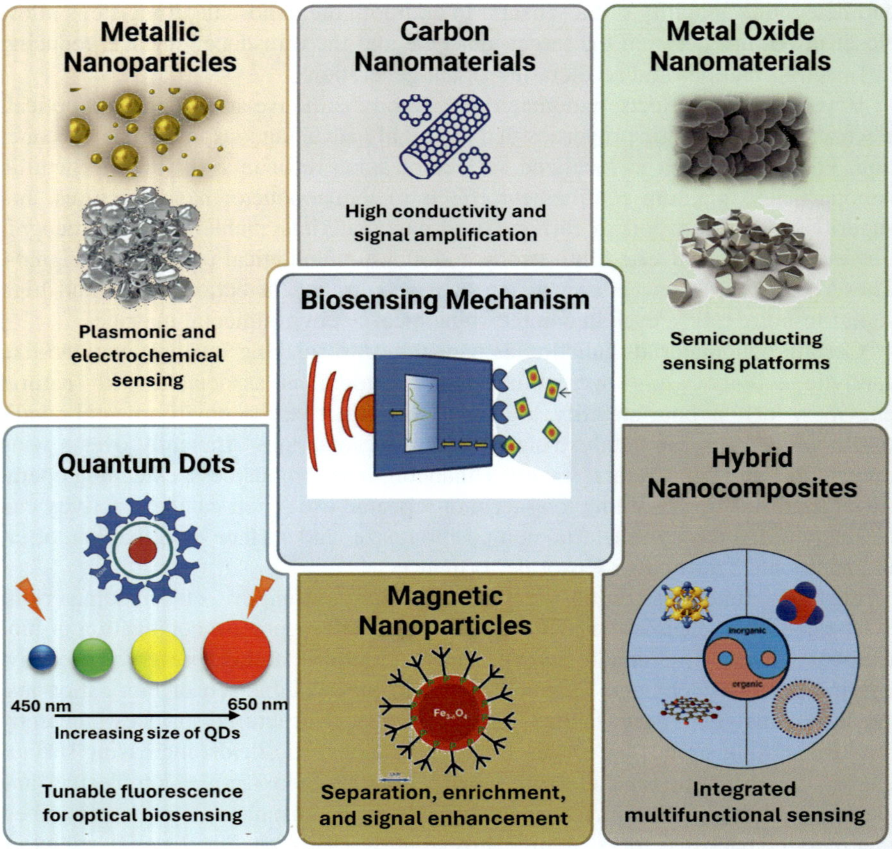

FIGURE 6.3 Overview of functional nanomaterials integrated into modern biosensor architectures.

Carbon Nanomaterials: Graphene, graphene oxide, carbon nanotubes, and carbon dots offer exceptional electrical conductivity, high mechanical strength, and good biocompatibility. These features promote rapid electron transport and stable biomolecule immobilization, thereby significantly improving the sensitivity and reliability of electrochemical biosensors.

Quantum Dots: Quantum dots are semiconductor nanocrystals characterized by size-dependent and tunable fluorescence emission along with high photostability. These properties enable simultaneous detection of multiple targets in multiplexed fluorescent biosensing platforms with minimal signal overlap.

Magnetic Nanoparticles: Magnetic nanoparticles enable selective capture, separation, and enrichment of target analytes through the application of external magnetic fields. This capability enhances detection sensitivity, particularly in complex biological samples, by facilitating efficient sample preconcentration.

Metal Oxide Nanomaterials: Metal oxides such as ZnO and TiO_2 provide high surface reactivity and catalytic activity, while also improving charge transfer characteristics at the sensor interface. These properties make them effective platforms for enhancing signal transduction in both optical and electrochemical biosensors.

Polymeric Nanomaterials: Conducting and functional polymers (e.g., polyaniline, polypyrrole, polymeric nanoparticles) offer mechanical flexibility, chemical stability, and easy functionalization. They are widely used to improve biocompatibility, signal stability, and integration into flexible or wearable biosensors.

6.4 RECENT DEVELOPMENTS IN NANO-BIOSENSING PLATFORMS

Technological advances in nanofabrication, materials engineering, and bio-interface design have driven the development of innovative nano-biosensing platforms with unprecedented performance metrics. Precise control over nanomaterial size, shape, and surface chemistry has enabled highly efficient biorecognition and signal transduction, resulting in markedly enhanced sensitivity and lower limits of detection. Concurrently, advances in micro- and nano-patterning techniques have improved sensor reproducibility and reliability by enabling uniform and well-defined sensing architectures. Integration of nanomaterials with advanced transduction mechanisms, such as electrochemical, optical, plasmonic, and FET-based systems, has further improved signal resolution, response speed, and real-time monitoring capability (Figure 6.2). In addition, progress in surface functionalization strategies has minimized nonspecific interactions, thereby enhancing selectivity even in complex biological matrices. Importantly, the convergence of nano-biosensors with microfluidics, flexible electronics, and data analytics has enabled miniaturized, multiplexed, and point-of-care platforms capable of rapid and accurate analysis. Collectively, these technological advancements have redefined biosensor performance benchmarks, positioning nano-biosensing platforms as powerful tools for next-generation diagnostics, environmental monitoring, and precision medicine.

6.4.1 Lateral Flow Assays Enhanced with Nanoparticles

Lateral flow assays (LFAs) are simple, paper-based immunoassays designed to provide rapid and user-friendly point-of-care detection without the need for complex instrumentation (Figure 6.2). They operate on capillary-driven fluid flow, enabling quick sample transport and on-site analysis. The incorporation of colloidal gold nanoparticles as signal reporters has become standard due to their intense color, stability, and ease of conjugation with antibodies, allowing direct visual readout of test results. This nanoparticle-based labeling enhances assay sensitivity while maintaining low cost, portability, and suitability for decentralized diagnostics.

Advances are given as follows:

- Dual-Mode LFAs: They integrate colorimetric nanoparticles with fluorescent reporters, such as combining gold nanoparticles with quantum dots. This design preserves rapid visual readout while enabling enhanced sensitivity and semiquantitative analysis through fluorescence measurement.

- Smartphone Integration: Coupling LFAs with smartphone-based imaging and analysis allows digital capture and processing of test results. Dedicated applications improve result interpretation, enable data storage and sharing, and facilitate on-site diagnostics, particularly in resource-limited or remote settings.
- Multiplexed LFAs: They employ distinct nanomaterial labels with unique optical signatures to detect multiple targets simultaneously. This capability is especially valuable for respiratory panel testing and pandemic screening, where rapid differentiation between pathogens is critical.
- Signal Amplification Strategies: Use of enzyme-loaded nanoparticles, nanozymes, or multilayer nanoparticle assemblies enhances signal intensity, significantly improving detection limits without increasing assay complexity.
- Magnetic-Assisted LFAs: Magnetic nanoparticles enable pre-concentration and guided transport of analytes prior to lateral flow, increasing assay sensitivity and improving performance in low-abundance targets.

6.4.2 Field-Effect Transistor Biosensors

Graphene and other 2D materials serve as highly effective conductive channels in FET biosensors due to their atomic-scale thickness, high carrier mobility, and exceptional sensitivity to surface charge variations. When charged biomolecules bind to the functionalized 2D surface, they induce measurable changes in the channel conductance, enabling direct, label-free electrical detection with ultrasensitive response.

Recent advances in 2D material–based FET biosensors are as follows:

- Ultrasensitive, Real-Time Detection: Demonstrated capability to detect viral antigens and nucleic acids in real time at femtomolar concentration levels, enabling early-stage infection diagnostics.
- Improved Surface Chemistry and Stability: Development of antifouling surface chemistries and optimized functionalization strategies that minimize nonspecific adsorption, signal drift, and background noise, thereby improving reliability.
- Multiplexed and Miniaturized Device Architectures: Integration of 2D FETs into compact, multiplexed arrays allows simultaneous detection of multiple biomarkers, supporting high-throughput and rapid diagnostic applications.

6.4.3 Surface-Enhanced Raman Scattering Biosensors

Surface-enhanced Raman scattering (SERS) substrates engineered with precisely controlled nanogaps, and high hotspot densities generate intense localized electromagnetic fields, dramatically amplifying Raman signals from analyte molecules. These optimized nanostructures enable ultrahigh sensitivity, often reaching single-molecule detection limits, while preserving the inherent molecular fingerprint specificity of Raman spectroscopy. Such characteristics make SERS particularly powerful for identifying chemically similar biomolecules and trace-level analytes. Integration of SERS platforms with machine learning (ML) algorithms further enhances analytical performance, especially for complex or heterogeneous samples. Advanced data-driven models enable efficient pattern recognition, background subtraction, and spectral classification, improving accuracy, robustness, and reproducibility. This combination facilitates reliable biomarker discrimination and disease diagnostics in real-world biological matrices where conventional spectral analysis is limited.

6.4.4 Electrochemical Biosensors

Nanostructured electrodes functionalized with metallic nanoparticles or carbon-based nanomaterials significantly enhance biosensor sensitivity by increasing the effective surface area and promoting efficient electron transfer at the electrode–electrolyte interface. These modifications enable improved immobilization of biorecognition elements and facilitate rapid signal transduction, resulting in lower detection limits for a wide range of targets, including metabolites, proteins, and nucleic acids. Integration of such nanostructured electrodes with microfluidic systems further advances biosensor performance by enabling precise control over sample handling, reduced reagent consumption, and automated assay workflows. Microfluidic miniaturization shortens analysis time and improves reproducibility, making these platforms highly suitable for rapid, high-throughput clinical diagnostics and point-of-care applications.

6.4.5 Emerging Platforms

6.4.5.1 Plasmonic and Photonic Biosensors

They leverage nanostructured metals and dielectric materials to generate strong electromagnetic field enhancements at the sensor surface. LSPR-based platforms enable label-free detection by translating biomolecular binding events into measurable shifts in resonance wavelength or intensity (Figure 6.2). These sensors offer rapid response times, high sensitivity, and real-time monitoring capability, making them particularly suitable for kinetic studies, early disease diagnostics, and low-abundance biomarker detection.

6.4.5.2 Wearable and Implantable Biosensors

Nanomaterials play a critical role in enabling wearable and implantable biosensors by providing mechanical flexibility, biocompatibility, and stable signal transduction under physiological conditions. Integration of nanostructures with soft substrates allows continuous monitoring of biochemical and biophysical parameters such as metabolites, ions, and biomarkers directly from bodily fluids. These devices support long-term, real-time health monitoring and personalized medicine by enabling minimally invasive or noninvasive sensing with high reliability.

6.5 APPLICATIONS IN MEDICAL DIAGNOSTICS

Nano-biosensors have found widespread applications across diverse medical fields owing to their high sensitivity, specificity, rapid response, and miniaturization potential, which collectively surpass the performance of conventional diagnostic platforms. By integrating nanomaterials, such as metal nanoparticles, quantum dots, carbon nanostructures, and lipid-based nanocarriers with biological recognition elements (antibodies, aptamers, enzymes, nucleic acids), nano-biosensors enable ultrasensitive, real-time, and often label-free detection of clinically relevant biomarkers.

In clinical diagnostics, nano-biosensors facilitate early detection of infectious diseases, cancer biomarkers, and metabolic disorders by identifying trace-level analytes (pico- to femtomolar concentrations), thereby supporting timely intervention and improved patient outcomes. In point-of-care and wearable healthcare systems, their compact size and low power requirements allow integration into portable devices and skin-mounted platforms for continuous monitoring of physiological parameters such as glucose, lactate, electrolytes, and stress hormones. Nano-biosensors also play a critical role in personalized medicine and therapeutic monitoring, enabling real-time assessment of drug levels, treatment efficacy, and disease progression. In neurodegenerative and cardiovascular disease management, they support sensitive detection of biomarkers associated with inflammation, oxidative stress, and neuronal damage. Furthermore, in immunology and oncology, multiplexed nano-biosensor arrays permit simultaneous detection of multiple cytokines or tumor markers, improving diagnostic accuracy and disease stratification.

Overall, the convergence of nanotechnology, biosensing, and microelectronics positions nano-biosensors as transformative tools in modern medicine, with strong potential to advance early diagnosis, continuous health monitoring, and precision therapeutics (Figure 6.4).

6.5.1 Infectious Disease Diagnostics

Nano-biosensors achieve rapid, sensitive detection of pathogens by combining nanomaterials (e.g., metallic nanoparticles, magnetic nanoparticles) with specific biorecognition elements. These enable point-of-care diagnosis with lower limits of detection and shorter assay times compared with conventional culture or PCR tests, making them valuable during outbreaks and routine screening. For example, a precisely electropolymerized molecularly imprinted polymer (MIP)-based electrochemical sensor incorporating an antibody-functionalized gold-polyaniline (Au-PAni) nanocomposite has been developed for the selective and ultrasensitive detection of dengue virus–like particles, achieving a detection limit as low as 180 fM, excellent selectivity against other viral particles, and reliable performance over multiple cycles, demonstrating its suitability for rapid viral diagnostics [12]. Additionally, functionalized magnetic nanoparticle–based sensors have been reported for the rapid detection of SARS-CoV-2 with nanomolar-level sensitivity, and electrochemical and optical nano-biosensors employing silver nanoparticles, gold nanoparticles, and quantum dots have shown enhanced sensitivity for *Mycobacterium tuberculosis* and other infectious biomarkers, highlighting the versatility and effectiveness of nanomaterial-enabled biosensing platforms in infectious disease diagnostics [13].

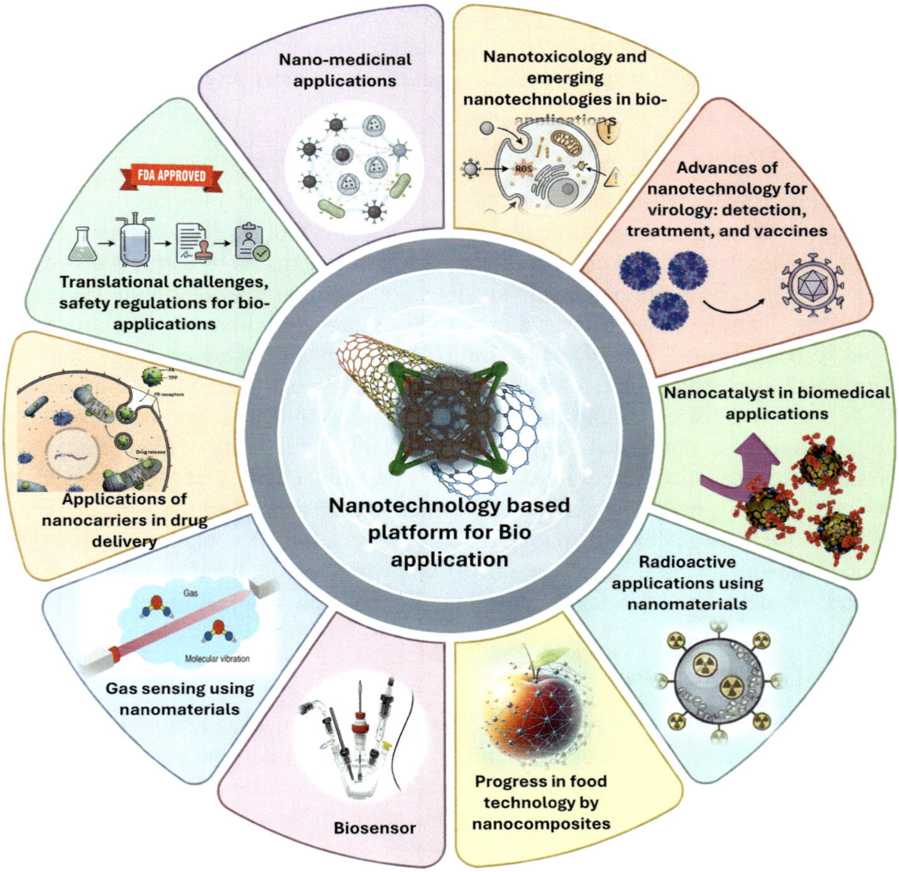

FIGURE 6.4 Clinical diagnostic landscape for biosensor applications in human health monitoring.

6.5.2 Cancer Biomarker Detection

Nano-biosensors facilitate early detection of cancer biomarkers (such as proteins, metabolites, or nucleic acids) at ultralow concentrations, enabling earlier treatment decisions and improved prognoses compared with traditional immunoassays. For instance, nanoparticle-enhanced sensors employing materials like carbon nanotubes and quantum dots have been used experimentally to detect markers associated with prostate, breast, lung, and pancreatic cancers with increased specificity and lower detection limits than conventional methods, demonstrating significant performance improvements in early-stage cancer diagnostics [14]. Moreover, recent research has developed innovative nanostructured platforms such as an Fe-doped Cu_3N nanocube–based electrochemical sensor that detects cancer-associated metabolic biomarkers (e.g., H_2O_2 released by cancer cells) with minute-scale response time and can distinguish cancerous tissue from normal controls, underlining the potential of nanomaterial-enabled sensing for rapid, point-of-care cancer screening [15].

6.5.3 Metabolic and Chronic Disease Monitoring

Nano-biosensors play a crucial role in metabolic disorder monitoring by enabling the highly sensitive and real-time detection of key metabolites such as glucose, lactate, cholesterol, urea, and uric acid, which are directly linked to metabolic homeostasis and disease progression. Owing to their large surface-to-volume ratio and enhanced electron/optical transport properties, nanomaterial-based sensors provide rapid response times, low detection limits, and high analytical accuracy, making them particularly well suited for the long-term management of chronic metabolic diseases such as diabetes, cardiovascular-associated dyslipidemia, and renal dysfunction. Furthermore, the miniaturization and mechanical flexibility of nano-biosensors facilitate their seamless integration into wearable, implantable, and continuous monitoring platforms, including skin patches, microneedle arrays, and flexible electronics. Such systems enable continuous tracking of metabolic fluctuations in biofluids (blood, interstitial fluid, sweat, or saliva), allowing personalized disease management, early detection of metabolic imbalance, and timely therapeutic intervention.

6.5.4 Genetic and Prenatal Testing

Nano-biosensors targeting specific DNA and RNA sequences enable highly specific and rapid mutation detection, pathogen genotyping, and gene expression profiling, which are critical components of precision medicine. By exploiting nanoscale transducers with tailored surface functionalization, these platforms achieve direct, label-free recognition of complementary nucleic acid targets with minimal sample processing and short assay times. For example, high-Q nanoantenna-based sensing platforms functionalized with nucleic acid fragments have demonstrated rapid, amplification-free, and ultrasensitive detection of gene targets by enhancing local electromagnetic fields, thereby allowing real-time genetic screening without the need for PCR amplification [16].

6.5.5 Neurological and Neurodegenerative Disease Detection

Nano-biosensors capable of detecting proteomic biomarkers such as amyloid-β, tau, and α-synuclein offer promising opportunities for the early diagnosis of neurodegenerative diseases including Alzheimer's and Parkinson's. By leveraging high-surface area nanomaterials and advanced transduction mechanisms, these platforms enable ultrasensitive and often label-free detection of disease-associated proteins from minimally invasive biofluids such as blood, saliva, or cerebrospinal fluid. Comprehensive studies and reviews emphasize that nano-biosensors significantly lower detection limits for neurological biomarkers compared with conventional assays, thereby facilitating earlier disease diagnosis, improved monitoring of disease progression, and more effective therapeutic intervention [17].

6.5.6 Immunological and Inflammatory Disorder Assessment

Nano-biosensors enable the sensitive quantification of cytokines, autoantibodies, and inflammatory biomarkers at very low concentrations, providing detailed insights into immune status and the dynamic progression of acute and chronic inflammatory conditions. By exploiting nanostructured transducers with large surface areas and enhanced signal amplification, these platforms support rapid analysis and simultaneous detection of multiple immune biomarkers within a single assay. Such multiplexed nano-biosensing approaches have been shown to achieve low limits of detection and fast response times for biomarker panels, thereby improving diagnostic accuracy, real-time immune-monitoring, and clinical decision-making in inflammatory and immune-mediated diseases [18].

6.5.7 Cardiovascular Disease Diagnostics

Nano-biosensors enable the early detection of key cardiac biomarkers such as troponins, B-type natriuretic peptide, and C-reactive protein with enhanced sensitivity and a broad dynamic range, which is crucial for the timely diagnosis of acute cardiovascular events. By leveraging nanostructured materials and advanced transduction mechanisms, these sensing platforms provide rapid and highly selective biomarker analysis and can be readily integrated into flexible, portable, and point-of-care formats for on-site testing. Comprehensive nano-sensor reviews highlight the strong potential of optical, electrochemical, paper-based, and pressure-based nano-biosensors in cardiovascular disease diagnostics, emphasizing their high selectivity, fast response, and suitability for early disease detection in clinical and emergency settings [19].

6.6 CHALLENGES AND INNOVATIONS IN BIOSENSOR TECHNOLOGY

6.6.1 Sensitivity vs. Specificity

Achieving ultrahigh sensitivity is a primary objective in modern biosensor design; however, increasing sensitivity often amplifies nonspecific interactions and background noise, which can compromise selectivity. Highly sensitive nanomaterials may respond to unintended analytes or environmental fluctuations, leading to false positives. Current innovations focus on improving surface chemistry, incorporating highly specific biorecognition elements (such as aptamers or MIPs), and employing signal-processing strategies to enhance target discrimination without sacrificing detection limits.

6.6.2 Reproducibility and Standardization

Reproducibility remains a major bottleneck, particularly in nano-biosensors, due to batch-to-batch variability in nanomaterial synthesis, size distribution, morphology, and surface functionalization. Minor inconsistencies can significantly affect sensor performance and signal output. To address this, efforts are being directed toward standardized fabrication protocols, scalable synthesis methods, and quality-controlled surface modification techniques, alongside the development of reference materials and calibration standards for cross-laboratory validation.

6.6.3 Sample Complexity and Matrix Effects

Biological samples such as blood, serum, saliva, and urine contain complex mixtures of proteins, salts, enzymes, and other interfering substances that can adsorb onto sensor surfaces and obscure target signals. These matrix effects reduce accuracy and reliability in real-world diagnostics. Innovations such as antifouling surface coatings, selective membranes, on-chip sample pretreatment, and microfluidic integration are being explored to minimize nonspecific adsorption and improve sensor performance in complex biological environments.

6.6.4 Device Stability and Shelf Life

Maintaining long-term stability of biosensors, especially those intended for field deployment or point-of-care use, is challenging due to degradation of biological recognition elements and nanomaterial instability over time. Temperature fluctuations, humidity, and mechanical stress can further deteriorate performance. Advances in sensor stabilization include the use of robust synthetic receptors, protective encapsulation layers, lyophilized reagents, and optimized storage conditions to extend shelf life without loss of sensitivity or specificity.

6.6.5 Cost and Scalability

While advanced nanomaterials and sophisticated fabrication techniques enhance biosensor performance, they often increase production costs and limit large-scale deployment. Achieving a balance between high analytical performance and affordability is critical for widespread clinical and public health applications. Emerging innovations emphasize low-cost nanomaterial synthesis, printable and roll-to-roll manufacturing, paper-based platforms, and integration with consumer electronics, aiming to deliver scalable, cost-effective biosensor technologies suitable for mass deployment.

6.7 INNOVATIONS AND FUTURE DIRECTIONS

Rapid progress in biosensor technology is being fueled by the increasing demand for highly sensitive, specific, and scalable diagnostic tools capable of operating in complex biological environments and real-world settings. While conventional biosensors have demonstrated significant utility, persistent challenges related to signal accuracy, multiplexing capability, data interpretation, and clinical translation have driven the exploration of advanced technological innovations. Recent research efforts increasingly focus on integrating nanomaterials with intelligent data processing, biomolecular engineering, and smart device architectures to overcome these limitations. Such advancements aim not only to enhance analytical performance, such as sensitivity, selectivity, and response time, but also to enable real-time monitoring, decentralized diagnostics, and seamless connectivity with digital health platforms. Collectively, these developments are shaping the evolution of next-generation biosensors that are more adaptive, robust, and suitable for precision medicine and population-scale health surveillance.

6.7.1 Artificial Intelligence and Machine Learning

Artificial intelligence (AI) and ML are increasingly being integrated into biosensor systems to enhance signal processing, pattern recognition, and interpretation of complex datasets. AI/ML algorithms can distinguish true target signals from noise, compensate for drift and variability, and analyze multiplexed outputs from multi-analyte sensors, thereby improving diagnostic accuracy and reliability. These approaches are particularly valuable for wearable and point-of-care biosensors, where real-time data analytics and decision support are essential.

6.7.2 CRISPR-Based Biosensors

Such biosensors exploit the inherent molecular specificity of CRISPR-Cas systems for nucleic acid recognition, combined with nanomaterial-enabled signal amplification. By coupling CRISPR-mediated target recognition with optical, electrochemical, or plasmonic nano-transducers, these platforms achieve highly selective and rapid detection of genetic material without the need for extensive amplification. Such systems show strong potential for pathogen detection, mutation analysis, and decentralized genetic diagnostics.

6.7.3 Integration with Digital Health

The integration of biosensors with digital health ecosystems through smartphones, wearable devices, and cloud-based data infrastructure, enables remote diagnostics, telemedicine, and real-time health monitoring. Wireless data transmission and cloud analytics allow continuous tracking of biomarkers at the population level, supporting early disease detection, personalized healthcare, and large-scale epidemiological surveillance, particularly in resource-limited or remote settings.

6.7.4 3D and 4D Biosensors

Advanced 3D and 4D biosensors utilize architecturally complex nanostructures that provide increased surface area, spatial control, and dynamic responsiveness. While 3D biosensors enhance sensitivity and multiplexing by offering hierarchical sensing interfaces, 4D biosensors incorporate time-dependent or stimuli-responsive behavior, allowing sensors to adapt to changing biological environments. These systems enable real-time, multiparameter detection in complex and dynamic biological settings.

6.7.5 Biomimetic Nanostructures

Biomimetic biosensors are designed to emulate natural biological recognition mechanisms, such as enzyme–substrate interactions, antibody–antigen binding, or cell membrane interfaces. By mimicking these systems using nanostructured materials, biosensors achieve improved specificity, reduced nonspecific interactions, and enhanced binding efficiency. Biomimetic nanostructures, including artificial receptors and membrane-inspired interfaces, represent a promising strategy for developing highly selective and robust biosensors for clinical diagnostics.

6.8 CONCLUSION

Biosensor technology has evolved into a cornerstone of modern diagnostics, driven by continuous advances in materials science, nanotechnology, microfabrication, and bio-interface engineering. This chapter has highlighted how the integration of nanomaterials fundamentally enhances biosensor performance by improving sensitivity, selectivity, signal transduction efficiency, and multiplexing capability. The unique physicochemical properties of nanomaterials—such as high surface-to-volume ratio, tunable optical and electrical behavior, catalytic activity, and versatile surface functionalization—have enabled the detection of biomolecules at ultralow concentrations, even within complex biological matrices. As a result, nano-enabled biosensors now surpass many conventional platforms in terms of analytical precision, response speed, and portability.

The classification of biosensors based on biorecognition elements and transduction mechanisms underscores the diversity and adaptability of sensing strategies available for a wide range of applications. Emerging platforms, including FET-based sensors, SERS substrates, wearable and implantable devices, and nanoparticle-enhanced LFAs, demonstrate how nanoscale engineering has expanded biosensing from laboratory settings to point-of-care, real-time, and continuous monitoring systems. These developments have had a particularly profound impact on medical diagnostics, enabling early detection of infectious diseases, cancer biomarkers, metabolic disorders, genetic abnormalities, and cardiovascular and neurodegenerative conditions, thereby supporting precision medicine and improved patient outcomes.

Despite these advances, challenges related to reproducibility, stability, cost, sample complexity, and large-scale clinical translation remain significant. Addressing these limitations requires standardized fabrication methods, robust surface chemistries, antifouling strategies, and scalable manufacturing approaches. Looking forward, the convergence of nano-biosensors with AI, digital health platforms, CRISPR-based recognition systems, and biomimetic designs is expected to further enhance diagnostic accuracy, data interpretation, and real-world applicability. Collectively, these innovations position nano-biosensors as transformative tools for next-generation healthcare, environmental monitoring, and global health surveillance, with strong potential to reshape how diseases are detected, monitored, and managed.

REFERENCES

1. V. Naresh, N. Lee, A review on biosensors and recent development of nanostructured materials-enabled biosensors, *Sensors*, 21(2021) 1109.
2. J. Wang, Glucose biosensors: 40 years of advances and challenges, *Sensors Update*, 10(2002) 107–19.

3. E. Morales-Narváez, C. Dincer, The impact of biosensing in a pandemic outbreak: COVID-19, *Biosensors & Bioelectronics*, 163(2020) 112274.
4. J. Kaur, S. Choudhary, R. Chaudhari, R. Jayant, A. Joshi, Enzyme-based biosensors, in: K. Pal, H.-B. Kraatz, A. Khasnobish, S. Bag, I. Banerjee, U. Kurugant (Eds.), *Bioelectronics and Medical Devices*, Woodhead Publishing, 2019, pp. 211–40.
5. G.S. Wilson, Y. Hu, Enzyme-based biosensors for in vivo measurements, *Chemical Reviews*, 100(2000) 2693–704.
6. L. Fang, X. Liao, B. Jia, L. Shi, L. Kang, L. Zhou, et al., Recent progress in immunosensors for pesticides, *Biosensors and Bioelectronics*, 164(2020) 112255.
7. J. Tang, D. Tang, Q. Li, B. Su, B. Qiu, G. Chen, Sensitive electrochemical immunoassay of carcinoembryonic antigen with signal dual-amplification using glucose oxidase and an artificial catalase, *Analytica Chimica Acta*, 697(2011) 16–22.
8. Q. Wu, Y. Zhang, Q. Yang, N. Yuan, W. Zhang, Review of electrochemical DNA biosensors for detecting food borne pathogens, *Sensors*, 19(2019) 4916.
9. P. Damborský, J. Švitel, J. Katrlík, Optical biosensors, *Essays in Biochemistry*, 60(2016) 91–100.
10. M. Pohanka, Overview of piezoelectric biosensors, immunosensors and DNA sensors and their applications, *M*aterials, 11(2018) 448.
11. M.D. Mukherjee, P. Gupta, V. Kumari, I. Rana, D. Jindal, N. Sagar, et al., Wearable biosensors in modern healthcare: emerging trends and practical applications, *Talanta Open*, 12(2025) 100486.
12. M. Ghosh, U. Dasgupta, P. Chakraborty, M.K. Sarangi, E.Y. Park, A.D. Chowdhury, Precisely electropolymerized molecularly imprinted polymer-based sensor electrode for selective detection of dengue virus-like particles, *Chemical Engineering Journal*, 529(2026) 172500.
13. A.U. Ibrahim, P.C. Pwavodi, M. Oszoz, B.B. Duwa, I. Irkham, Y.W Hartati. Nano-modified biosensors for detection of pathogenic diseases: the prospect of smart, multiplex and point-of-care testing: review article, *ADMET and DMPK*, 13(2025) 2799.
14. A. Gdowski, A.P. Ranjan, A. Mukerjee, J.K. Vishwanatha, Nanobiosensors: role in cancer detection and diagnosis, in: R. Adhikari, S. Thapa (Eds.), *Infectious Diseases and Nanomedicine I*, Springer India, 2014, pp. 33–58.
15. U. Dasgupta, M. Ghosh, S.S. Singh, V.K. Mishra, S. Maji, M. Das, et al., Cu_3N–Fe nanocube-based electrochemical sensing of cancer metabolites with minute-scale response time, *Materials Horizons*, 13(2026).
16. J. Hu, F. Safir, K. Chang, S. Dagli, H.B. Balch, J.M. Abendroth, et al., Rapid genetic screening with high quality factor metasurfaces, *Nature Communications*, 14(2023) 4486.
17. S. Prasad, Nanobiosensors: the future for diagnosis of disease?, *Nanobiosensors in Disease Diagnosis*, 3(2014) 1–10.
18. D. Sagar, N. Raghavendra, S.G. Prakash, G. Buduru, Nanobiosensors: concepts and emerging clinical applications, *Pharmaceutical Nanotechnology*, 12(2024) 197–205.
19. C. Sejuti Ray, G. Sourav, R. Monosiz, D. Srabona, Advancing precision medicine with nanosensor: emerging technologies for early diagnosis of heart disease, *Current Nanomedicine*, 15(2025) 546–60.

7 Gas Sensing Using Nanomaterials

Tamara V. Basova and Darya Klyamer

7.1 INTRODUCTION

The ability to detect and monitor gases with high precision has become indispensable in addressing pressing global challenges that span environmental sustainability, industrial safety, food quality assurance, and medical diagnostics. Toxic and hazardous gases such as carbon monoxide (CO), nitrogen oxides (NO_x), sulfur dioxide (SO_2), ammonia (NH_3), hydrogen sulfide (H_2S), and volatile organic compounds (VOCs) are routinely released from vehicles, fossil fuel combustion, agricultural activities, and industrial processes. Their presence in the atmosphere not only contributes to environmental degradation through phenomena like smog formation and acid rain but also poses direct health risks ranging from respiratory illnesses and neurological disorders to cancer. Beyond environmental concerns, gases have gained clinical importance as biomarkers like exhaled human breath contain hundreds of VOCs whose concentrations vary with metabolic and pathological states. For example, acetone levels in breath correlate with blood glucose in diabetes, nitric oxide serves as a marker for asthma and chronic obstructive pulmonary disease (COPD), and VOCs such as benzene and formaldehyde are linked to lung cancer. These insights highlight the dual role of gas sensing at the intersection of environmental protection and noninvasive healthcare. Nanotechnology has revolutionized this field by enabling the design of sensing materials with unprecedented sensitivity, selectivity, and miniaturization. The unique physicochemical properties of nanomaterials such as their exceptionally high surface-to-volume ratios, tunable band structures, and surface functionalization capabilities allow them to interact strongly and selectively with trace levels of gases. One-dimensional (1D) nanowires and nanotubes, two-dimensional sheets like graphene and MoS_2, noble metal nanoparticles, quantum dots, and hybrid nanocomposites have all been engineered into sensing platforms capable of detecting gases at concentrations as low as parts per billion (ppb), often at room temperature. This chapter explores the fundamental principles of nanomaterial-enabled gas sensing and their application across different domains. It discusses how chemiresistive, field-effect transistor (FET), optical, and piezoelectric mechanisms are enhanced by nanostructuring, and examines the deployment of nanomaterials for detecting toxic and hazardous gases in environmental monitoring. The emerging role of gas sensors in noninvasive medical diagnostics through breath analysis is highlighted with examples ranging from acetone-based diabetes monitoring to VOC detection in cancer. The integration of nanomaterial-based sensors into flexible, wearable, and portable devices is also examined, showing their potential

DOI: 10.1201/9781003725930-7

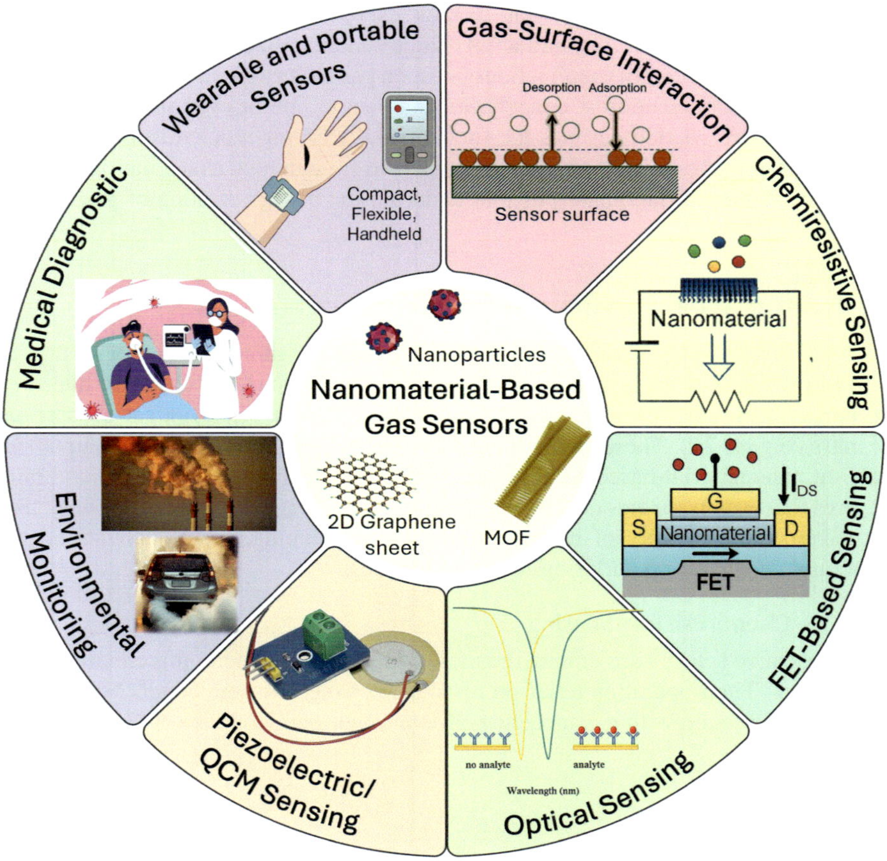

FIGURE 7.1 Conceptual illustration of nanomaterial-based gas sensing mechanisms and their applications in environmental and biomedical monitoring.

for real-time monitoring in both clinical and industrial settings. Finally, the chapter addresses critical challenges including selectivity, stability, humidity interference, and scalability, and considers future prospects where nanotechnology-driven gas sensors will form part of intelligent sensor networks for personalized healthcare, and next-generation industrial automation (Figure 7.1).

7.2 PRINCIPLES OF GAS SENSING USING NANOMATERIALS

Gas sensing plays a critical role in human health, protecting the environment, and ensuring industrial and domestic safety. From detecting toxic gases such as carbon monoxide and nitrogen dioxide in urban air, to monitoring VOCs in food storage facilities, to diagnosing diseases through exhaled breath analysis, the need for accurate, sensitive, and selective gas sensors has been growing exponentially. The emergence of nanomaterials has transformed this field by enabling sensors that are smaller, faster, and efficient. Owing to their exceptionally high surface-to-volume ratio, tunable band structures, and ability to be functionalized with chemical receptors, nanomaterials amplify interactions between gas molecules and sensing elements, thus allowing for detection at concentrations down to ppb or even parts-per-trillion (ppt) range. This section outlines the fundamental working mechanisms of gas sensors, highlights the unique advantages conferred by nanomaterials, and introduces the major classes of nanomaterials that underpin the next generation of gas sensing devices.

7.2.1 Basic Working Mechanism of Gas Sensors

Each gas sensor is based on the interaction between gas molecules and a surface of a sensitive material. When molecules adsorb onto this surface, they can alter key properties such as electrical conductivity, thermal conductivity, optical absorption, or mass (Figure 7.2). These changes are then transduced into measurable output signals. In nanomaterial-based sensors, the exceptionally high surface-to-volume ratio ensures that even trace amounts of gas can cause significant shifts in sensor response. Moreover, the tunability of nanomaterials through doping, functionalization, and structural design allows tailoring for specific gases.

7.2.1.1 Chemiresistive Sensing

Chemiresistive sensors are among the most widely studied and commercially viable gas sensors. Their operation relies on resistance changes in semiconducting materials upon interaction with gas molecules. Metal oxide semiconductors such as SnO_2,

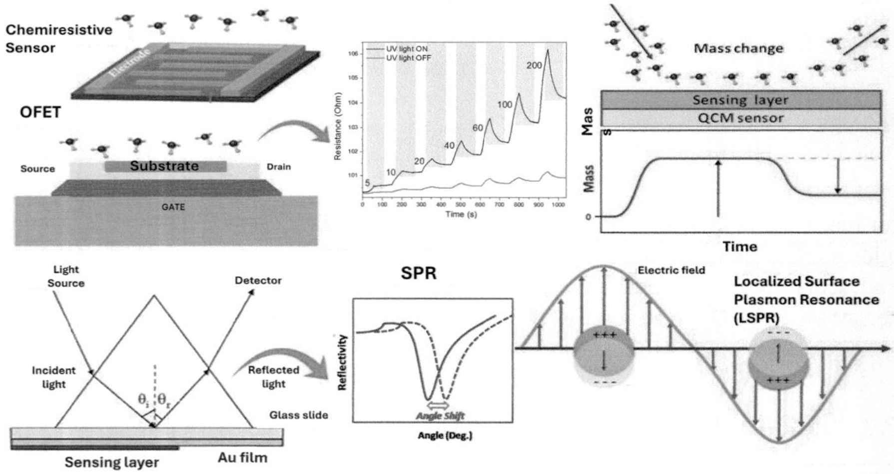

FIGURE 7.2 Schematic illustration of major gas sensing mechanisms: chemoresistive sensing based on resistance modulation upon gas adsorption, chronoamperometric detection via time-dependent current response under applied potential, quartz crystal microbalance (QCM) piezoelectric sensing through mass-induced frequency shifts, and surface plasmon resonance (SPR) sensing based on refractive index variations at the metal-dielectric interface.

ZnO, WO_3, and TiO_2 are classic examples. In air, oxygen molecules adsorb on their surfaces, capturing electrons from the conduction band and forming an electron depletion layer. When exposed to reducing gases such as CO, H_2, or NH_3, the reaction with adsorbed oxygen releases electrons back to the conduction band, decreasing resistance. Conversely, oxidizing gases like NO_2 or O_2 further withdraw electrons, increasing resistance. The sensitivity of these devices can be drastically improved using nanostructures. SnO_2 nanowires have been shown to detect CO concentrations as low as 5 ppm with sub-second response times. Similarly, ZnO nanorods synthesized by hydrothermal methods have demonstrated excellent ethanol sensitivity, making them ideal for applications such as alcohol breath analyzers and fermentation monitoring in food industries. Doping provides another dimension of enhancement. For example, Pd-doped SnO_2 nanofibers exhibit superior selectivity for hydrogen detection due to the catalytic dissociation of H_2 on Pd sites. In environmental applications, In_2O_3 nanoparticles have been used to detect NO_2 in polluted urban air, offering detection down to 10 ppb. These examples underscore how structural engineering and chemical modification of nanomaterials significantly refine chemiresistive performance. In addition to metal oxides, conductive polymers [1,2], as well as polyaromatic molecules, such as metal porphyrins (MPor) and phthalocyanines (MPc) [3,4], whose films can behave like p- and n-semiconductors, are also widely used as active layers of chemiresistive gas sensors. Their surface is also modified with metal or metal oxide nanoparticles to increase sensitivity and selectivity. For example, the modification of cobalt phthalocyanine (CoPc) surface with Au nanoparticles has allowed the development of sensors for ammonia and nitric oxide with limits of detection (LODs) of 0.1 ppm and 4 ppb, respectively [5].

7.2.1.2 Field-Effect Transistor Sensors

FET-based gas sensors represent another class of highly sensitive devices, often employing 1D (carbon nanotubes [CNTs], nanowires) or two-dimensional (graphene, MoS_2, WS_2) semiconductors as the channel material. Gas adsorption alters the local charge distribution, shifting the threshold voltage or modulating channel conductance. Because the active channel can be only a few atoms thick, even a single adsorbed gas molecule can cause measurable electrical perturbations. Graphene-based FET sensors have detected NO_2 at concentrations below 100 ppb at room temperature, owing to graphene's extraordinary carrier mobility. MoS_2 nanosheet FETs have shown sensitivity toward NH_3 and SO_2, both of which are relevant for monitoring industrial emissions and indoor air quality. In medical contexts, single-walled carbon nanotube (SWCNT)-based FETs have been engineered to detect acetone in exhaled breath at sub-ppm levels, which is of clinical relevance for noninvasive diabetes monitoring. Their operation at room temperature and ultralow power requirements make FET sensors particularly suitable for portable and wearable diagnostic devices.

7.2.1.3 Optical Sensors

Optical gas sensors exploit changes in absorption, refractive index, fluorescence, or scattering that occur upon gas–material interactions. Surface plasmon resonance (SPR) sensors are widely used for gas detection [6,7]. SPR occurs when light excites electron density waves (plasmons) at a metal surface—typically nanostructured gold or silver—under total internal reflection. This causes a sharp drop in reflected light intensity. The resonance angle depends on the refractive index (n) of the material near the metal surface. Even tiny changes in n alter the SPR signal, allowing sensitive detection of surface-bound substances by monitoring reflected light. Due to their strong localized surface plasmon resonances (LSPRs), metal nanoparticles coated with gas-selective receptors (e.g., polymers, metal oxides, or ligands) that selectively adsorb or react with target gases (e.g., H_2, CO, NO_x, NH_3, VOCs) are also utilized for the creation of sensitive gas sensors. Gas adsorption alters the dielectric environment of these nanostructures, causing measurable spectral shifts. For example, gold nanoparticles (AuNPs) functionalized with thiol groups have been used to detect H_2S, where exposure to the gas induces nanoparticle aggregation and a visible red-to-blue color change. Carbon quantum dots have been employed as fluorescent probes for ammonia detection, with NH_3 quenching their emission intensity. A striking example of optical sensing is the detection of explosive vapors: surface-enhanced Raman scattering (SERS) substrates made of silver nanostructures can identify trace levels of trinitrotoluene (TNT) vapor, providing a molecular fingerprint with unparalleled sensitivity. In the food sector, fluorescent graphene quantum dots have been reported for monitoring ethylene emissions from ripening fruit, offering a noninvasive tool for postharvest quality control.

7.2.1.4 Piezoelectric Sensors

Piezoelectric sensors, particularly quartz crystal microbalance (QCM) devices, detect gases by monitoring shifts in resonance frequency caused by molecular adsorption on a coated crystal surface. Nanostructured coatings amplify the response by providing higher adsorption capacities. For example, ZnO nanorod–coated QCM sensors have been shown to detect acetone vapors at clinically relevant concentrations for diabetes diagnostics. Similarly, polymer-nanoclay composites deposited on QCM substrates enabled formaldehyde detection at sub-ppm levels, making them suitable for indoor air quality monitoring. Other innovations include graphene oxide (GO)-coated surface acoustic wave (SAW) devices, which have demonstrated remarkable sensitivity toward VOCs like benzene and toluene.

7.2.1.5 Thermal Conductivity Sensors

Although less common, thermal conductivity sensors also benefit from nanomaterials. These devices measure changes in the rate of heat dissipation caused by gas adsorption. Nanoporous materials such as mesoporous silica and metal–organic frameworks (MOFs) have been employed to enhance selectivity by selectively adsorbing certain gases. For instance, MOF-coated thermal sensors have been used to distinguish between CH_4 and CO_2 mixtures in environmental monitoring.

7.3 TYPES OF NANOMATERIALS USED IN GAS SENSING

A wide variety of nanomaterials (Figure 7.3) have been investigated for gas sensing applications, each offering unique advantages depending on the target gas, operating temperature, and deployment environment.

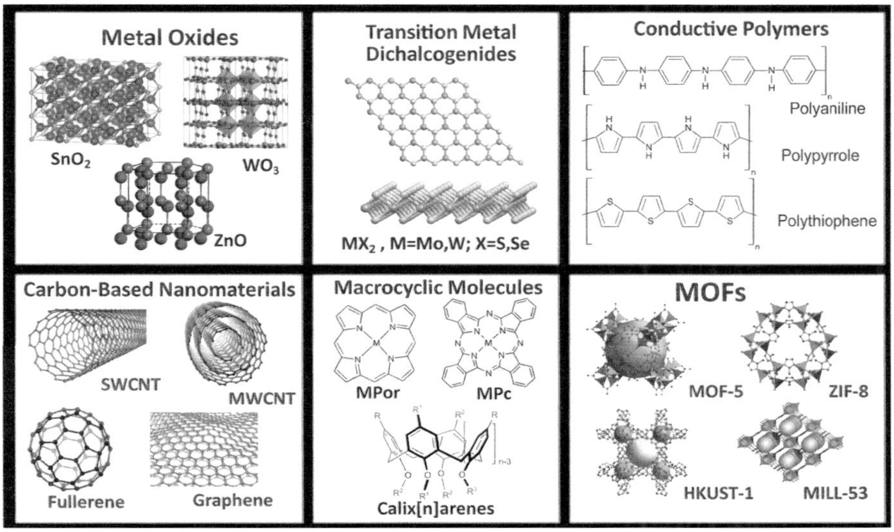

FIGURE 7.3 Representative classes of widely used gas-sensing materials, including metal oxides (e.g., SnO_2, WO_3, ZnO), transition metal dichalcogenides (MX_2; M = Mo, W; X = S, Se), conductive polymers (polyaniline, polypyrrole, polythiophene), carbon-based nanomaterials (SWCNTs, multi-walled carbon nanotubes [MWCNTs], fullerene, graphene), macrocyclic molecules (metalloporphyrins, metallophthalocyanines, calix[n]arenes), and metal–organic frameworks (MOF-5, ZIF-8, HKUST-1, MIL-53).

7.3.1 Metal Oxide Nanostructures

Metal oxide semiconductors remain the backbone of gas sensing technology due to their robustness, affordability, and strong surface reactivity with many gases. When engineered into nanostructures such as nanoparticles, nanorods, nanofibers, hollow spheres, or hierarchical 3D frameworks, their high surface area significantly enhances adsorption and catalytic activity. ZnO nanorods have been successfully employed in ethanol sensing for portable breath analyzers, detecting concentrations as low as 10 ppm, relevant for law enforcement in drunk-driving checks. SnO_2 nanofibers fabricated via electrospinning have demonstrated superior performance in detecting CO and CH_4, both of which are critical in mine safety, where early detection can prevent lethal explosions. Similarly, TiO_2 nanotubes decorated with platinum nanoparticles have been optimized for hydrogen sensing, offering rapid response and recovery times essential for monitoring leakage in hydrogen fuel cells. Other notable examples include WO_3 nanostructures for NO_x detection in urban air pollution monitoring and In_2O_3 nanoparticles for ozone sensing, highlighting the versatility of metal oxides across different gases. Their main drawback, however, is often the need for elevated operating temperatures (>200°C), though strategies like noble metal doping and UV activation have enabled lower-temperature operation.

7.3.2 Transition Metal Dichalcogenides

Two-dimensional transition metal dichalcogenides (TMD) such as MoS_2, WS_2, and WSe_2 are an emerging class of nanomaterials for gas sensing. Their atomically thin structures ensure maximum exposure of surface atoms, while their tunable bandgaps and semiconducting behavior allow integration into FET sensors. MoS_2 nanosheets have demonstrated high selectivity for NH_3 at room temperature, making them attractive for medical breath analysis and industrial emission control. WS_2 thin films have shown strong sensitivity toward NO_2, relevant for air quality monitoring in polluted cities. Furthermore, flexible and transparent TMD-based sensors have been fabricated on polymer substrates, opening possibilities for wearable electronics capable of continuous personal air monitoring. Functionalization with polymers or nanoparticles further enhances selectivity, for example, Pt-decorated MoS_2 nanosheets have been tailored for H_2 detection in hydrogen economy applications.

7.3.3 Carbon-Based Nanomaterials

Carbon nanostructures such as CNTs, graphene, GO, and reduced GO are attractive for gas sensing due to their high conductivity, large surface area, and ability to function at room temperature. Their sp^2-hybridized frameworks provide strong π–π interactions with gas molecules, while functionalization introduces chemical selectivity. CNT-based chemiresistors have achieved ppb-level NH_3 detection, making them promising platform for medical breath diagnostics for liver or kidney dysfunction patients. GO, rich in oxygen-containing groups, has been used for humidity sensing in grain storage silos, helping prevent fungal contamination. Au-decorated CNTs exhibit selective H_2S sensing for industrial leak detection, while Ag-decorated graphene significantly improves NO_x sensing performance in urban environments. Importantly, carbon-based sensors operate efficiently at room temperature, offering advantages for wearable health monitors and low-power IoT devices.

7.3.4 Conductive Polymers

Conductive organic polymers such as polypyrrole (PPy), polyaniline (PANI), polythiophene, poly(3,4-ethylenedioxythiophene), and polyacetylene have emerged as promising candidates for gas sensor development [2,8]. Their appeal stems from their ability to operate effectively at ambient temperatures and their compatibility with flexible, bendable substrates—making them ideal for next-generation wearable or conformable sensing devices.

Among the various target gases, ammonia stands out as the most extensively investigated analyte using PPy- and PANI-based platforms. A critical factor influencing sensor efficiency is the material's surface architecture, especially when engineered at the nanoscale. For instance, 1D nanostructured conducting polymers, such as nanowires, nanotubes, or nanofibers, offer significantly increased surface-to-volume ratios, which facilitate more efficient gas molecule adsorption and diffusion. This structural advantage translates directly into improved sensing metrics. However, it should be noted that their sensor response is still lower than that of sensors based on semiconductor oxides. One promising approach to improving sensor performance while maintaining room temperature operation is to combine a conducting polymer with another material, such as a metal oxide, metal nanoparticles, carbon, or another polymer [9].

7.3.5 Phthalocyanine, Porphyrins, and Other Polycyclic Molecules

MPor and MPc are particularly well suited for detecting gaseous analytes due to their intense coloration and accessible metal coordination sites, which readily interact with analyte molecules. Moreover, both the benzene rings of the phthalocyanine macrocycle and the axial positions of the molecules can be functionalized with various substituents. These groups can serve as active sites that enhance interactions with analyte molecules, thereby improving the sensor sensitivity and selectivity. Additionally, certain MPor and phthalocyanines display electrochromic properties, undergoing visible color changes during redox processes [10]. Moreover, MPor and MPc are readily processable into uniform thin films using techniques such as physical vapor deposition, spin-coating, Langmuir–Blodgett deposition, or drop-casting.

Numerous studies in the literature have explored metal porphyrin and metal phthalocyanine thin films for use in optical [7,11], chemiresistive, [4] and organic field-effect transistor (OFET) [12] sensors to detect gases such as ammonia, hydrogen sulfide, nitrogen oxides, carbon monoxide, and vapors of VOCs. Notably, NO_2 detection using these films can reach sub-ppm levels, even down to the ppb range [13]. It has been established that incorporating electron-withdrawing substituents enhances sensitivity toward electron-donating gases like ammonia and amines. For instance, fluoro-substituted phthalocyanines can achieve ammonia detection limits as low as 0.01–0.1 ppm [14]. Importantly, such materials can selectively detect ammonia even in the presence of interfering species like CO_2 and VOCs, and under conditions of relatively high relative humidity, highlighting their potential for noninvasive ammonia monitoring in exhaled breath. Moreover, functionalizing porphyrin and phthalocyanine macrocycles with alkyl or aryl groups bearing diverse functional moieties enhances their responsiveness to VOCs [15]. However, the detection limits for VOCs generally remain higher than those achieved for ammonia and nitrogen oxides.

Beyond their use as standalone sensing layers, porphyrins and phthalocyanines are frequently employed as structural building blocks in covalent organic frameworks (COFs) [16]. Incorporation into COFs can further improve their porosity, stability, and analyte accessibility, thereby expanding their utility and performance in advanced gas sensing applications.

Calixarenes are macrocyclic compounds featuring a well-defined central cavity, readily synthesized through a variety of established chemical methodologies. This intrinsic cavity enables them to reversibly form host–guest complexes with a range of inorganic gases and organic vapors. Their structural versatility allows for precise control over ring size and facile functionalization with diverse chemical groups, making them ideal candidates for tailored molecular recognition. This tenability combined with high thermal and chemical stability permits fine adjustment of cavity dimensions, binding affinity, and selectivity. Their porous architecture facilitates rapid analyte diffusion, enhancing response kinetics in sensing applications. In this chapter, we highlight the integration of calixarene-based receptors into a range of transduction platforms, including SPR, SAW, QCM, and fiber-optic sensing systems [17]. The synergy between the robust, selective recognition properties of calixarenes and these sensitive detection modalities has enabled the development of reliable, high-performance sensors for the detection and monitoring of hazardous gases and VOCs.

7.3.6 Metal–Organic Frameworks

MOFs, featuring structural diversity, large specific surface area, controllable pore size/geometry, and host–guest interactions, hold great promises for fabricating various MOF-based devices for diverse applications including gas sensing [18]. Tremendous progress has been made in the past decade on the fabrication of MOF-based sensors with elevated sensitivity and selectivity toward various analytes due to their preconcentrating and molecule-sieving effects. MOFs enable versatile and sensitive gas detection on multiple platforms, including chemiluminescence, gravimetry, electrochemistry, photoluminescence, and SERS. While there are still challenges to overcome, such as stability, selectivity, and low-concentration gas detection, MOF-based sensors have strong potential for environmental monitoring and medical diagnostics.

MOF-based sensors are widely tested for the detection of VOCs. A chemiluminescent sensor based on MOF-5 has been developed to detect isobutanol with a LOD of 3.7 mg/L [19]. Later, core–shell CeO_2@ZIF-8 nanoparticles improved the response speed by 5× and the recovery by 3× for propanal, but thermal instability remains a challenge. Despite this, the potential of cataluminescence (CTL)-MOFs is high [20].

MOFs such as HKUST-1, ZIF-8, and MOF-5 allow for sensitive VOC detection through mass changes [21]. Electrosprayed HKUST-1 films achieve LODs of 10–50 ppm, and HKUST-1 shows high selectivity for benzene homologues (e.g., *p*-xylene at 400 ppb) through Cu^{2+} interactions. ZIF-69 microresonators boost the sensitivity by 150× for isopropanol and CO_2 [22]. Despite the poor conductivity of MOFs, composites such as MOF/graphene and MOF/CNT/M enable chemiresistive sensing. For example, MIL-53(Cr-Fe)/Ag/CNT detected alcohols at concentrations as low as ~30 ppm [23]. Room temperature sensors such as MOF/graphene for breath biomarker detection are emerging [24]. Capacitive sensors are limited but are growing. For example, Cu-BTC, ZIF-8, and MIL-96(Al) sensors have been used to detect formaldehyde, ethanol, and methanol at room temperature based on dielectric changes. Ln-MOFs with Eu^{3+} and Tb^{3+} offer sharp emissions that allow the creation of photoluminescent sensors for vapor detection of dimethylformamide (DMF), formaldehyde, and biogenic amines [25]. EuMOF-FITC films enable smartphone-based visual monitoring of freshness in fish (LOD: 2.17 mg/L of histamine) [26]. MIL-100(Fe) can act as a SERS substrate without the need for noble metals [27]. The sensor can detect toluene at 2.5 ppm, acetone at 20 ppm, and chloroform at 92.7 ppm and has the potential for lung cancer diagnosis through breath biomarkers.

MOF-based sensors are also utilized for the detection of inorganic gases. ZIF-8 enabled room-temperature I_2 sensing via impedance spectroscopy but showed irreversible responses [28]. Later, MFM-300(X) (X = Al, Fe, In, Sc) offered improved reversibility—MFM-300(Fe) and (Sc) maintained performance over cycles, demonstrating that MOF metal centers can be tuned for reversible, sensitive

I_2 detection [29]. Cu-containing nanoscale coordination particles (LOD: 2 ppm) [30], $Zr(TBAPy)_5(TCPP)$ (LOD: 30 ppb) [31], and MIL-100(In)@Eu^3/Cu^{2+} film were shown to demonstrate the response to H_2S. QCM sensors based on fluorinated MOFs (KAUST-7/8) and luminescent sensors based on amino-functionalized MOF-5-NH_2 (LOD: 0.05 ppm) were used for sulfur dioxide (SO_2) determination [32]. Nitrogen oxides (NO_2/NO) were detected using a colorimetric sensor prepared using calixarene-based Zr-MOF, [33] while a PDVT-10/porphyrin-MOF heterojunction OFET sensor achieved ultrahigh NO_2 sensitivity (LOD: 8.25 ppb) [34].

7.3.7 Metal Nanoparticles

Noble metal nanoparticles such as gold (Au), silver (Ag), and palladium (Pd) are widely incorporated into gas sensors as catalytic or plasmonic enhancers. They accelerate surface reactions, reduce activation energy, and amplify signal transduction. Palladium nanoparticles are especially valuable for hydrogen sensing, as Pd readily absorbs H_2, forming PdH_x and inducing large changes in electrical resistance. For example, the modification of the surface of CoPc with Pd and $Pd_{0.8}Au_{0.2}$ nanoparticles has been shown to lead to a more than 10-fold increase in the sensitivity of the heterostructures toward hydrogen [35]. This principle underlies several commercial hydrogen leak detectors used in automotive and aerospace applications.

Silver nanoparticles embedded in polymer films have been employed for colorimetric sensing of ammonia, where visible color shifts allow detection without instrumentation. AuNPs supported on TiO_2 or ZnO improve VOC sensing via LSPR, enabling sensitive optical detection of acetone, formaldehyde, and toluene. These examples demonstrate how metal nanoparticles, while often used in small amounts, play critical roles in boosting sensitivity and enabling rapid, selective detection.

7.3.8 Hybrid Nanocomposites

Combining nanomaterials often yields synergistic effects, overcoming the limitations of individual components. Hybrids can exploit the catalytic activity of metals, the conductivity of carbon nanostructures, and the high surface area of metal oxides or porous frameworks. SnO_2-graphene hybrids combine the high sensitivity of SnO_2 with the superior electron transport of graphene, enabling ultralow detection limits for CO and NO_x. CNT-polymer composites enhance selectivity by leveraging specific polymer–gas interactions, useful for distinguishing VOCs in indoor environments. CNTs can be effectively functionalized with phthalocyanines through both covalent and non-covalent strategies. The resulting CNT-phthalocyanine hybrid materials combine the high surface area, excellent conductivity, and mechanical strength of CNTs with the selective gas-binding capabilities and redox activity of phthalocyanines. These synergistic properties make the hybrids particularly well suited for gas sensing applications. Indeed, they have demonstrated high sensitivity and selectivity toward a range of hazardous or environmentally relevant gases, including ammonia (NH_3), nitrogen dioxide (NO_2), hydrogen sulfide (H_2S), and chlorine (Cl_2) [36]. Such sensors are promising for use in environmental monitoring, industrial safety, and medical diagnostics, where reliable and real-time detection of trace gases is critical.

MOF with nanoparticle hybrids is particularly exciting, as MOFs provide tailored porosity and selective adsorption channels, while nanoparticles provide rapid signal transduction. A striking case is the detection of formaldehyde at sub-ppm levels using ZnO/MOF hybrid nanocomposites, where the MOF pores concentrate the gas for the ZnO to sense. More recently, Cu_3N-Fe nanocomposites have shown promising catalytic activity for electrochemical sensing of H_2O_2 released from cancer cells. Although still under exploration, such multifunctional hybrids are now being extended to volatile gases, demonstrating how sensor development is moving toward integrated platforms capable of detecting both environmental pollutants and biological markers.

7.4 NANOMATERIALS FOR DETECTION OF TOXIC GASES AS ENVIRONMENTAL MONITORING

The monitoring of toxic gases in the environment is a matter of urgent importance for public health, occupational safety, and ecological balance. Rapid urbanization and industrialization have significantly increased emissions of harmful gases, many of which are colorless and odorless, making them imperceptible without technological intervention. Chronic exposure to low concentrations of such gases can have serious health consequences, while acute exposure to high levels may be life-threatening. Nanomaterial-based sensors offer new opportunities to detect these gases at trace levels, enabling early warning systems and preventive measures. Several toxic gases are of particular concern due to their prevalence, toxicity, and environmental impact. Carbon monoxide (CO), produced by incomplete combustion of fossil fuels in vehicles, stoves, and furnaces, binds strongly to hemoglobin with an affinity 200 times greater than oxygen, leading to hypoxia and life-threatening poisoning; even low levels of 10–50 ppm cause headaches and dizziness, while higher concentrations are often fatal. Nitrogen oxides (NO_x), primarily generated from vehicle exhausts and power plants, are key contributors to photochemical smog and acid rain; exposure to NO_2 above 200 ppb induces lung inflammation and worsens chronic respiratory conditions such as asthma and COPD. Sulfur dioxide (SO_2), released during the burning of coal, oil, and other sulfur-rich fuels, irritates the respiratory system and is a well-known asthma trigger; in the environment, it oxidizes to form sulfuric acid, a major cause of acid rain. Ammonia (NH_3), while essential in fertilizer production and widely used in agriculture, poses occupational hazards in enclosed environments, where chronic inhalation leads to eye damage and respiratory illness among agricultural and industrial workers. VOCs such as benzene, toluene, and formaldehyde are prevalent in indoor environments and industrial effluents; benzene is a well-documented carcinogen. Hydrogen sulfide (H_2S), with its characteristic "rotten egg" odor at trace levels, is deceptively dangerous since olfactory fatigue occurs quickly, leaving workers unaware of exposure; at higher concentrations it inhibits cytochrome oxidase, halting cellular respiration and leading to rapid collapse or death, a risk particularly acute in petroleum refineries, wastewater plants, and geothermal fields. Collectively, these toxic gases underscore the urgent need for reliable nanomaterial-based sensors capable of ultrasensitive, selective, and real-time detection to safeguard human health and mitigate environmental hazards.

7.4.1 Metal Oxide Nanomaterials for Toxic Gas Detection

Semiconducting metal oxides have long been the backbone of commercial gas sensors due to their robustness, tunable surface chemistry, and strong responses to a wide variety of gases. Nanoscale engineering significantly amplifies these properties by increasing surface area and exposing active crystal facets. ZnO nanowires represent one of the most studied nanostructures for CO and NO_x sensing. Their 1D morphology provides direct electron transport pathways, minimizing grain boundary effects and enhancing response speed. For instance, vertically aligned ZnO nanowire arrays grown on substrates have been used to detect NO_x at sub-ppm levels with response times of only a few seconds. Doping with elements like Al or Ga further enhances sensitivity by increasing carrier concentration. SnO_2 nanoparticles are widely used in commercial CO sensors, including those installed in household alarms. Their catalytic surface facilitates reactions between CO molecules and adsorbed oxygen ions, releasing electrons back into the conduction band and decreasing resistance. In research contexts, Pt- or Pd-decorated SnO_2 nanofibers have demonstrated detection of hydrogen down to 10 ppm at reduced operating temperatures, highlighting the role of catalytic nanoparticles in boosting performance. TiO_2 nanotubes and nanorods offer unique advantages for photocatalytic sensing. When illuminated with UV light, TiO_2 generates electron–hole pairs that interact strongly with adsorbed gases, producing a photo-enhanced sensing effect. This photocatalytic self-cleaning property ensures long-term sensor stability by preventing fouling from surface contaminants. For example, TiO_2 nanotube sensors have shown effective detection of formaldehyde and acetone vapors, relevant for indoor air quality monitoring. Metal oxide sensors, while powerful, traditionally require elevated operating temperatures (200°C–400°C), which increases energy consumption. However, nanostructuring and noble-metal doping are gradually pushing these sensors toward room-temperature operation, making them more compatible with portable and wearable systems.

7.4.2 Carbon-Based Nanomaterials

Carbon-based nanomaterials, including CNTs, graphene, and their derivatives, have emerged as attractive alternatives to traditional oxides due to their ability to function at room temperature with high sensitivity. Their π-conjugated structures provide excellent electrical conductivity, and their surfaces are highly responsive to charge transfer from adsorbed gas molecules. Graphene sensors exploit the fact that every atom is exposed to its two-dimensional surface. When gases like NO_2 adsorb on graphene, they act as electron acceptors, reducing carrier density and sharply increasing resistance. Reports have shown that graphene sensors can detect NO_2 at concentrations as low as 50 ppb. To improve selectivity, amine-modified GO selectively detects CO_2 by forming reversible carbamate bonds.

CNT networks also demonstrate strong gas sensitivity, with performance influenced by chirality, diameter, and functionalization. A classic example is the detection of NH_3 using single-walled CNTs, where NH_3 acts as an electron donor, reducing hole concentration in p-type CNTs and thereby increasing resistance. CNT-based sensors have been integrated into flexible substrates, leading to wearable environmental monitors capable of tracking workplace exposure to toxic gases in real time. Hybridization with polymers enhances both stability and selectivity. PANI-coated CNTs, for instance, show remarkable sensitivity to NH_3 at room temperature, owing to synergistic interactions between the polymer and the gas. Such composites are increasingly being explored for low-power, portable sensing devices. Sensors based on phthalocyanines and their hybrids with carbon nanomaterials are increasingly deployed in urban air quality networks, industrial emission control systems, and early-warning devices for hazardous gas leaks. CNTs modified with metallophthalocyanines exhibit strong interactions with Cl_2, enabling detection at ppb levels [37]. Certain hybrids show reversible and selective responses to NH_3, useful for monitoring indoor air quality and livestock environments [38].

7.4.3 Hybrid Nanocomposites

While single-component nanomaterials exhibit excellent sensing properties, hybrid systems often outperform them by combining complementary functionalities. Metal oxides provide strong chemical reactivity but poor conductivity, whereas graphene or CNTs offer excellent conductivity but limited intrinsic selectivity. Together, they form synergistic composites with superior performance. A striking example is the development of Pd-decorated SnO_2/graphene sensors for hydrogen detection. In this system, Pd nanoparticles dissociate H_2 molecules into atomic hydrogen, which then spills over onto the SnO_2 surface, enhancing electron transfer. Meanwhile, graphene provides a conductive network that accelerates charge transport, enabling detection at room temperature with fast response and recovery times. Similarly, ZnO-graphene composites have demonstrated high sensitivity toward NO_x, leveraging ZnO's strong adsorption capacity and graphene's electrical conductivity. Other hybrids include AuNPs–decorated TiO_2 nanotubes, which combine plasmonic enhancement with photocatalytic activity for VOC detection. Another exciting class is MOFs integrated with nanoparticles, which allow highly selective gas adsorption through their tunable porous structures. MOF-CNT hybrids, for example, have been used to detect benzene and toluene at trace concentrations, opening doors for advanced VOC monitoring in indoor and industrial environments.

7.5 APPLICATIONS IN MEDICAL DIAGNOSTICS AND EARLY DISEASE DETECTION

The use of gas sensing technologies in medicine is rapidly transforming how diseases are identified and monitored. Human breath, long regarded as a simple physiological function, is now recognized as a rich and noninvasive diagnostic medium. It contains lots of VOCs, as well as inorganic gases such as nitric oxide, ammonia, and carbon monoxide, each reflecting underlying metabolic and pathological processes (Figure 7.4). Importantly, changes in breath chemistry often occur earlier than clinical symptoms, making breath analysis a promising approach for early disease detection.

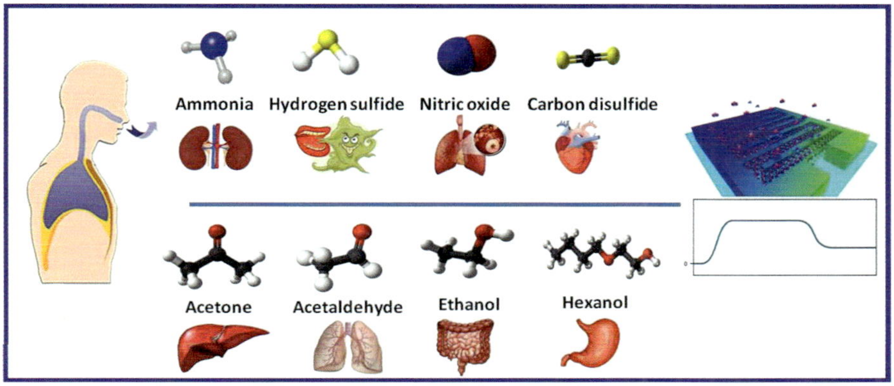

FIGURE 7.4 Various gas sensors for breadth analysis targeting different gases as biomedical disease markers.

7.5.1 Breath Analysis for Disease Diagnosis

Breath analysis is one of the most mature fields where nanomaterial-based gas sensing has demonstrated remarkable progress. Traditional diagnostic techniques like blood assays or imaging, while reliable, are invasive, expensive, and unsuitable for continuous monitoring. In contrast, nanomaterial-based gas sensors enable real-time, low-cost, and highly sensitive detection of disease biomarkers at concentrations as low as ppb. Such capabilities have opened the door to applications in chronic disease monitoring, cancer screening, infection detection, and wearable healthcare devices.

7.5.1.1 Diabetes Monitoring

Acetone is a well-established biomarker for diabetes. In healthy individuals, breath acetone levels are typically below 0.9 ppm, but in diabetic patients, especially during ketoacidosis, levels can exceed 1.8 ppm. Detecting acetone therefore provides a noninvasive alternative to frequent blood glucose monitoring. Metal oxide nanostructures have been widely explored for this application. ZnO nanowire sensors have shown sub-ppm acetone detection, with rapid response times suitable for real-time monitoring. Similarly, SnO_2 nanofibers decorated with Pd nanoparticles have achieved acetone detection down to 0.2 ppm, offering both sensitivity and selectivity in the presence of interfering VOCs. In one notable study, a nanostructured WO_3 sensor demonstrated the ability to distinguish between healthy individuals and diabetic patients by selectively responding to exhaled acetone, laying the foundation for noninvasive diabetes breathalyzers.

7.5.1.2 Lung Cancer Screening

Lung cancer is often diagnosed late due to the absence of clear early symptoms. Breath biomarkers such as benzene, toluene, formaldehyde, and ethylbenzene have been linked to lung cancer metabolism. Nanomaterial-based "electronic nose" (e-nose) systems have shown promise in detecting these signatures. In a recent study, arrays of gold nanoparticles functionalized with organic ligands were able to differentiate breath samples from lung cancer patients and healthy controls with high accuracy. In another study, GO-SnO_2 composites demonstrated selective sensing of formaldehyde at ppb levels, a compound elevated in lung cancer breath profiles. Clinical trials have tested multi-sensor e-nose platforms using nanomaterials, with encouraging results in distinguishing early-stage cancer patients from smokers and nonsmokers.

7.5.1.3 Asthma and Chronic Obstructive Pulmonary Disease

Exhaled nitric oxide (NO) is an accepted biomarker for airway inflammation, making it valuable for monitoring asthma and COPD. Patients with asthma often show elevated NO levels, sometimes exceeding 50 ppb compared to under 20 ppb in healthy individuals. Nanomaterial-based biosensors are pushing the boundaries of NO detection. Graphene-gold nanoparticle hybrids have achieved sub-ppb detection of NO, offering high precision for monitoring disease progression. MOF-based sensors have also been reported to capture and detect trace NO molecules with remarkable selectivity. In practice, such sensors could enable asthma patients to self-monitor airway inflammation at home, reducing reliance on hospital-based spirometry.

7.5.1.4 Other Metabolic Disorders

Beyond these major diseases, breath sensors have also been tested for renal failure, where elevated ammonia in breath reflects impaired urea metabolism. CNT-based sensors functionalized with PANI have been developed to selectively detect ammonia at ppb levels, showing potential for kidney disease monitoring. Similarly, TiO_2 nanotube sensors have been explored for acetone and isoprene detection, which are associated with oxidative stress and lipid metabolism disorders.

7.5.2 Infection Detection

Infectious diseases also alter the chemical composition of exhaled breath, providing diagnostic opportunities. *Helicobacter pylori*, a bacterium linked to gastric ulcers and cancer, produces urease that converts urea to ammonia. Elevated breath ammonia has therefore been used as a diagnostic marker. Traditional urea breath tests rely on isotope labeling, but nanomaterial-based ammonia sensors now provide a simpler alternative. For instance, CNT networks coated with PANI detected ammonia levels correlating with *H. pylori* infection, enabling rapid, noninvasive diagnosis. Respiratory infections such as tuberculosis (TB) produce characteristic VOCs, including methyl nicotinate and cyclohexane. Gold nanoparticle arrays in e-nose platforms have successfully distinguished TB patients' breath from healthy individuals' with diagnostic accuracy exceeding 80%. Similarly, ZnO nanowire sensors have been applied to detect volatile metabolites from *Pseudomonas aeruginosa*, a common cause of lung infections in cystic fibrosis patients. Sepsis is associated with increased breath concentrations of nitric oxide and certain VOCs. Experimental studies using GO sensors have demonstrated potential for early detection of such infection-related gases, which could be critical for timely intervention in intensive care settings.

7.5.3 Integration with Wearable Electronics

One of the most exciting frontiers is the integration of nanomaterial-based gas sensors into wearable electronics for continuous health monitoring. Advances in flexible substrates, low-power operation, and wireless connectivity have enabled sensors that can be embedded into masks, skin patches, or textiles. For example, CNT-based flexible gas sensors integrated into face masks have been used to continuously monitor exhaled acetone and NO, offering real-time data for diabetic and asthmatic patients. Another demonstration involved graphene sensors printed onto flexible substrates, which could be incorporated into patches worn on the skin near the nose or mouth to analyze breath VOCs in ambulatory patients. Wearable devices can also combine multiple sensing modalities. A prototype integrated a graphene-based NO sensor with temperature and humidity sensors into a single platform, enabling comprehensive monitoring of both environmental exposures and breath biomarkers. Such devices are envisioned as part of future telemedicine frameworks, where patients can transmit real-time health data to healthcare providers for early intervention.

7.6 CHALLENGES IN DEVELOPING EFFICIENT GAS SENSORS

Despite the rapid progress and promising results achieved by nanomaterial-based gas sensors, several fundamental challenges remain before these technologies can achieve widespread deployment in real-world applications. Among the foremost issues is selectivity. Many gases, particularly VOCs and inorganic pollutants, produce overlapping responses on similar sensing materials, making it difficult to distinguish one target analyte in the presence of others. For example, both ethanol and acetone can induce comparable resistance changes in ZnO nanowire sensors, complicating the reliable detection of diabetes-related acetone in the presence of alcohol vapors. Strategies such as surface functionalization, catalytic nanoparticle decoration, and sensor arrays functioning as "electronic noses" have been explored to improve selectivity, but achieving consistent, real-time discrimination of gases in complex ambient mixtures continues to be a major hurdle. Operating temperature presents another limitation. Many widely used semiconducting metal oxide sensors, such as SnO_2 or TiO_2, exhibit their highest sensitivity only at elevated temperatures above 200°C. This requirement not only increases power consumption but also restricts portability, as additional heating elements are necessary for operation. Such constraints are problematic for wearable or battery-powered devices intended for healthcare or environmental monitoring. Considerable research has gone into lowering the activation energy for surface reactions, for example by doping SnO_2 with palladium or platinum nanoparticles to enable hydrogen detection at near-room temperature. Two-dimensional materials such as graphene and MoS_2 also offer the advantage of room-temperature operation, but their large-scale stability and reproducibility remain under investigation. Long-term stability and repeatability of sensor performance represent further challenges. Nanomaterial surfaces, while highly reactive and sensitive, are also prone to degradation, poisoning, or irreversible surface reactions. Sulfur compounds such as H_2S can irreversibly bind to catalytic sites on Pd-decorated sensors, rendering them inactive after repeated exposure. Similarly, environmental pollutants or dust can make strong interference on sensor surfaces, reducing their effective lifetime. Self-cleaning photocatalytic materials such as TiO_2 nanotubes offer partial solutions, but ensuring consistent operation over months or years is still difficult, particularly for industrial and environmental sensors deployed in harsh conditions.

Another complication arises from the influence of humidity. Water vapor is the most common interference in real-world environments, and its adsorption can drastically interfere with sensing signals by competing with target gases for active sites. This is particularly problematic in medical breath analysis, where exhaled breath is almost fully saturated with water vapor. Therefore, the detection of ammonia or acetone in breath using metal oxide sensors often requires complex compensation algorithms or preconditioning of samples to remove humidity interference. While hydrophobic coatings, humidity filters, and sensor array approaches have been tested, none provides a fully reliable solution under varying atmospheric conditions.

Conductive polymer and phthalocyanine-based sensors have seen significant development over the past decade. Unlike metal oxide sensors, they function efficiently without external heating, enabling low-power and portable devices. Apart from this, they can be easily deposited as thin films on flexible or unconventional substrates using low-cost techniques like spin-coating or inkjet printing. By combining the strengths of these two material families, researchers create versatile, inexpensive, and highly sensitive sensing platforms that are finding increasing use in real-world applications. These sensors are poised to play a crucial role in the next generation of smart, interconnected environmental and health monitoring systems.

Taken together, these challenges highlight that while nanomaterial-based gas sensors provide unprecedented sensitivity and the promise of portable, real-time detection, major hurdles in selectivity, operating conditions, stability, humidity tolerance, and manufacturing scalability must be addressed to enable widespread adoption. Future progress will depend not only on continued innovation in nanomaterials but also on interdisciplinary integration with sensor design, electronics, and data analytics to build robust, reliable, and commercially viable gas sensing platforms.

REFERENCES

1. Y. Wang, A. Liu, Y. Han, T. Li, Sensors based on conductive polymers and their composites: a review, *Polymer International*, 69(2020) 7–17.
2. Y. Yan, G. Yang, J.-L. Xu, M. Zhang, C.-C. Kuo, S.-D. Wang, Conducting polymer-inorganic nanocomposite-based gas sensors: a review, *Science and Technology of Advanced Materials*, 21(2020) 768–86.
3. D. Klyamer, R. Shutilov, T. Basova, Recent advances in phthalocyanine and porphyrin-based materials as active layers for nitric oxide chemical sensors, *Sensors*, 22(2022) 895.
4. D. Klyamer, D. Bonegardt, T. Basova, Fluoro-substituted metal phthalocyanines for active layers of chemical sensors, *Chemosensors*, 9(2021) 133.
5. S.I. Dorovskikh, D.D. Klyamer, E.A. Maksimovskiy, V.V. Volchek, S.M. Zharkov, N.B. Morozova, et al., Heterostructures based on cobalt phthalocyanine films decorated with gold nanoparticles for the detection of low concentrations of ammonia and nitric oxide, *Biosensors*, 12(2022) 476.

6. S. Ahamed, K.K. Venkatesan, S.A. Jalaludeen, A review on various surface plasmon resonance-based sensors, *Plasmonics*, (2025) 1–17.
7. T. Basova, Phthalocyanine and porphyrin derivatives and their hybrid materials in optical sensors based on the phenomenon of surface plasmon resonance, *Chemosensors*, 12(2024) 56.
8. Y.C. Wong, B.C. Ang, A. Haseeb, A.A. Baharuddin, Y.H. Wong, Conducting polymers as chemiresistive gas sensing materials: a review, *Journal of the Electrochemical Society*, 167(2020) 037503.
9. G. Zamiri, A. Haseeb, Recent trends and developments in graphene/conducting polymer nanocomposites chemiresistive sensors, *Materials*, 13(2020) 3311.
10. T. Wang, W. Zhang, T. Li, Q. Xia, S. Yang, J. Weng, et al., Electrochromic smart window based on transition-metal phthalocyanine derivatives, *Inorganic Chemistry*, 63(2024) 3181–90.
11. E.V. Ermakova, A. Bessmertnykh-Lemeune, The optical sensing of volatile organic compounds using porphyrins, *Chemosensors*, 12(2024) 253.
12. S. Demir, S. Akbay, B. Canımkurbey, F. Yuksel, Novel copper (II) phthalocyanines as semiconductor layer in organic field effect transistors: synthesis and investigation of electrical properties, *Journal of Molecular Structure*, 1308(2024) 137981.
13. H. AlQahtani, M. Alshammari, A.M. Kamal, M. Grell, Copper phthalocyanine chemiresistors as industrial NO_2 alarms, *Sensors*, 25(2025) 2955.
14. D. Klyamer, D. Bonegardt, P. Krasnov, A. Sukhikh, P. Popovetskiy, T. Basova, Tetrafluorosubstituted metal phthalocyanines: study of the effect of the position of fluorine substituents on the chemiresistive sensor response to ammonia, *Chemosensors*, 10(2022) 515.
15. X. Duan, Y. Zhang, H. Wang, F. Dai, G. Yang, Y. Chen, A phthalocyanine sensor array based on sensitivity and current changes for highly sensitive identification of three toxic gases at ppb levels, *New Journal of Chemistry*, 44(2020) 13240–8.
16. Y. Chang, M. Chen, Z. Fu, R. Lu, Y. Gao, F. Chen, et al., Building porphyrin-based MOFs on MXenes for ppb-level NO sensing, *Journal of Materials Chemistry A*, 11(2023) 6966–77.
17. F. Davis, S.P. Higson, O.N. Oliveira Jr, F.M. Shimizu, Calixarene-based gas sensors, *Functional Nanomaterials: Advances in Gas Sensing Technologies*, S. Thomas, N. Joshi, V.K. Tomer (eds.), Springer, 2020, pp. 433–62.
18. Y.M. Jo, Y.K. Jo, J.H. Lee, H.W. Jang, I.S. Hwang, D.J. Yoo, MOF-based chemiresistive gas sensors: toward new functionalities, *Advanced Materials*, 35(2023) 2206842.
19. X. Wan, H. Song, D. Zhao, L. Zhang, Y. Lv, A Y-doped metal-organic framework-based cataluminescence gas sensor for isobutanol, *Sensors and Actuators B: Chemical*, 201(2014) 413–9.
20. X. Huang, S. Yan, D. Deng, L. Zhang, R. Liu, Y. Lv, Novel strategy for engineering the metal-oxide@ MOF core@ shell architecture and its applications in cataluminescence sensing, *ACS Applied Materials & Interfaces*, 13(2021) 3471–80.
21. E. Haghighi, S. Zeinali, Nanoporous MIL-101 (Cr) as a sensing layer coated on a quartz crystal microbalance (QCM) nanosensor to detect volatile organic compounds (VOCs), *RSC Advances*, 9(2019) 24460–70.
22. Y. Hwang, H. Sohn, A. Phan, O.M. Yaghi, R.N. Candler, Dielectrophoresis-assembled zeolitic imidazolate framework nanoparticle-coupled resonators for highly sensitive and selective gas detection, *Nano Letters*, 13(2013) 5271–6.
23. M. Ghanbarian, S. Zeinali, A. Mostafavi, A novel MIL-53 (Cr-Fe)/Ag/CNT nanocomposite based resistive sensor for sensing of volatile organic compounds, *Sensors and Actuators B: Chemical*, 267(2018) 381–91.

24. T.T. Tung, M.T. Tran, J.-F. Feller, M. Castro, T. Van Ngo, K. Hassan, et al., Graphene and metal organic frameworks (MOFs) hybridization for tunable chemoresistive sensors for detection of volatile organic compounds (VOCs) biomarkers, *Carbon*, 159(2020) 333–44.
25. H. Che, Y. Li, X. Tian, C. Yang, L. Lu, Y. Nie, A versatile logic detector and fluorescent film based on Eu-based MOF for swift detection of formaldehyde in solutions and gas phase, *Journal of Hazardous Materials*, 410(2021) 124624.
26. J. Wang, D. Li, Y. Ye, Y. Qiu, J. Liu, L. Huang, et al., A fluorescent metal–organic framework for food real-time visual monitoring, *Advanced Materials*, 33(2021) 2008020.
27. J.H. Fu, Z. Zhong, D. Xie, Y.J. Guo, D.X. Kong, Z.X. Zhao, et al., SERS-active MIL-100 (Fe) sensory array for ultrasensitive and multiplex detection of VOCs, *Angewandte Chemie*, 132(2020) 20670–9.
28. L.J. Small, T.M. Nenoff, Direct electrical detection of iodine gas by a novel metal–organic-framework-based sensor, *ACS Applied Materials & Interfaces*, 9(2017) 44649–55.
29. L.J. Small, R.C. Hill, J.L. Krumhansl, M.E. Schindelholz, Z. Chen, K.W. Chapman, et al., Reversible MOF-based sensors for the electrical detection of iodine gas, *ACS Applied Materials & Interfaces*, 11(2019) 27982–8.
30. C. Zong, X. Liu, H. Sun, G. Zhang, L. Lu, A new type of nanoscale coordination particles: toward modification-free detection of hydrogen sulfide gas, *Journal of Materials Chemistry*, 22(2012) 18418–25.
31. L. Guo, M. Wang, D. Cao, A novel Zr-MOF as fluorescence turn-on probe for real-time detecting H_2S gas and fingerprint identification, *Small*, 14(2018) 1703822.
32. M. Tchalala, P. Bhatt, K. Chappanda, S. Tavares, K. Adil, Y. Belmabkhout, et al., Fluorinated MOF platform for selective removal and sensing of SO_2 from flue gas and air, *Nature communications*, 10(2019) 1328.
33. M. Schulz, A. Gehl, J. Schlenkrich, H.A. Schulze, S. Zimmermann, A. Schaate, A calixarene-based metal–organic framework for highly selective NO_2 detection, *Angewandte Chemie International Edition*, 57(2018) 12961–5.
34. S. Yuvaraja, S.G. Surya, V. Chernikova, M.T. Vijjapu, O. Shekhah, P.M. Bhatt, et al., Realization of an ultrasensitive and highly selective OFET NO_2 sensor: the synergistic combination of PDVT-10 polymer and porphyrin–MOF, *ACS Applied Materials & Interfaces*, 12(2020) 18748–60.
35. N.S. Nikolaeva, D.D. Klyamer, S.M. Zharkov, A.R. Tsygankova, A.S. Sukhikh, N.B. Morozova, et al., Heterostructures based on Pd–Au nanoparticles and cobalt phthalocyanine for hydrogen chemiresistive sensors, *International Journal of Hydrogen Energy*, 46(2021) 19682–92.
36. T. Basova, M. Polyakov, Hybrid materials based on carbon nanotubes and polyaromatic molecules: methods of functionalization and sensor properties, *Macroheterocycles*, 13(2020) 91–112.
37. A.K. Sharma, A. Mahajan, R. Saini, R. Bedi, S. Kumar, A. Debnath, et al., Reversible and fast responding ppb level Cl_2 sensor based on noncovalent modified carbon nanotubes with Hexadecafluorinated copper phthalocyanine, *Sensors and Actuators B: Chemical*, 255(2018) 87–99.
38. V. Ivanova, D. Klyamer, P. Krasnov, E.N. Kaya, I. Kulu, S.T. Kostakoğlu, et al., Hybrid materials based on pyrene-substituted metallo phthalocyanines as sensing layers for ammonia detection: Effect of the number of pyrene substituents, *Sensors and Actuators B: Chemical*, 375(2023) 132843.

8 Applications of Nanocarriers in Drug Delivery

Purvi Kishore, Anushka Roy, and Amit Ranjan Maity

8.1 INTRODUCTION

Drug delivery is a strategic approach to administering therapeutic agents in a controlled and efficient manner to improve efficacy, safety, and patient compliance. Modern drug delivery systems (DDSs) aim to optimize pharmacokinetics, enhance bioavailability, enable controlled release, and achieve site-specific targeting. The performance of a DDS is largely influenced by the route of administration and the encapsulation strategy, where drugs are protected within carriers to prevent degradation and enable targeted distribution. Advances in formulation science and biomedical engineering have enabled DDS to overcome limitations of conventional therapies, such as poor solubility, instability, and rapid clearance, while supporting the delivery of sensitive biomolecules including mRNA and siRNA [1].

Recent progress in nanotechnology has propelled drug delivery toward precision medicine by enabling modulation of drug behavior at tissue, cellular, and subcellular levels (Figure 8.1). Targeted drug delivery (TDD) strategies focus on directing therapeutics specifically to diseased sites, minimizing systemic toxicity and reducing required doses. Nanocarriers (NC) play a central role by coordinating the drug, carrier, and biological target to enhance therapeutic efficiency. Nanomedicine, integrating nanoscale materials with biomedical science, has emerged as a powerful platform for this purpose. Typically ranging from 1 to 1,000 nm, NCs are engineered from biocompatible materials and can incorporate drugs through encapsulation or surface attachment, enabling controlled release and improved stability [2].

Nanomedicine employs both passive and active targeting mechanisms. Passive targeting utilizes the enhanced permeability and retention (EPR) effect, while active targeting relies on ligand–receptor interactions to promote selective cellular uptake [3]. Despite its promise, nanomedicine must overcome biological barriers such as the blood–brain barrier (BBB) and the tumor microenvironment. By tailoring size, surface charge, and responsiveness to physiological cues, NCs can enhance barrier penetration and therapeutic localization. Overall, nanomedicine represents a transformative approach that addresses the shortcomings of conventional therapies and enables safer, more effective targeted treatments.

DOI: 10.1201/9781003725930-8

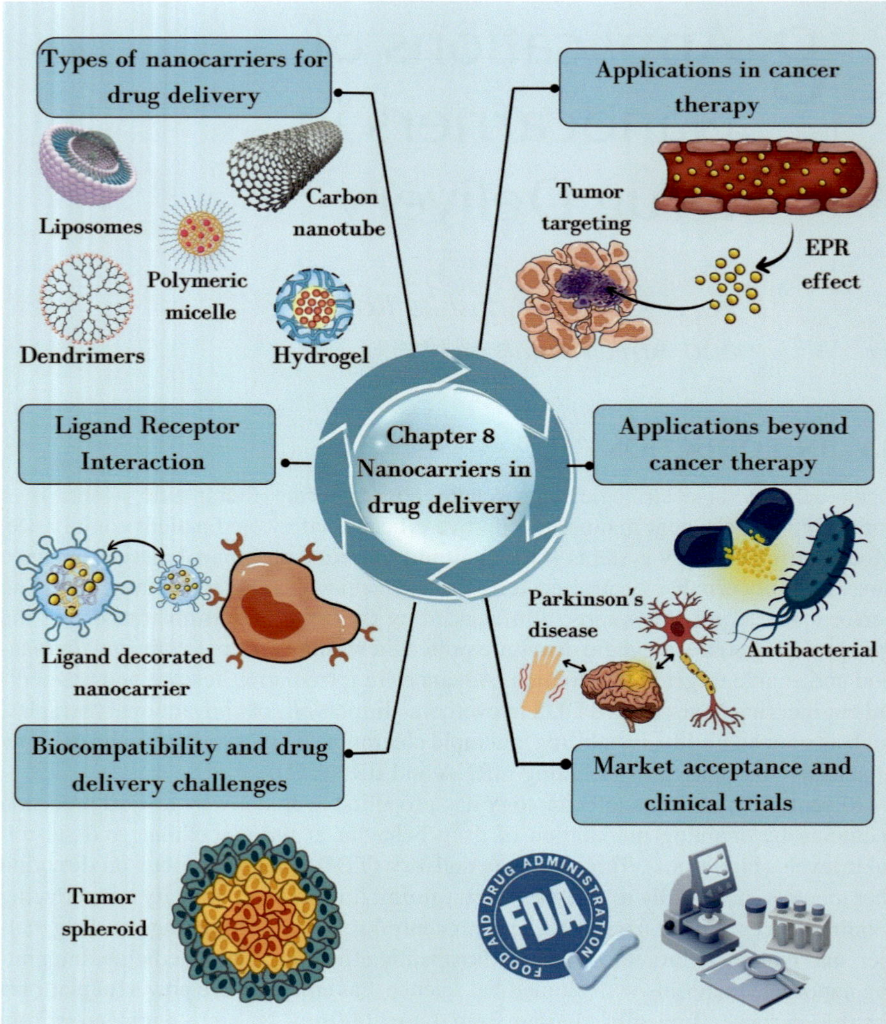

FIGURE 8.1 Schematic overview of nanocarriers in drug delivery, highlighting major carrier types (liposomes, polymeric micelles, dendrimers, hydrogels, and carbon nanotubes), ligand–receptor-mediated targeting strategies, applications in cancer therapy (including tumor targeting via the EPR effect), emerging uses beyond oncology (e.g., antibacterial and neurodegenerative disease treatment), and key considerations such as biocompatibility, translational challenges, market acceptance, and clinical evaluation.

8.2 TYPES OF NANOCARRIERS IN DRUG DELIVERY

Nanocarriers are nanoscale delivery systems, typically within the size range of 10–1,000 nm in diameter, engineered to transport drugs precisely to specific sites of action. Their minute size and large population enable them to accumulate

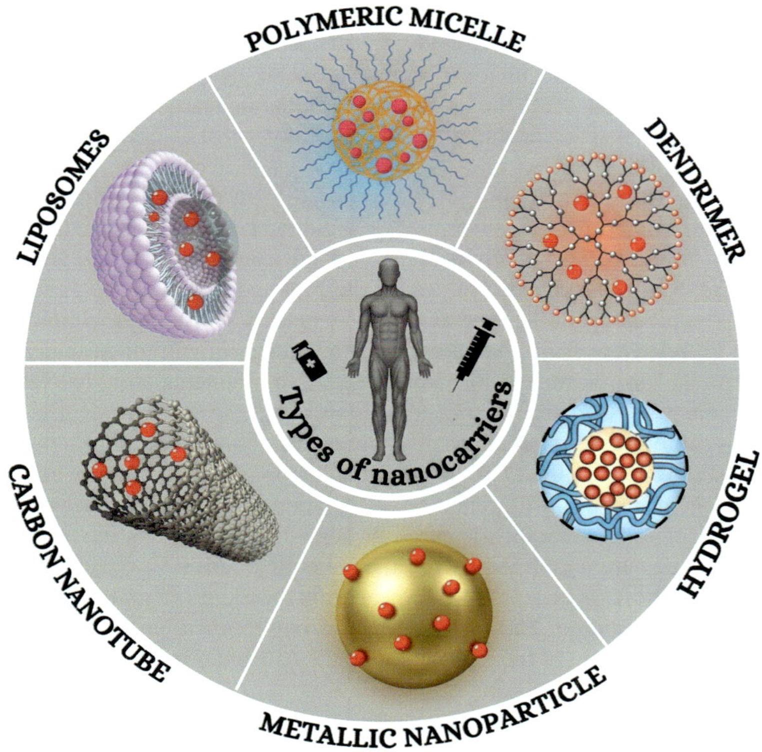

FIGURE 8.2 Different types of nanocarriers for drug delivery applications.

efficiently within diseased tissues such as tumors, inflamed regions, or infected cells (Figure 8.2). Beyond site-specific targeting, NCs enhance drug solubility, prolong systemic circulation, and protect bioactive compounds from enzymatic or chemical degradation. To ensure colloidal stability under physiological conditions, NCs are often functionalized through the grafting or adsorption of polymeric surfactants or other surface modifiers. This surface engineering forms a protective steric layer that generates repulsive electrostatic and hydrophilic forces, thereby preventing particle aggregation and maintaining dispersion stability.

Based on their composition and structural organization, NCs are broadly classified into three major categories: vesicular NCs, polymeric NCs, and inorganic NCs, each possessing distinct physicochemical properties and therapeutic advantages.

8.2.1 Liposomes in Drug Delivery Application

Liposomes are closed, spherical vesicular systems consisting of one or multiple concentric phospholipid bilayers that encloses an internal aqueous core. Their formation is driven by the amphiphilic nature of phospholipids, which possess hydrophilic polar head groups and hydrophobic acyl chains. When dispersed in an aqueous medium, these molecules spontaneously self-assemble into bilayer structures, orienting their hydrophilic heads toward the surrounding water where the hydrophobic tails orient toward the interior, reducing their exposure to the surrounding aqueous environment. This configuration represents the lowest thermodynamic energy state, resulting in a structurally stable vesicle capable of therapeutic molecules of both hydrophilic and hydrophobic nature.

Structurally, liposomes are primarily composed of phospholipids and cholesterol, which together determine the membrane's rigidity, permeability, surface charge, and overall stability. Phosphatidylcholine, derived from either natural source (e.g., egg yolk, soybean) or synthetic routes, is the most commonly used lipid component due to its biocompatibility and zwitterionic nature. While phospholipid bilayers alone can be relatively fluid and susceptible to leakage of entrapped materials, the inclusion of cholesterol imparts mechanical strength by intercalating between phospholipid molecules. Cholesterol enhances bilayer packing density, decreases membrane permeability to water-soluble substances, and stabilizes the liposome near the phase transition temperature (T_c). This fine regulation of bilayer fluidity and rigidity is crucial for optimizing drug retention, circulation half-life, and release kinetics. Liposomes encapsulate therapeutic cargo through distinct localization mechanisms: hydrophilic drugs are entrapped within the aqueous interior, whereas hydrophobic molecules and those with amphiphilic properties become integrated into the surrounding lipid membrane. The resulting hybrid environment enables liposomes to carry a diverse spectrum of bioactive compounds like small molecule of drugs, proteins, or nucleic acids.

Drug transport through liposomal systems occurs via either passive or active targeting strategies. In the passive mode, liposomes take advantage of the EPR phenomenon, which results from the defective vasculature and inadequate lymphatic clearance typically found in tumor or inflamed tissues. Such a physiological mechanism promotes the selective deposition of liposome-based formulations in pathological regions. In contrast, active targeting is accomplished by decorating the liposomal surface with ligands including antibodies, peptides, folic acid (FA), or aptamers. These ligands selectively recognize and bind to overexpressed receptors on target cells, promoting receptor-mediated endocytosis (RME) and intracellular drug delivery. The release of encapsulated therapeutics can occur through diffusion across the lipid membrane or by employing stimuli-responsive liposomes that react to stimuli encompassing alterations in pH, thermal conditions, enzyme activity, or redox potential. Advanced liposomal designs include pH-sensitive, thermosensitive, cationic, fusogenic, magnetoliposomes, photosensitive, and PEGylated (stealth) liposomes. Among these, PEGylated liposomes coated with polyethylene glycol (PEG) are particularly significant, as the hydrophilic polymeric layer sterically reduces opsonization and uptake by the mononuclear phagocyte system, thereby prolonging circulation time and enhancing pharmacokinetic behavior.

Liposomes have multiple advantages that have advanced their application in nanomedicine and targeted drug delivery. They improve the solubility and bioavailability of poorly soluble therapeutics while reducing systemic toxicity, enable sustained and controlled drug release, and protect labile biomolecules such as nucleic acids and proteins from enzymatic degradation. Consequently, liposomal formulations have been successfully applied in oncology, antimicrobial therapy, vaccine delivery, gene therapy, and transdermal as well as ocular drug delivery. Clinically approved liposomal drugs such as Doxil® (liposomal doxorubicin) and Ambisome® (liposomal amphotericin B) demonstrate their translational success and therapeutic superiority over conventional formulations.

Despite their extensive potential, challenges remain in terms of large-scale manufacturing, long-term stability, reproducibility, and immunogenicity. The high cost of production and the complexity of lipid–drug interactions further complicate commercialization. Nevertheless, continuous advancements in lipid chemistry, scalable formulation techniques, and surface functionalization have positioned liposomes as one of the most mature and clinically relevant NC systems in modern targeted drug delivery [4,5].

8.2.2 Polymeric Micelles in Drug Delivery Application

Polymeric micelles are nanoscale colloidal systems that arise from the self-organization behavior of amphiphilic block copolymers under aqueous conditions. Typically exhibiting sizes between 10 and 100 nm in diameter, these micelles possess a core–shell architecture, comprising a hydrophobic inner core and a hydrophilic outer corona. This unique structure provides a versatile platform enabling the incorporation of drugs with poor aqueous solubility within the hydrophobic domain, while the hydrophilic shell stabilizes the system, prevents aggregation, and enhances circulation in physiological media. The nanoscale dimension and excellent stability of polymeric micelles tend to concentrate preferentially in tumor and inflamed sites via the EPR phenomenon, underscoring their potential in targeted therapeutic delivery.

Structurally, polymeric micelles are nanoscale assemblies constructed from amphiphilic block copolymers composed of both hydrophilic and hydrophobic units that dictate their self-assembly behavior and performance. The hydrophobic core is typically composed of biodegradable polymers such as poly(ε-caprolactone), polylactic acid, poly(lactic-co-glycolic acid), polyethers, or poly(amino acids). This core functions as a nanoscale reservoir for hydrophobic drugs, where encapsulation occurs through hydrophobic interactions, stabilized by non-covalent forces including van der Waals interactions, π–π stacking, and hydrogen bonds. The hydrophilic shell, commonly constructed from PEG, provides steric stabilization, improves biocompatibility, and ensures colloidal stability and stealth properties by reducing protein adsorption and opsonization by the reticuloendothelial system (RES) which ensures prolonged systemic circulation.

Despite its well-recognized benefits, PEGylation may trigger the accelerated blood clearance effect after multiple doses, primarily due to the development of anti-PEG antibodies. To mitigate this, alternative hydrophilic polymers such as poly(2-oxazoline), poly(amino acids), or natural polysaccharides like dextran, heparin, chitosan, and hyaluronic acid have been employed to achieve comparable stability and biocompatibility. The physicochemical properties of polymeric micelles including size, stability, drug-loading efficiency, and release kinetics are influenced by several factors. These include the molecular weight of the copolymer blocks, the critical micelle concentration, and the intensity of intermolecular interactions between the polymer matrix and the loaded drug molecules. Crosslinking either the core or shell regions enhances mechanical stability, minimizes premature disassembly under dilution, and enables stimuli-responsive drug release triggered by pH, temperature, redox potential, or enzymatic activity. This responsiveness allows precise drug liberation within pathological microenvironments such as tumors or inflamed tissues.

Polymeric micelle delivery can be refined through two distinct mechanisms: passive targeting, which utilizes the EPR effect to exploit leaky tumor vasculature and poor lymphatic drainage for natural accumulation, and active targeting, which involves decorating the micelle surface with specific ligands (like antibodies or peptides). Such ligands interact selectively with overexpressed receptors on target cells, initiating RME and enhancing intracellular drug accumulation. In addition, positively charged micelles interact electrostatically with anionic cell membranes and mucosal surfaces, resulting in enhanced binding, prolonged retention, and greater uptake efficiency. The versatility of polymeric micelles has enabled their application across diverse therapeutic domains. They have shown remarkable potential in oncology, gene and protein delivery, mucosal drug administration, and anti-inflammatory therapy. Their ability to improve solubility, prolong systemic exposure, and provide controlled release enhances both therapeutic efficacy and patient compliance. Moreover, advanced micellar architectures such as unimolecular micelles, core-crosslinked micelles, and shell-crosslinked micelles have been developed to further improve drug stability, prolong circulation, and fine-tune release behavior.

Despite their success at the preclinical and early clinical stages, challenges persist, including limited large-scale reproducibility, complex manufacturing processes, protein corona formation, and variability in in vivo performance. Addressing these issues through advances in polymer chemistry, controlled polymerization, and scalable formulation technologies will be critical for the successful translation of polymeric micelles into clinical therapeutics.

In summary, polymeric micelles represent a highly adaptable and biocompatible class of NCs that combine the benefits of structural tunability, sustained release, and targeting precision. Their multifunctional design continues to evolve, positioning them as a cornerstone of modern nanomedicine and an indispensable platform for next-generation DDSs [6,7].

8.2.3 Dendrimers in Drug Delivery Application

Dendrimers are highly ordered, nanosized macromolecules possessing a branched, tree-like structure originating from a central core. The word "dendrimer" comes from the Greek *dendron*, meaning "tree," reflecting their systematic, layer-by-layer branching pattern. Typically range between 1 and 15 nm in diameter, dendrimers possess a multigenerational, three-dimensional (3D) framework that provides exceptional control over size, shape, surface functionality, and molecular weight, which are rarely achieved in conventional polymer systems. Structurally, dendrimers consist of three essential components: (i) a central core, which serves as the origin of molecular growth; (ii) interior branching units (dendrons), which extend outward in successive generations; and (iii) terminal surface groups, which can be chemically modified to introduce desired functionalities. Each generation of branching exponentially increases the number of terminal groups, resulting in a densely packed, globular nanostructure with a high degree of surface functionality and internal cavities suitable for drug encapsulation or molecular conjugation. The monodispersed and well-defined architecture of dendrimers make them highly reproducible and predictable in biological performance compared to linear polymers.

Dendrimers are typically synthesized using two principal approaches, divergent and convergent. In the divergent method, growth proceeds outward from a multifunctional core through iterative reaction steps, producing a complete dendritic structure with multiple reactive termini. Conversely, the convergent method involves synthesizing individual dendrons from the periphery toward the core, followed by their attachment to a central nucleus. The divergent approach is more efficient for producing large quantities, whereas the convergent strategy allows greater structural precision and easier purification of intermediate generations. These methods provide remarkable flexibility in tailoring the physicochemical and biological characteristics of dendrimers for specific biomedical applications. The mechanism of drug loading and release in dendrimers depends on their structural configuration and surface chemistry. Therapeutic molecules can be entrapped within the internal voids of the dendrimer through hydrophobic, electrostatic, hydrogen-bonding, or π–π interactions, or they may be covalently conjugated to surface functional groups to form stable prodrugs. Accordingly, two principal release mechanisms are recognized: (i) endo-release, where the encapsulated drug diffuses or is displaced from internal cavities in response to environmental stimuli including alterations in pH, ionic strength, or temperature; and (ii) exo-release, where drugs conjugated to surface groups are released following cleavage of chemical linkages, often mediated by enzymatic or hydrolytic processes. Such tunable release kinetics allow dendrimers to act as controlled and targeted NCs, minimizing systemic toxicity while maximizing local therapeutic concentration.

Among the various dendritic systems developed, poly(amidoamine), poly(propylene imine), and polyethyleneimine dendrimers are the most widely explored in pharmaceutical and biomedical research. Their amine-rich surface facilitates further functionalization with PEG, specific ligands, or targeting groups to enhance solubility, minimize immune recognition, and prolong circulation time in vivo. The PEGylation or glycosylation of dendrimers also enhances their stealth properties and biocompatibility, mitigating rapid clearance by the mononuclear phagocyte system.

Dendrimers have demonstrated substantial potential across multiple therapeutic and diagnostic domains. In cancer therapy, surface-functionalized dendrimers achieve active targeting by attaching ligands such as FA, antibodies, or aptamers that specifically bind to receptors overexpressed on tumor cells, thereby promoting receptor-mediated internalization and selective cytotoxic action. Additionally, dendrimer-based formulations improve the solubility and bioavailability of hydrophobic chemotherapeutics while reducing off-target effects. In gene therapy, cationic dendrimers serve as efficient nonviral vectors capable of complexing with DNA, siRNA, or mRNA through electrostatic interactions, promoting cellular uptake and endosomal escape. Similarly, in infectious disease treatment, dendrimer–antibiotic conjugates and antimicrobial dendrimers disrupt microbial membranes and biofilms, providing a powerful tool against multidrug-resistant pathogens.

Beyond therapeutic delivery, dendrimers also function as diagnostic and theranostic agents. Surface modification with imaging probes such as gadolinium, fluorophores, or radionuclides enables their use in magnetic resonance imaging (MRI), computed tomography (CT), or nuclear imaging, offering simultaneous diagnosis and therapy (theranostics). Notably, maltose-modified dendrimers have shown the capability to cross the BBB, offering new opportunities aimed at the therapeutic intervention of neurodegenerative disorders such as Alzheimer's and Parkinson's diseases by inhibiting amyloid-β or α-synuclein aggregation. Moreover, dendrimer–antigen conjugates are being explored as vaccine adjuvants, capable of eliciting robust immune responses with improved antigen presentation and durability. Despite their extensive advantages, dendrimers face several challenges in clinical translation, including cytotoxicity associated with cationic surface groups, potential immunogenicity, and complexities in large-scale synthesis and purification. Recent advances in biodegradable dendritic polymers, surface engineering, and stimuli-responsive designs aim to overcome these limitations, enabling safer and more effective NCs for precision medicine.

In summary, dendrimers represent a paradigm of precision-engineered NCs, combining architectural uniformity, high functional versatility, and tunable biocompatibility. Their multifunctional framework allows for simultaneous imaging, targeting, and therapy placing dendrimers at the forefront of next-generation nanomedicine and personalized DDSs [8].

8.2.4 Hydrogel in Drug Delivery Application

Hydrogels represent a versatile class of polymer-based NCs widely utilized in biomedical and pharmaceutical sciences for controlled and targeted drug delivery. They are composed of a 3D crosslinked polymeric network that can absorb and retain large volumes of water or biological fluids without dissolving, owing to the presence of hydrophilic functional groups. In their nanoscale form, typically between 1 and 1,000 nm, hydrogels offer exceptional tunability in mechanical properties, porosity, and responsiveness to physiological cues, positioning them as promising materials for advanced therapeutic applications.

Structurally, hydrogels can be synthesized through physical or chemical crosslinking of natural or synthetic polymers. Physical crosslinking forms polymer networks through non-covalent interactions such as hydrogen bonding, electrostatic attractions, or hydrophobic associations. These reversible interactions result in biocompatible and stimuli-responsive gels, making them especially useful for biomedical and drug delivery applications. In contrast, chemical crosslinking forms covalent linkages among polymer chains, providing enhanced structural integrity, stability, and controlled degradation. The resulting polymeric network forms an interconnected system of nanoscale pores, enabling encapsulation and diffusion-controlled release of bioactive molecules. The swelling behavior of hydrogels arises from the balance between osmotic pressure and the elasticity of the polymeric network, allowing them to expand several hundred times their dry weight in aqueous environments while maintaining structural coherence.

The physicochemical and biological properties of hydrogels are dictated largely by their polymeric composition. Synthetic polymers such as PEG, poly(vinyl alcohol), poly(acrylic acid), and poly(N-isopropylacrylamide) provide precise control over mechanical strength, porosity, and degradation rates, making them suitable for consistent and controlled DDSs. Nonetheless, their poor bioactivity and limited natural compatibility with biological environments often call for surface functionalization or integration with biopolymers such as chitosan, alginate, hyaluronic acid, dextran, and gelatin. These naturally sourced polymers provide excellent biocompatibility and biodegradability, and non-immunogenic, thereby improving the overall biological performance of the material by enabling better interaction with cells and tissues. For instance, chitosan-based pH-responsive nanohydrogels have demonstrated significant efficacy in topical and transdermal applications, including improved skin integrity and enhanced therapeutic outcomes in melanoma treatment models.

Drug encapsulation and release mechanisms in hydrogels depend on both polymer composition and network density. Drugs can be incorporated during gel formation via in situ polymerization and crosslinking or loaded post-synthetically through diffusion into preformed hydrogels. Encapsulation mechanisms include physical entrapment within the polymeric matrix, electrostatic complexation, or covalent conjugation to functional groups along the polymer backbone. Controlled release occurs through three principal mechanisms: (i) diffusion, where drug molecules migrate through the swollen network; (ii) polymer degradation, where hydrolysis or enzymatic breakdown liberates the active agents; and (iii) swelling-controlled release, where expansion of the matrix facilitates diffusion. Furthermore, incorporation of stimuli-responsive elements allows hydrogels to allow dynamic response to environmental stimuli such as pH, temperature, ionic strength, enzymes, or redox potential enabling on-demand and site-specific drug release in response to pathological conditions. The biomedical applications of nanohydrogels are broad and continually expanding. They have been employed as drug and gene delivery platforms, wound-healing scaffolds, tissue-engineering matrices, and biosensors. Their hydrophilic nature and soft, tissue-like consistency make them particularly suitable for ocular, transdermal, and mucosal delivery systems, where they minimize irritation and enhance bioavailability. In cancer therapy, hydrogel-based NCs enable localized and sustained release of chemotherapeutic agents, leading to reduced systemic side effects and improved therapeutic outcomes. Moreover, hydrogels serve as biomimetic scaffolds that support cell growth and differentiation, facilitating regeneration of skin, cartilage, and bone tissues.

Despite these advantages, several challenges impede the clinical translation of hydrogel-based NCs. The synthesis of chemically crosslinked hydrogels often requires harsh reaction conditions or toxic reagents that may compromise biocompatibility or residual solvent safety. Synthetic hydrogels, though mechanically robust, may lack biodegradability, while natural polymer–based hydrogels, though biocompatible, can suffer from weak mechanical strength and poor stability in physiological environments. Addressing these limitations requires the development of hybrid hydrogels, combining the mechanical resilience of synthetic polymers with the bifunctionality of natural macromolecules. Additionally, nanocomposite hydrogels incorporating NCs or bioactive agents have shown promise in enhancing mechanical strength, conductivity, and therapeutic functionality.

In summary, hydrogels constitute a dynamic and multifunctional platform in nanomedicine, capable of responding intelligently to biological cues while maintaining structural integrity and biocompatibility. Their adaptability for diverse therapeutic modalities from controlled drug delivery to regenerative medicine positions hydrogels as key enablers of precision and personalized healthcare in the era of advanced nanotherapeutics [9].

8.2.5 Inorganic Nanocarriers in Drug Delivery Application

Inorganic NCs represent a rapidly advancing class of nanoscale delivery platforms characterized by their structural rigidity, tunable physicochemical properties, and multifunctional behavior. Unlike organic NCs, which are primarily polymer- or lipid-based, inorganic systems such as metallic nanocarriers (MNCs), silica NCs, quantum dots, and carbon-based nanostructures offer distinctive mechanical, optical, and magnetic attributes that are important for precisely tuning them for therapeutic and diagnostic purposes. Their unique ability to integrate drug delivery, imaging, and therapeutic functions within one integrated platform, termed theragnostic, has positioned inorganic NCs at the forefront of precision nanomedicine.

MNCs, particularly those composed of gold (Au), silver (Ag), iron oxide (Fe_3O_4), palladium (Pd), copper (Cu), and platinum (Pt), have emerged as highly versatile NCs for targeted and controlled drug delivery. Their nanoscale dimensions (10–100 nm) and large surface-to-volume ratio enable efficient interaction with biomolecules and cellular membranes, facilitating selective uptake and minimal off-target effects. Structurally, MNCs are crystalline or amorphous cores stabilized by organic or inorganic capping agents that prevent aggregation and provide a surface for further functionalization. Surface modification through PEG (PEGylation), polysaccharides, or biocompatible ligands enhances colloidal stability, reduces immune clearance, and improves systemic circulation time. The surfaces can also be modified with targeting ligands including antibodies, peptides, aptamers, or small molecules to facilitate RME at specific pathological sites. Drug loading on MNCs occurs through adsorption, covalent conjugation, or encapsulation within polymeric coatings. Drug release mechanisms are often governed by stimuli-responsive cues including pH changes, enzyme activity, temperature, or redox gradients which enable site-specific and on-demand delivery in pathological microenvironments. For instance, the acidic environment of tumors or endosomes can trigger the cleavage of acid-labile linkers, resulting in selective drug release while minimizing systemic toxicity.

Different metallic cores impart unique functional advantages. Gold nanocarriers (AuNCs) exhibit excellent biocompatibility and tunable optical properties due to their surface plasmon resonance (SPR) effect, making them ideal for both photothermal therapy and photoacoustic imaging. Upon laser irradiation, AuNCs convert absorbed light into localized heat, effectively ablating cancer cells without damaging surrounding tissues. Silver NCs possess potent antimicrobial and antiviral activity, primarily by inducing the formation of reactive oxygen species that compromise bacterial cell membranes, while iron oxide NCs exhibit superparamagnetic properties that enable magnetic field–guided targeting and imaging via MRI. Platinum and palladium NCs function as catalytic carriers for prodrug activation and oxidative stress modulation in tumor environments, whereas copper NC are gaining attention as cost-effective alternatives with intrinsic antimicrobial and photothermal properties.

The synthesis of MNCs generally follows two fundamental strategies: (i) top-down approaches, such as laser ablation, milling, or electrochemical dispersion, that reduce bulk metal into nanosized fragments, and (ii) bottom-up approaches, including chemical reduction, sol–gel synthesis, microemulsion, and thermal decomposition, that assemble NCs from atomic or molecular precursors. The latter offers greater control over particle size, morphology, and surface functionality, essential for achieving reproducibility and uniformity in biomedical applications. In therapeutic practice, MNCs exhibit dual roles as carriers and therapeutic agents. Their integration into theranostic systems allows real-time tracking of drug distribution and therapeutic response through imaging modalities such as MRI, positron emission tomography, fluorescence, or CT. For example, gold nanorods conjugated with doxorubicin not only deliver the drug efficiently to tumor tissues but also enable optical imaging and photothermal destruction of malignant cells. Likewise, superparamagnetic iron oxide NCs serve as both contrast agents and magnetically steerable carriers for cancer imaging and hyperthermia-based therapy.

Despite their broad potential, there are several limitations that prevent the clinical translation of MC-based NCs. These include cytotoxicity due to metal ion release, immune recognition, long-term biodistribution, and clearance issues, particularly for particles larger than the renal excretion threshold (~6 nm). Additionally, large-scale synthesis with consistent particle characteristics remains difficult, and regulatory concerns surrounding the long-term safety of metallic residues persist. Addressing these limitations demands green synthesis approaches, biodegradable coatings, and comprehensive toxicological evaluation to ensure clinical compatibility.

Overall, MNCs provide a versatile and multifunctional platform suitable for targeted drug delivery, molecular imaging, and photothermal or photodynamic therapeutic applications. Their tunable optical, electronic, and magnetic properties, combined with the capacity for surface modification and controlled release, make them indispensable in advancing next-generation nanotheranostic systems [10].

8.2.6 Carbon Nanotube in Drug Delivery Application

Carbon nanotubes (CNTs) are hollow, cylindrical nanostructures consisting of carbon atoms arranged in a hexagonal lattice pattern, representing one of the most promising NC systems for advanced biomedical applications. Possessing exceptional tensile strength, electrical conductivity, and a large surface-to-volume ratio arising from their elongated tubular structure, CNTs provide a highly efficient platform for the transport of drugs, imaging agents, and biomacromolecules. Their combined physicochemical stability and molecular tunability enable precise modulation of drug loading, release behavior, and targeting efficiency, making CNTs an essential tool in TDD and nanotheranostic research.

Structurally, CNTs are divided into two principal types: single-walled carbon nanotubes (SWCNTs) and multi-walled carbon nanotubes (MWCNTs). SWCNTs are formed by rolling a single graphene sheet into a continuous cylindrical structure, typically exhibiting diameters between 0.4 and 2 nm, while MWCNTs comprise several concentric graphene layers, with diameters generally ranging from 2 to 100 nm. The layered architecture of MWCNTs provides superior mechanical robustness and greater drug-loading capacity, while SWCNTs offer improved dispersibility and easier surface modification, making each type suitable for distinct biomedical purposes. CNTs possess hollow interiors and extensive π-electron systems, which enable the encapsulation and diagnostic agents, including small molecules, peptides, proteins, nucleic acids, and imaging probes. Drug molecules can be integrated into CNTs through three primary strategies:

1. Encapsulation within the internal cavity for physical entrapment and protection against degradation.
2. Adsorption onto the outer surface via π–π stacking, hydrophobic interactions, or van der Waals forces.
3. Covalent functionalization, involving the attachment of drug molecules or targeting ligands through amide, ester, or disulfide linkages, which could be engineered to cleave under defined physiological environment.

Functionalization serves as a key factor which affects the biocompatible nature, solubility, and pharmacokinetics of CNT-based systems. Pristine CNTs are inherently hydrophobic and tend to aggregate in aqueous media, which limits their biomedical applicability. To overcome this limitation, surface modification through oxidation, carboxylation, PEGylation, or polymer coating introduces hydrophilic groups that enhance dispersion, reduce cytotoxicity, and prevent nonspecific interactions with biological components. Furthermore, bioconjugation with targeting agents such as antibodies, peptides, aptamers, or FA facilitates active targeting toward specific cell receptors, enabling selective uptake via RME. Mechanistically, CNTs exhibit an inherent advantage in cellular internalization owing to their elongated, needle-like morphology. This geometry allows them to pierce cellular membranes through energy-independent nanopenetration or endocytosis, resulting in efficient intracellular delivery of therapeutic cargo. Once internalized, the release of encapsulated agents can be triggered by pH, redox potential, enzymatic activity, or thermal stimuli, depending on the type of linker or encapsulation strategy employed. In addition, CNTs are designed to facilitate both light-induced thermal and dynamic therapies, where they act as near-infrared absorbers that transform light into localized thermal energy, effectively inducing cancer cell apoptosis without harming surrounding healthy tissues.

In biomedical research and clinical translation, CNTs have demonstrated a wide spectrum of applications. In oncology, CNT-based NCs are employed for site-specific delivery of chemotherapeutics such as doxorubicin, paclitaxel, and cisplatin, achieving high drug accumulation in tumors while minimizing systemic toxicity. In gene therapy, CNTs serve as efficient vectors for the transport of plasmid DNA, siRNA, and miRNA across cellular barriers, offering a safer and more stable alternative to viral systems. Moreover, functionalized CNTs have been utilized in biosensing and diagnostic imaging, exploiting their conductive and optical properties for the detection of biomolecules and tumor biomarkers. In tissue engineering, CNTs are incorporated into scaffolds to enhance mechanical strength, electrical conductivity, and cellular adhesion, facilitating regeneration in cardiac, neural, and bone tissues.

Despite these promising attributes, the clinical translation of CNT-based NCs faces several critical challenges. The cytotoxicity and bio persistence of CNTs, primarily arising from their hydrophobicity, metal impurities, and oxidative stress induction, remain major safety concerns. Furthermore, issues related to biodegradability, long-term clearance, and immune response must be systematically addressed before widespread clinical use. To mitigate these limitations, current research focuses on developing biodegradable CNT composites, employing green synthesis routes, and integrating surface coatings with biomimetic polymers or proteins to enhance their biocompatibility and clearance profiles [11].

In summary, CNTs represent a multifunctional and adaptable NC platform that combines structural precision, tunable chemistry, and unique physicochemical properties for advanced therapeutic applications. Through continued innovation in surface engineering, safety optimization, and targeted design, CNTs hold substantial promise for next-generation drug delivery, regenerative medicine, and precision nanomedicine.

8.3 LIGAND–RECEPTOR INTERACTION IN DRUG DELIVERY: THE KEY MECHANISM

This strategy operates on the principle of specific molecular recognition and high binding affinity between a ligand conjugated to a drug molecule or its carrier and a receptor that is overexpressed on target cells, particularly cancer cells. A key design parameter for an optimal ligand–receptor-mediated targeted drug delivery systems (TDDSs) is receptor overexpression on diseased cells. The interaction begins when a targeting molecule, such as an antibody, peptide, or small molecule, interact with its corresponding receptor on the plasma membrane. The high-affinity and specific binding ensures that the ligand associates preferentially with its cognate receptor rather than with unrelated sites. In cancer therapeutics, receptor overexpression is especially critical, as malignant cells typically express these receptors at levels several times higher than healthy counterparts. The expression ratio between diseased and normal cells is a major determinant of therapeutic safety and selectivity. Generally, a minimum of a threefold increase in receptor expression in diseased cells is sufficient to achieve targeted accumulation while limiting collateral toxicity [12]. A list of various NCs is presented in Table 8.1 along with their characteristic properties for drug delivery.

Ligand–receptor interaction forms the cornerstone of TDDSs, enabling site-specific localization of drugs at diseased sites with reduced off-target toxicity. However, receptor expression is not always exclusive to diseased cells, which can compromise targeting specificity. To achieve efficient delivery, the extent of receptor overexpression must be sufficient to promote preferential binding and penetration of NC-encapsulated drugs into diseased cells relative to healthy tissues. The biodistribution of the therapeutic agent thus mirrors the relative receptor density. For highly potent drugs, the dosing must be optimized to ensure selective delivery, whereas for less toxic compounds, a lower receptor expression differential may be acceptable.

Several receptors have been identified as promising targets for ligand-mediated delivery. Folate receptors (FRs), particularly FRα, a cell-surface glycoprotein, shows

TABLE 8.1
Different Types of Nanocarriers Used for Targeting

Type of NC	Component	Size (nm)	Characteristic properties
Liposome	Phospholipids (mainly phosphatidylcholine) and cholesterol forming the bilayer membrane	100–150	Spherical, self-assembled vesicles with amphiphilic bilayer, aqueous core, encapsulate hydrophilic and hydrophobic drugs, biocompatible, and stable
Polymeric micelle	Amphiphilic block copolymers with hydrophilic (PEG or polysaccharides) and hydrophobic parts	10–100	Amphiphilic aggregates with hydrophobic core and hydrophilic shell, high drug loading, controlled release, biocompatible
Dendrimers	Central-core, repetitive branching units (dendrons) and terminal functional groups	1–15	Branched, tree-like structure with internal cavities, uniform size and shape capable of encapsulating drugs
Hydrogel	Crosslinked polymeric network made of synthetic or natural polymer	1–1,000	3D hydrophilic network, capable of swelling in water
Metallic NP	Metals such as gold, silver, palladium, copper, and platinum	4–20	High surface area-to-volume ratio, optical (SPR) and magnetic properties
Carbon nanotubes	Cylindrical nanocarriers made of carbon atoms arranged in a hexagonal lattice and exist as SWCNTs or MWCNTs	0.4–100	Cylindrical, hollow, needle-like structure with high surface area

elevated expression levels in malignancies such as breast, lung, ovarian, colon, or renal carcinomas. Functionalization of NCs with FA has demonstrated enhanced cancer cell uptake, with studies reporting up to 50% greater internalization compared to unmodified carriers. Similarly, integrin αvβ3 receptors, which mediate cell adhesion to the extracellular matrix, are overexpressed in several solid tumors including brain cancers. The arginine-glycine-aspartic acid (RGD) peptide motif is widely utilized for targeting αvβ3 integrins, facilitating selective tumor localization. Other receptor systems such as CD44, CXCR4, and interleukin receptors also play pivotal roles in receptor-mediated targeting. For instance, CD44 is abundantly expressed on cancer stem cells and is associated with metastasis; its inhibition via NC-mediated delivery has been shown to suppress tumor progression. Similarly, CXCR4 and interleukin receptors have been successfully exploited for targeted delivery using receptor-specific NCs [13].

Targeting ligands function as molecular navigation systems, guiding therapeutic payloads to their intended cellular destinations and enhancing treatment efficacy, a key limitation in conventional therapies. These ligands display high specificity and affinity toward receptors that are upregulated on diseased cells. Upon conjugation to NCs, they form the structural and functional basis of ligand-directed TDDSs.

The role of targeting ligands in NC-mediated drug delivery can be summarized in four interrelated functions:

1. Specific recognition of overexpressed receptors on diseased cells.
2. Selective binding with high affinity to minimize off-target accumulation.
3. Facilitation of internalization via RME.
4. Optimization of therapeutic efficacy while minimizing systemic toxicity.

A broad range of molecules can serve as targeting ligands, including small molecules, carbohydrates, peptides, aptamers, and antibodies, each with unique structural and functional advantages. Proper ligand design ensures high receptor specificity, enabling NCs to distinguish malignant from healthy cells, enhance local drug concentration, and leads to increased overall therapeutic efficacy and safety profile of the delivery system.

Following ligand–receptor recognition, cellular uptake proceeds predominantly via RME. In this process, ligand binding induces clustering of receptors and formation of ligand–receptor complexes, which are internalized through clathrin-mediated endocytosis, the most common pathway. The internalized NCs are trafficked into early endosomes, where subsequent sorting determines the intracellular fate, either being trafficked to the plasma membrane or degradation in lysosomes. The intrinsic properties of the receptor–ligand complex, such as receptor oligomerization, binding strength, and pH sensitivity govern the efficiency and directionality of endocytosis. Once internalized, the therapeutic payload may be released into the cytosol or localized within specific organelles, depending on carrier design and environmental triggers. These trafficking pathways, both clathrin-dependent and clathrin-independent, are critical for ensuring precise intracellular localization and controlled release of the therapeutic agent. Notably, some receptors internalized via non-clathrin routes are recycled back to the membrane, while others are targeted for lysosomal degradation, underscoring the complexity and dynamic nature of intracellular trafficking [14].

RME thus functions not only as an uptake mechanism but also as a biological signaling process that links extracellular recognition with intracellular therapeutic action. The efficiency of this mechanism directly influences drug bioavailability, localization, and therapeutic outcomes.

8.4 LIGAND DECORATION AND DUAL-TARGETING STRATEGIES

Ligand decoration, also referred to as surface functionalization, is a key engineering strategy for enhancing NC specificity and targeting efficiency. In this approach, various drug molecules or carrier surfaces are functionalized with ligands that facilitate multivalent interactions binding simultaneously to multiple receptor domains or receptor subunits, as listed in Table 8.2. Fine-tuning the ligand density on the NC surface is critical: an insufficient number of ligands can lead to weak binding and poor internalization, whereas excessive decoration may induce steric hindrance or promote nonspecific interactions.

The bioconjugation chemistry underlying ligand attachment plays a vital role in achieving controlled drug release. Most NCs employ cleavable linkers such as ester,

TABLE 8.2
Different Types of Ligands Used for Targeting in Drug Delivery

Ligand Type	Receptor Molecule	Location	Action Mechanism	Example	Associated Diseases
Small molecules	Folate receptor (FR), sigma receptors, asialoglycoprotein receptor, PSMA, integrin αvβ3	Cancer cell surface, hepatocytes	Receptor-mediated endocytosis, specific binding, modulation of protein activity, nonenzymatic methylation	Folic acid, anisamide, benzamides, carbohydrates (e.g., galactose), PSMA targeting molecules (e.g., N-acetyl-L-Asp-L-Glu analogues)	Ovarian, lung, breast, and gastrointestinal cancers; melanoma; inflammatory diseases; autoimmune diseases; neurodegenerative diseases
Peptide	Integrins (e.g., αvβ3, α4β1, α4β7), interleukin-4 receptor, HER2, G-coupled receptors, nucleolin, HDM2 protein, TIM-3, EphA4	Cancer cell surface, tumor vasculature, intracellular (e.g., nucleus), extracellular matrix	Receptor-mediated endocytosis, specific binding, modulation of cell signaling, inhibition of protein–protein interactions, tumor penetration	RGD peptide, iRGD peptide, IL4RPep-1, GA5 peptide, PNC27, TIM-3 binding peptide, pH (low) insertion peptides (pHLIP), Tat peptide	Cancer (tumor vasculature, lung tumors), inflammatory disorders (multiple sclerosis, inflammatory bowel diseases, dry eye disease, asthma), cardiovascular diseases, autoimmune diseases, osteoporosis
Antibody	HER2, CD20, CD40, EGFR, FRα, CD38, CTLA4, PD1, PD-L1, α4β7 integrin, integrin αvβ3, αLβ2	Soluble ligands, immune cells, tumor cells	Receptor blockade, immune-mediated cytotoxicity (ADCC, CDC), agonistic activity, inhibition of dimerization, direct cell toxicity, modulation of protein activity	Trastuzumab (anti-HER2), rituximab (anti-CD20), anti-EGFR antibodies (e.g., cetuximab), ChiLob 7/4 (anti-CD40), anti-FRα antibodies, daratumumab (anti-CD38), anti-CTLA-4 antibodies, anti-PD1/PD-L1 antibodies, vedolizumab (anti-α4β7 integrin)	Cancer (breast, ovarian, lung, gastrointestinal, gynecological, squamous cell head and neck cancers, melanoma), cardiovascular diseases, autoimmune diseases (rheumatoid arthritis, systemic lupus erythematosus, multiple sclerosis), inflammatory bowel diseases, dry eye disease

(Continued)

TABLE 8.2 (*Continued*)
Different Types of Ligands Used for Targeting in Drug Delivery

Ligand Type	Receptor Molecule	Location	Action Mechanism	Example	Associated Diseases
Aptamers nucleic acid	Nucleolin, PSMA, tenascin-C, VEGF, PDGF-beta, thrombin, factor VIIa, ATP	Cancer cell surface, nucleus, extracellular matrix, intracellular	Specific binding, inhibition of protein activity, conformational changes, induction of autophagy, targeted transport	AS1411 (anti-nucleolin), GBI-10 (anti-tenascin-C), Macugen (anti-VEGFR), DNA aptamers (e.g., anti-PSMA), RNA aptamers (e.g., anti-VEGFR)	Cancer, diseases with abnormal neovascularization (ocular disorders, diabetes, multiple sclerosis)
Protein domain	VEGF receptor, integrin $\alpha v\beta 3$, EGFR, HER2, CD40, zinc fingers, kinase domain	Cancer cell surface, intracellular	Specific binding, conformational changes, dimerization, allosteric inhibition, zinc ejection, modulation of protein function	FN3-based ligands (monobody), Z domain–based ligands (affibody), DARPin-based ligands, transferrin, neurotoxin, histidine-rich glycoprotein (HRGP330)	Cancer, neurodegenerative diseases

hydrazone, or disulfide bonds that degrade under specific physiological conditions, particularly within acidic or reductive environments. For instance, pH-sensitive linkers remain stable in systemic circulation but cleave within the acidic microenvironment of tumors or endosomes, ensuring spatiotemporally controlled release of the drug. This responsiveness enhances intracellular trafficking and therapeutic selectivity. To further improve targeting precision, dual-ligand functionalization has emerged as an advanced strategy. In this design, two different ligands are conjugated to the same NC, one for cell surface recognition and the other for subcellular organelle targeting. For example, a NC may utilize FA or transferrin to bind receptors overexpressed on cancer cell membranes (facilitating uptake), while a second ligand such as triphenylphosphonium (TPP) directs the carrier to mitochondria, lysosome-targeting peptides guide delivery to degradative compartments, or nuclear localization signal (NLS) peptides promote nuclear transport. This dual-targeting approach integrates cellular- and organelle-level precision, enhancing therapeutic outcomes while minimizing off-target toxicity, a critical advancement in the development of next-generation TDDS [15].

In essence, ligand–receptor interactions serve as the molecular foundation of targeted drug delivery, dictating specificity, selectivity, and efficiency. Through strategic ligand design, receptor recognition, and fine-tuned conjugation chemistry, NCs can achieve controlled, site-specific, and intracellular delivery of therapeutics. Emerging innovations in ligand engineering such as dual-targeting and stimuli-responsive linkers continue to elevate the precision and efficacy of nanomedicine, bringing TDDS closer to clinical realization in personalized cancer therapy and beyond.

8.5 TUMOR-DIRECTED DELIVERY: PASSIVE AND ACTIVE STRATEGIES

The advancement of nanomedicine in cancer therapy is fundamentally driven by a unique biological hallmark feature of solid tumors known as the EPR effect. This phenomenon describes the enhanced localization of nanoscale therapeutics within tumor tissues relative to normal counterparts and serves as the biological basis for passive tumor targeting (Figure 8.3). Although the EPR effect exhibits certain limitations, it remains a central concept guiding the design and optimization of NC-based DDSs. Conventional chemotherapeutic agents are often limited by nonspecific biodistribution, rapid systemic clearance, and severe off-target toxicity. Nanomedicine seeks to address these drawbacks by enabling site-specific drug accumulation and controlled release, thereby improving therapeutic efficacy and reducing systemic side effects. The EPR effect underpins this selectivity by exploiting distinct structural and physiological abnormalities inherent to tumor vasculature [16].

In healthy tissues, blood vessels are characterized by a tight endothelial barrier, supported by pericytes and a well-organized basement membrane. These components tightly regulate the transvascular movement of macromolecules, maintaining homeostasis and minimizing leakage. In contrast, the vasculature of tumor tissues is profoundly aberrant. The rapid and disordered angiogenesis associated with tumor growth driven by regulatory growth proteins such as vascular endothelial growth factor (VEGF), fibroblast growth factor, and platelet-derived growth factor (PDGF)

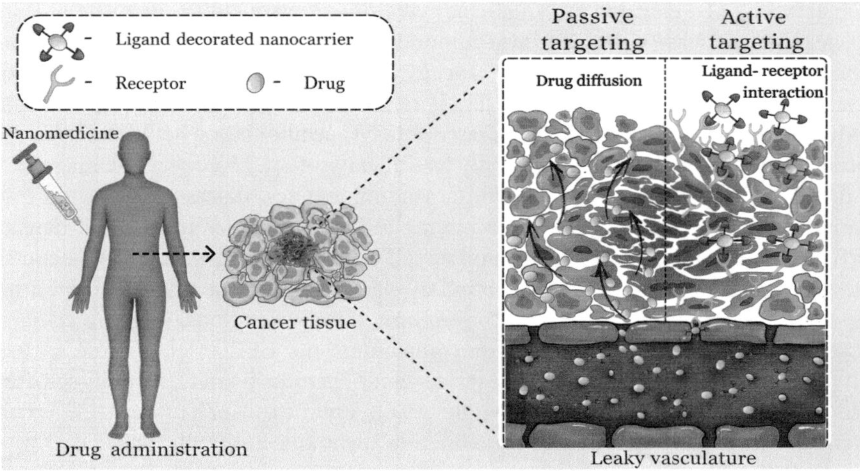

FIGURE 8.3 Schematic representation of passive and active targeting mechanisms of nanocarriers in cancer therapy, enhancing cellular uptake and localized drug delivery.

produces dilated, tortuous vessels with incomplete endothelial linings and discontinuous basement membranes. These irregularities create inter-endothelial gaps ranging from 100 nm to several micrometers, allowing NCs to readily extravasate into the tumor interstitium.

An equally critical factor contributing to the EPR effect is the deficiency of functional lymphatic drainage within tumors. While normal tissues efficiently clear excess macromolecules and interstitial fluid via an intact lymphatic network, tumor tissues lack effective lymphatic clearance. Consequently, once NCs infiltrate the tumor microenvironment, they remain retained for extended durations, leading to progressive accumulation. Collectively, these two features leaky vasculature (enhanced permeability) and impaired lymphatic drainage (retention) constitute the mechanistic basis of the EPR effect. When NC-based drugs are administered intravenously, their biodistribution and therapeutic success depend primarily on circulation time and vascular accessibility. NCs that evade rapid clearance by the RES or renal filtration remain in systemic circulation long enough to exploit the vascular abnormalities characteristic of tumors. To prolong blood residence time and minimize immune recognition, surface modification strategies, particularly PEGylation, are widely utilized. The efficiency of EPR-mediated accumulation further depends on NC size, surface charge, hydrophobicity, and stability. Particles that are too small (<10 nm) are typically filtered by the kidneys, whereas larger particles (>200 nm) are sequestered by the liver and spleen. Thus, an optimal balance often within the 50–150 nm range is essential to maximize tumor penetration while minimizing off-target accumulation.

Once within the tumor microenvironment, NCs undergo passive targeting, wherein they accumulate in the tumor tissue without requiring specific ligand–receptor interactions. These NCs may then release their therapeutic payloads either gradually by diffusion or via some external factors responsive to local microenvironmental stimuli, such as acidic pH, elevated enzymatic activity, or oxidative stress. This site-specific and regulated release enhances intra-tumoral drug concentration, reduces systemic exposure, and improves therapeutic efficacy compared to conventional chemotherapy. Despite its promise, the EPR effect is not universally consistent. Experimental studies have demonstrated that the difference in NC accumulation between tumor and normal tissues is often modest, typically less than two-fold. Moreover, the magnitude of the EPR effect varies significantly across tumor types, disease stages, and even spatial regions within a single tumor, owing to heterogeneities in vascular density, perfusion rate, and interstitial fluid pressure. These factors can restrict NC penetration and hinder uniform drug distribution throughout the tumor mass, thereby limiting overall therapeutic outcomes. To overcome these limitations, ongoing research focuses on strategies that enhance or complement the EPR effect. These include active targeting approaches employing receptor-specific ligands, stimuli-sensitive delivery systems that release therapeutic agents upon exposure to tumor microenvironmental factors, and vascular modulation techniques aimed at normalizing or transiently increasing tumor vessel permeability. Such combinatorial strategies aim to achieve more predictable and efficient NC delivery [17].

Clinically, several nanomedicines have successfully exploited the EPR effect for improved tumor targeting. Among them, Doxil® (PEGylated liposomal doxorubicin) remains one of the most notable examples, demonstrating prolonged circulation, reduced cardiotoxicity, and enhanced tumor accumulation compared to free doxorubicin. Although the efficacy of EPR-based delivery varies between patients and tumor types, the phenomenon continues to serve as a cornerstone during the development of nanomedicine for tumor targeted therapy and a guiding principle in developing next-generation, adaptive DDSs.

8.6 IN VITRO MODELS USED IN DRUG DELIVERY: A QUICK VALIDATION OF NANOCARRIER FORMULATIONS

In the recent decades, drug delivery has progressed through biomedical engineering and technology-driven innovations that result in enhanced drug efficiency and stability. Drug delivery intends to manage the pharmacokinetics of the drug through three levels of body, i.e., tissue, cellular, and organelle level, thereby facilitating optimized drug delivery. These developments have led to better therapeutic outcomes and have improved quality of life by addressing challenges such as poor solubility, limited bioavailability, and premature degradation. These levels address the distinct biological barriers and opportunities to improve drug localization and action. Tissue-level targeting (level 1) responds to the passive strategy of targeting, which facilitates enhanced accumulation of NCs with drugs within the cancer tissues. The targeting strategy at this level is primarily based on physiological difference between healthy and cancer cells driven by the EPR effect. These leaky vasculatures along with the lymphatic drainage leads to reduced clearance of macromolecules from the interstitial space. The combination of these characteristics facilitates the targeted NC to extravasate from the systemic circulation into the cancer cells and undergo prolonged vascular retention. However, in normal tissues, their integrity remains intact and efficient lymphatic drainage shows no accumulation. Furthermore, the tissue-level delivery system utilizes unique physiochemical characteristics of tumors like acidic tumor microenvironment to enhance drug localization in the cancer tissues. The cellular-level targeting or level 2 is based on the phenomenon of active targeting. It involves directing DDS toward specific cellular population. This strategy is achieved through surface modification of the NC with specific ligands for recognition of overexpressed cellular receptors on the cancer cells. These recognition elements comprise monoclonal antibodies, peptides, aptamers, or small-molecule ligands such as folate, cRGD, or transferrin. Ligand–receptor interaction is followed by RME for selective uptake of NCs by the cancer cells. This cellular-level targeting enhances the therapeutic index, which leads to maximizing efficacy and reducing off-target toxicity. At the subcellular-level NC delivers drug inside specific organelles or compartment within the target cell. Upon internalization by the target cell, it localizes within the endosome through endocytosis. The strategies for subcellular targeting involve designing NC that can escape endosomes or those which can incorporate specific localization signals like nucleus- or mitochondria-targeting ligands to guide the drug to its final destination. To further enhance the targeting strategy through ligand decoration and surface modification, it offers dual-ligand decoration on the surface of single DDS. In this, the two ligands target different receptors on the same cell. Ligand 1 (e.g., FA for FR overexpressed on the cancer cells, transferrin for overexpressed transferrin receptors, etc.) targets the receptors on the cell surface and enhances cellular uptake into the target cell. Alternatively, ligand 2 directs the internalized carrier toward specific organelle. These ligands are small molecules or peptides with characteristic features to target organelle. Cellular organelles like mitochondrion are typically targeted with lipophilic cations like TPP, lysosome through peptide that interacts with its membrane protein and nucleus is targeted via NLS peptide. Therefore, dual targeting strategy contributes to the overall cellular targeting and holds immense priority for TDD, particularly for organelle-targeted therapies with fewer side effects. Effective subcellular targeting is essential for optimizing the therapeutic efficacy and to ensure localization at specific site of action within the cell rather than being degraded or isolated in active vesicles.

To evaluate this targeted delivery strategy, various in vitro models are used. Models like 2D cell culture offer controlled environment for mechanistic studies of cellular uptake and trafficking and 3D spheroid models offer accurate replica of the in vitro tumor microenvironment. These 3D models, especially multicellular tumor spheroids, offer advanced experimental platforms that mimic the structural formation, physiological behavior, and tumor microenvironment of solid tumor in vitro. Traditional 2D monolayer cell cultures provide preliminary cytotoxicity assessment but fail to capture the intricate cell interactions, nutrients, and oxygen gradients along with drug diffusion. In contrast, 3D models mimic physiological features such as hypoxia, acidic pH, and nutrient deprivation that affect cell proliferation, kinetics, gene regulation, and drug response. A spheroid generally consists of an outer proliferation zone, middle quiescent layer, and a necrotic core which mimics the heterogenicity found in vascular tumor region. This spheroid configuration facilitates realistic evaluation of drug diffusion, by passing barriers, oxygen, nutrient gradient, and metabolic zonation which provides critical insights into the distribution, transport, and physiological behavior of the NC with solid tumor. The characteristic features of 3D models provide quantitative assessment of NCs, internalization, endosomal release, intracellular trafficking, and cytotoxic potency which provides insights prior to in vitro validation or animal experimentation. From an ethical point of view, 3D models provide 3Rs—replacement, reduction, and refinement, which reduces the dependence on animal studies, reducing research cost and high-throughput screening of drug formulations. Apart from the limitations like long-term stability, batch variability, and standardization difficulties, the ongoing advancements like microfluidics tumor-on-a chip have extended the physiological accuracy of 3D models. Therefore, the 3D in vitro spheroid models provide an indispensable bridge between 2D cell culture and in vivo animal models, which provides a biomimetic reproducible and ethically sustainable platform for tumor biology, nanomedicine research, and personalized cancer therapy treatment [18,19].

8.7 APPLICATIONS OF NANOCARRIERS BEYOND CANCER THERAPY

Beyond oncology, NC has demonstrated remarkable potential in the diagnosis, management, and mitigation of several noncancerous diseases, including neurodegenerative, cardiovascular, and infectious disorders. By exploiting the unique physicochemical properties of nanoscale materials, NCs enhances drug delivery precision, improves therapeutic efficacy, and minimizes systemic toxicity across a broad spectrum of pathological conditions.

8.7.1 Nanomedicine in Neurodegenerative Disorders

One of the most significant applications of nanomedicine lies in the management of neurodegenerative diseases, where it addresses the long-standing challenge of therapeutic delivery to the central nervous system (CNS). The primary limitation in treating CNS disorders is the BBB, a highly selective physiological barrier that limits the entry of therapeutic molecules into brain tissue.

Engineered NCs, typically with diameters around 100 nm, have shown the ability to traverse the BBB by leveraging their optimized size, surface chemistry, and adaptability. This innovation has enabled progress in the management of neurodegenerative diseases like Alzheimer's disease and Parkinson's disease, where site-specific drug delivery within distinct brain regions is essential. Various nanomaterials such as biologically engineered NCs, liposomal NCs, polymeric micelles, and quantum dots are currently under investigation to enhance CNS drug penetration. These advanced TDDSs improve drug pharmacokinetics, enable sustained release, and facilitate region-specific modulation of disease pathways, including inhibition of protein aggregation, delivery of neuroprotective agents, and modulation of oxidative stress in neural tissues. Collectively, nanomedicine offers a transformative strategy to overcome BBB-associated barriers and improve therapeutic outcomes in neurodegenerative disorders.

8.7.2 Nanomedicine in Cardiovascular Diseases

Heart and vascular diseases continue to be a predominant cause of death globally, and nanomedicine offers innovative tools for diagnosis, targeted treatment, and real-time monitoring. NC-mediated TDD has proven effective in managing disorders such as atherosclerosis, restenosis, and myocardial infarction, where localized drug deposition is essential to prevent systemic toxicity. Perfluorocarbon-based NCs have emerged as efficient platforms for targeted imaging and therapy, facilitating precise localization and controlled release of cardiovascular drugs. Additionally, nanocoated drug-eluting stents have significantly improved the efficacy and safety of vascular interventions by reducing restenosis and enhancing re-reendothelialization.

Nanomedicine also plays a crucial role in mitigating drug-induced cardiotoxicity, such as that caused by anthracycline-based chemotherapeutics like doxorubicin. Moreover, the development of nano-biosensors has revolutionized cardiovascular diagnostics by enabling high affinity and specificity–based detection of cardiac biomarkers, thereby improving early disease diagnosis and prognosis monitoring. Collectively, nanomedicine in cardiology offers a powerful framework for precise diagnostics, targeted therapy, and improved clinical outcomes.

8.7.3 Nanomedicine in Infectious Diseases

Nanomedicine has also emerged as a promising approach in combating infectious diseases caused by bacteria, viruses, and fungi. The distinctive physical properties, including magnetic, optical, and electrical traits of NCs facilitate rapid and selective detection of pathogens, enhancing diagnostic accuracy and speed. A variety of NC platforms including polymeric micelles, liposomes, lipid-based NCs, and dendrimers have been designed to improve the pharmacokinetic and pharmacodynamic profiles of antimicrobial agents. These systems enhance solubility, stability, absorption, and controlled release, addressing the major limitations of conventional antimicrobial therapies, such as drug resistance, dose-dependent toxicity, and poor biodistribution. Nanomedicine provides promising solutions to multidrug-resistant infections, enabling targeted delivery across biological barriers, prolonged systemic circulation, and reduced adverse effects. Injectable NC-based antiretroviral formulations have improved HIV management by reducing dosing frequency and improving therapeutic adherence, while also serving as potential prophylactic interventions. In vaccine development, NC systems have played a transformative role. Cationic lipid NCs, for instance, served as the delivery vehicles for mRNA-based COVID-19 vaccines, demonstrating the clinical viability of nanotechnology in vaccinology. Beyond vaccine delivery, nanomedicine also exhibits intrinsic antimicrobial activity, and is capable of inducing oxidative stress, releasing metal ions, and disrupting microbial membranes. These mechanisms provide novel means to overcome antibiotic resistance and enhance antimicrobial efficacy.

Thus, nanomedicine represents a multifunctional and transformative platform for the management of infectious diseases integrating pathogen detection, targeted therapy, vaccine design, and antimicrobial action. Through these synergistic mechanisms, NC-based systems offer a next-generation solution to global infectious disease challenges, supporting both precision medicine and public health resilience [20].

8.8 ROADMAP FOR CLINICAL TRANSLATION

The successful clinical transition of NCs into real-world therapeutics, i.e., bench to clinical application is a complex, multistage process that requires rigorous preclinical validation, strategic clinical trial design, and meticulous navigation through regulatory frameworks. Unlike conventional small-molecule therapeutics, NCs face unique translational challenges stemming from their structural complexity, formulation diversity, and novel mechanisms of action.

The translational journey begins with robust preclinical research aimed at establishing the safety, efficacy, and predictability of nanomedicines before advancing to human studies. This stage demands comprehensive characterization of physicochemical properties including particle size, morphology, surface charge, and chemical modification, since these attributes critically determine biodistribution, pharmacokinetics, and therapeutic efficacy. Preclinical studies employ appropriate animal models and advanced in vitro systems, such as patient-derived organoids and organ-on-chip platforms, which more accurately replicate human physiology and tissue-level interactions. Such models provide valuable insights into NC behavior, including systemic circulation, stability, and target tissue interactions.

In this phase, safety, biodistribution, pharmacokinetics, and proof-of-concept efficacy must be demonstrated to support an Investigational New Drug (IND), filing with the regulatory authorities like the U.S. Food and Drug Administration (FDA). Following IND approval, clinical development progresses through phased human trials, where nanomedicines are evaluated for safety, toxicity, dose optimization, and therapeutic effectiveness in patient populations. To enhance in vivo performance, surface engineering strategies such as PEGylation, zwitterionic coatings, and biomimetic camouflage are often applied to minimize immune-mediated clearance and enhanced systemic circulation, ensuring that NCs reach their intended targets efficiently. The incorporation of Quality by Design (QbD) along with essential parameters during the design of formulation enables systematic control over key parameters, improving reproducibility and facilitating large-scale manufacturing. This approach also ensures that NCs maintain stability and desired bioactivity in the final formulation. A significant bottleneck in clinical translation lies in verifying the biocompatibility and biodegradability of NCs. Metallic, carbon-based, and polymeric NCs must demonstrate minimal cytotoxicity and negligible accumulation in vital organs. Chronic exposure studies are required to assess potential immunogenicity and inflammatory responses. Continuous surface optimization through hydrophilic coatings can mitigate these risks while improving pharmacological profiles [21].

Following preclinical validation, regulatory alignment and standardization become critical. Early consultation with the governing authorities like the FDA and the European Medicines Agency helps clarify data requirements, acceptable quality parameters, and testing standards. Implementation of Good Manufacturing Practice–like procedures during research and development (R&D) promotes scalability and compliance, reducing delays during clinical trials. Regulatory focus is placed on critical quality attributes, which includes factors like particle size, surface chemistry, drug encapsulation efficiency, and stability, all of which determine product consistency and patient safety. Globally, organizations such as CEN, ISO, ASTM, and VAMAS are working toward harmonizing testing methods and reference materials for nanomedicines. While global standardization remains fragmented, initiatives such as "The International Standardization Roadmap for Nanomedicine" have begun establishing unified frameworks for quality assurance and safety evaluation. The adoption of well-defined standard operating procedures at the laboratory level ensures data reproducibility and fosters regulatory confidence, key prerequisites for patient safety, and clinical acceptance.

Personalized nanomedicine represents the next frontier in clinical translation. Tailoring nanoscale therapeutics to an individual's genetic makeup, tumor microenvironment, and metabolic profile integrates nanotechnology with genomic and proteomic data, leading to precision therapies that adapt to patient-specific pathophysiology. Patient variability, particularly in metabolism, immune response, and disease microenvironment, profoundly affects NC performance and must be incorporated into clinical design.

In essence, translating nanomedicine into clinical reality requires a balance between innovation and regulatory discipline. The process extends beyond material design to include rigorous preclinical validation, safety assurance, scalable manufacturing, and precision personalization. Only through this integrated framework can nanomedicine evolve from experimental potential to clinically reliable, patient-ready therapeutic solutions.

8.9 MARKET ACCEPTANCE

Alongside clinical translation, the market acceptance of nanomedicine represents a defining factor in its integration into mainstream healthcare. Despite offering superior therapeutic precision and patient outcomes compared to conventional treatments, widespread adoption is constrained by manufacturing complexity, regulatory cost, and economic scalability. The financial dynamics of nanomedicine are multifaceted, encompassing expenses related to R&D, production, and comparative cost-effectiveness relative to traditional therapies. While nanomedicine aims to achieve enhanced therapeutic efficacy and reduced side effects, its high development costs remain a critical barrier to market penetration. The design and production of nanoscale formulations require extensive interdisciplinary collaboration, integrating nanotechnology, materials science, and biotechnology, and necessitating deep understanding of nano–bio interactions, biodistribution, immunogenicity, and long-term toxicity. Each of these factors contributes substantially to elevated R&D expenditure.

Moreover, clinical trials for nanomedicines, though often shorter or more targeted than those for biologics, still represent a major financial commitment. Recent analyses indicate that the average cost of nanomedicine clinical trials corresponds to approximately 47% of that for biologics or new molecular entities within comparable timeframes. This cost efficiency is partially attributed to nanomedicine's inherent ability to improve drug delivery, widen therapeutic windows, and reduce adverse events, thereby streamlining development cycles. Nevertheless, high upfront investment, combined with uncertainty surrounding long-term clinical benefits and reimbursement models, continues to restrict broad market adoption. Addressing these economic challenges requires advances in material synthesis and scalable production technologies. Emerging methods such as simple conjugation chemistries, microfluidic synthesis, and continuous manufacturing have shown promise in reducing production costs while maintaining product quality and reproducibility. The integration of QbD principles further enhances process consistency and regulatory compliance. Despite current economic hurdles, nanomedicine continues to represent a paradigm shift in precision therapeutics offering a balance between clinical efficacy and financial feasibility. Ongoing efforts to streamline manufacturing, reduce costs, and improve scalability are expected to expand accessibility and foster greater confidence among stakeholders, including clinicians, patients, and regulatory agencies.

Ultimately, the market success of nanomedicine will depend on the convergence of scientific innovation, cost-effective production, and clear reimbursement strategies. By leveraging cutting-edge synthesis technologies and market-driven optimization, nanomedicine stands poised to transform modern healthcare with affordable, targeted, and high-efficacy therapeutic solutions.

8.10 CONCLUSION

Nanomedicine has emerged as a transformative paradigm in the field of TDDSs, offering innovative strategies to address the challenges inherent in the conventional therapeutics. By addressing these drawbacks related to poor bioavailability, systemic toxicity, and inadequate target specificity, nanomedicine has redefined the landscape of precision medicine. Among its many advancements, ligand–receptor-mediated targeting represents a pivotal breakthrough, enabling functionalized NCs to selectively identify and interact with the target receptors highly expressed on diseased cells. This specific interaction facilitates enhanced cellular uptake, minimizes off-target effects, and markedly improves therapeutic efficacy. When integrated with the passive localization pathways, particularly the EPR phenomenon, nanomedicine achieves exceptional precision in drug localization and controlled release, surpassing the capabilities of traditional formulations. Furthermore, diverse NC platforms including liposomes, polymeric NCs, dendrimers, solid lipid NCs, MNCs, and carbon-based nanostructures offer unique physicochemical advantages such as structural stability, high drug-loading capacity, and tunable surface functionality. Beyond drug delivery, many of these systems also exhibit theranostics potential, combining diagnostic imaging with therapeutic intervention to facilitate real-time tracking of therapeutic response.

REFERENCES

1. A. Tewabe, A. Abate, M. Tamrie, A. Seyfu, E. Abdela Siraj, Targeted drug delivery—from magic bullet to nanomedicine: principles, challenges, and future perspectives, *Journal of Multidisciplinary Healthcare*, 14(2021) 1711–24.
2. M. Hashida, Role of pharmacokinetic consideration for the development of drug delivery systems: a historical overview, *Advanced Drug Delivery Reviews*, 157(2020) 71–82.
3. Y.H. Bae, K. Park, Targeted drug delivery to tumors: myths, reality and possibility, *Journal of Controlled Release*, 153(2011) 198–205.
4. F. Farooque, M. Wasi, M.M. Mughees, Liposomes as drug delivery system: an updated review, *Journal of Drug Delivery and Therapeutics*, 11(2021) 149–58.
5. M. Ghosh, U. Dasgupta, S. Barman, A. Ray, B.P. Chatterjee, A. Chakraborty, et al., Cancer cell detection and precision targeting drug delivery by covalently functionalized liposome, *ACS Applied Bio Materials*, 8(2025) 8285–96.
6. S. Barman, S.M. Roy, P. Kishore, M. Ghosh, P. Bag, A.K. Sarkar, et al., Concurrent targeted delivery of doxorubicin and curcumin to the cancer cells using simple and versatile ligand-installed multifaceted chitosan-based nanoconjugates, *Journal of Materials Chemistry B*, 13(2025) 2490–503.

7. A.R. Maity, N.R. Jana, Chitosan–cholesterol-based cellular delivery of anionic nanoparticles, *The Journal of Physical Chemistry C*, 115(2011) 137–44.
8. A.K. Sarkar, S. Jana, G. Kaur, H. Arora, S. Barman, N. Mukherjee, et al., Chemically designed functional nanomicelles for blood–brain barrier crossing, *Nano Letters*, 25(2025).
9. S. Saha, R. Kar, K. Sikder, D. Manna, R.R. Pal, S. Chakraborti, et al., Deciphering the inhibitory mechanism of antimicrobial peptide pexiganan conjugated with sodium-alginate chitosan-cholesterol nanoparticle against the opportunistic pathogen *Acinetobacter baumannii*, *Journal of Drug Delivery Science and Technology*, 101(2024) 106305.
10. S. Parveen, R. Misra, S.K. Sahoo, Nanoparticles: a boon to drug delivery, therapeutics, diagnostics and imaging, *Nanomedicine in Cancer*, L. Balogh (ed.), Taylor & Francis, 2017, pp. 47–98.
11. H. Zare, S. Ahmadi, A. Ghasemi, M. Ghanbari, N. Rabiee, M. Bagherzadeh, et al., Carbon nanotubes: Smart drug/gene delivery carriers, *International Journal of Nanomedicine*, (2021) 1681–706.
12. A.R. Maity, D. Stepensky, Delivery of drugs to intracellular organelles using drug delivery systems: analysis of research trends and targeting efficiencies, *International Journal of Pharmaceutics*, 496(2015) 268–74.
13. S.M. Roy, V. Garg, S.P. Sivaraman, S. Barman, C. Ghosh, P. Bag, et al., Overcoming the barriers of nuclear-targeted drug delivery using nanomedicine-based strategies for enhanced anticancer therapy, *Journal of Drug Delivery Science and Technology*, 83(2023) 104408.
14. S.M. Roy, S. Barman, A. Basu, T. Ghatak, S.K. Pore, S.K. Ghosh, et al., Amine as a bottom-line functionality on DDS surface for efficient endosomal escape and further subcellular targets, *Journal of Drug Delivery Science and Technology*, 71(2022) 103303.
15. P. Kishore, S. Barman, R. Dey, A. Jana, M. Ghosh, P. Bag, et al., Delivering drugs to cancer cells and inside the mitochondria using a dual-ligand installed targeted drug delivery system, *ACS Applied Nano Materials*, 8(2025) 19668–78.
16. A.R. Maity, D. Stepensky, Limited efficiency of drug delivery to specific intracellular organelles using subcellularly "targeted" drug delivery systems, *Molecular Pharmaceutics*, 13(2016) 1–7.
17. S. Maitra Roy, S. Barman, P. Kishore, B. Chatterjee, P. Bag, T. Ghatak, et al., Acidic pH-triggered release of doxorubicin from ligand-decorated polymeric micelles potentiates efficacy against cancer cells, *ACS Applied Nano Materials*, 6(2023) 18988–98.
18. S.M. Roy, P. Kishore, D. Saha, P. Ghosh, R. Kar, S. Barman, et al., 3D multicellular tumor spheroids used for in vitro preclinical therapeutic screening, *Journal of Drug Delivery Science and Technology*, 86(2023) 104636.
19. S.M. Roy, V. Garg, S. Barman, C. Ghosh, A.R. Maity, S.K. Ghosh, Kinetics of nanomedicine in tumor spheroid as an in vitro model system for efficient tumor-targeted drug delivery with insights from mathematical models, *Frontiers in Bioengineering and Biotechnology*, 9(2021) 785937.
20. S. Barman, A. Chakraborty, S. Saha, K. Sikder, S. Maitra Roy, B. Modi, et al., Efficient synergistic antibacterial activity of α-MSH using chitosan-based versatile nanoconjugates, *ACS Omega*, 8(2023) 12865–77.
21. K. Abdullah, G. Sharma, A.P. Singh, J.A. Siddiqui, Nanomedicine in cancer therapeutics: current perspectives from bench to bedside, *Molecular Cancer*, 24(2025) 169.

9 Nano-Medicinal Applications

Doddy Irawan Setyo Utomo

9.1 INTRODUCTION

Nanomedicine has rapidly emerged as one of the most transformative frontiers in modern healthcare, offering solutions that were once considered unachievable with conventional medicine. Unlike traditional drugs or diagnostic tools, many nanomaterials can be engineered to cross biological barriers, deliver therapeutic agents with subcellular precision, and provide real-time monitoring of biological processes. This convergence of nanotechnology with medicine has given rise to a wide spectrum of applications, ranging from targeted drug delivery and regenerative medicine to neural therapeutics and point-of-care (POC) diagnostics. One of the most promising areas of nanomedicine lies in stem cell research and tissue engineering, where nanoparticles and nanostructured scaffolds not only enable precise tracking of stem cells after transplantation but also provide extracellular matrix (ECM)-like cues that direct their differentiation into specific lineages. In regenerative medicine, nanofibrous scaffolds designed through electrospinning or self-assembly mimic natural tissue environments, enhancing cell adhesion, proliferation, and repair. Nanomaterial-based approaches are now widely explored for bone, vascular, and neural tissue regeneration, where conductive or bioactive nanostructures stimulate osteogenesis, angiogenesis, or neuronal signaling. At the same time, nanomedicine is playing a crucial role in addressing neurological disorders, a field long limited by the impermeability of the blood–brain barrier (BBB). Parallel advances in gene therapy have leveraged nanocarriers like dendrimers, liposomes, and gold nanoparticles (AuNPs) for the safe and targeted delivery of nucleic acids, including small interfering RNA (siRNA) and CRISPR systems. Additionally, from quantum dot (QD)-based multiplex assays and AuNP–enhanced lateral flow strips to lab-on-a-chip microfluidic devices, these platforms enable rapid detection of disease biomarkers, early diagnosis, and personalized treatment strategies. Such technologies are particularly impactful in low-resource settings, where conventional diagnostic infrastructure may be limited.

Nanomedicine integrates therapeutic, diagnostic, and regenerative approaches at the nanoscale, opening pathways toward precision medicine, improved patient outcomes, and sustainable healthcare systems. As schematically presented in Figure 9.1, this chapter reviews key advances in stem cell engineering, regenerative scaffolds, tissue repair, neurological therapeutics, diagnostics, and biosensors, while also considering the regulatory and ethical landscapes that shape their future.

DOI: 10.1201/9781003725930-9

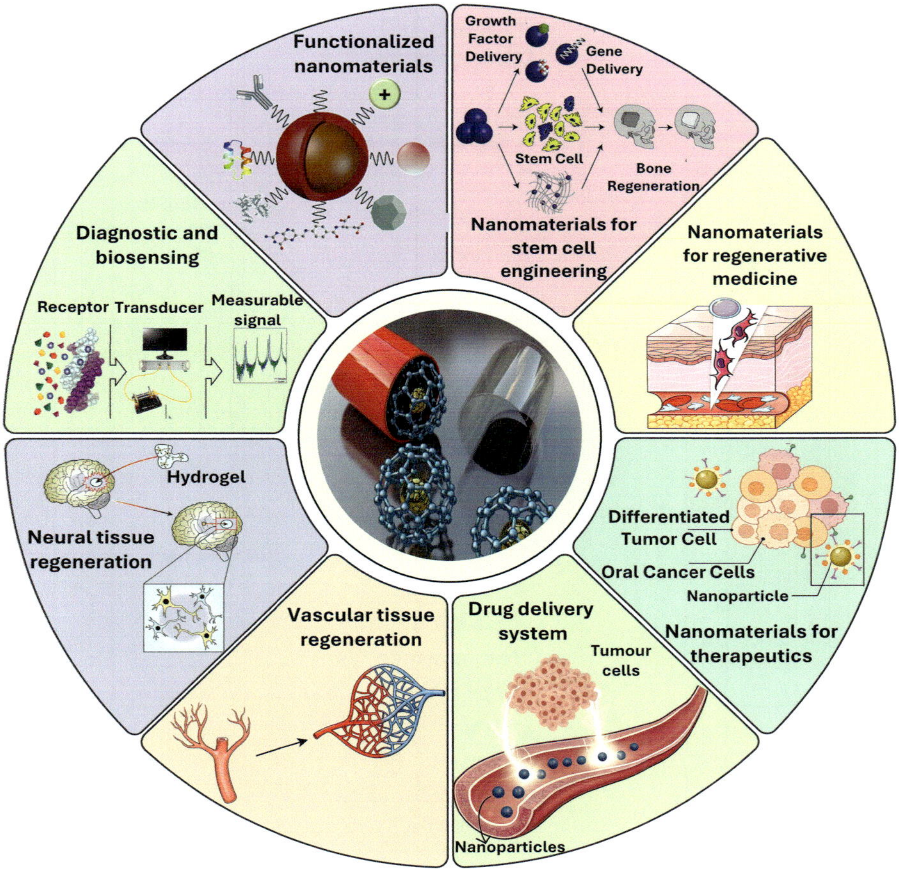

FIGURE 9.1 Overview of functionalized nanomaterials and their multifunctional roles in nanomedicine.

9.2 NANOMATERIALS FOR STEM CELL RESEARCH AND ENGINEERING

Stem cell research and regenerative medicine rely heavily on the ability to track, control, and guide stem cell behavior after transplantation. Two key areas (Figure 9.2) where nanomaterials play a transformative role are tracking transplanted stem cells in vivo to monitor their migration, survival, and integration, and creating nano-engineered environments that mimic the ECM to direct their controlled differentiation into functional cell lineages.

9.2.1 Nanoparticle-Based Stem Cell Tracking

Tracking stem cells in vivo is crucial to ensure their therapeutic efficacy and safety. Nanoparticles have become indispensable tools for this purpose because of their

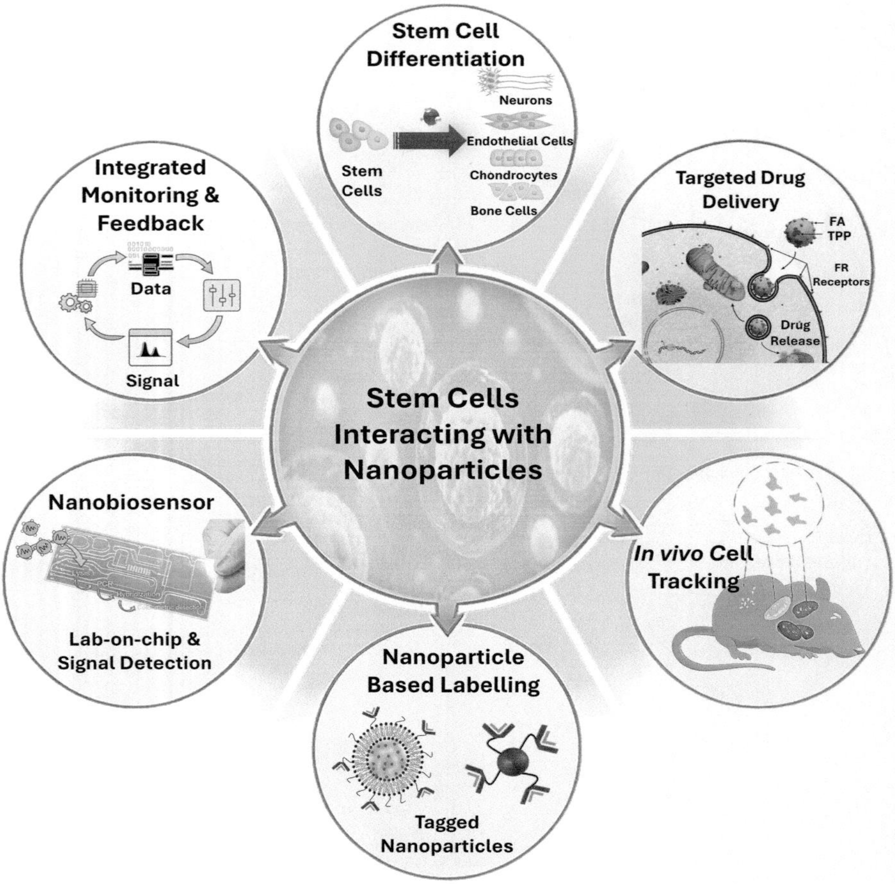

FIGURE 9.2 Stem cells interfacing with nanomaterials for sensing, tracking, differentiation, and therapeutic control.

unique optical, magnetic, and acoustic properties. QDs are colloidal semiconductor nanocrystals that exhibit size-tunable fluorescence, high photostability, and broad excitation with narrow emission spectra, offering distinct advantages over traditional fluorophores. QDs made of cadmium selenide, cadmium sulfide, or indium phosphide can be tuned to emit across a wide spectral range (525–800 nm), enabling multiplex imaging of different stem cell populations using a single excitation source. For example, embryonic stem cells labeled with QDs of varying sizes can be simultaneously tracked within a host organism, offering insight into how different cell lineages migrate and differentiate in vivo. However, the reliance on heavy metals in conventional QDs poses cytotoxicity risks, including disruption of cell viability and embryonic development, which limits their clinical translation due to long-term toxicity and regulatory concerns. Superparamagnetic iron oxide nanoparticles (SPIOs) have been extensively explored for stem cell tracking due to their ability to act as strong contrast agents in magnetic resonance imaging (MRI). When coated with biocompatible polymers such as dextran, chitosan, or gelatin, SPIOs show improved stability and cellular uptake. Mesenchymal stem cells (MSCs) labeled with dextran-coated SPIOs have been tracked in vivo to evaluate homing efficiency in injured tissues. However, challenges such as poor endocytosis, generation of reactive oxygen species (ROS), and toxicity potentially arising from iron ion release following nanoparticle degradation. Strategies such as coating SPIOs with poly-L-lysine or gold shells have been used to reduce toxicity and enhance MRI contrast. Dual labeling approaches combining SPIOs with gadolinium chelates have further improved tracking accuracy, allowing live and dead stem cells to be distinguished during MRI imaging [1]. AuNPs offer another versatile platform for stem cell tracking, particularly in photoacoustic imaging. A dual system has been developed in which MSCs were labeled with gold nanorods, while macrophages were labeled with gold nanospheres. Because nanorods absorb strongly in the near-infrared region, while nanospheres exhibit distinct scattering properties, the two cell types could be distinguished in vivo using photoacoustic signals. This approach was especially useful in cardiac ischemia studies, where both transplanted MSCs and infiltrating macrophages needed to be tracked simultaneously to assess immunological responses. The unique shape- and size-dependent optical properties of AuNPs thus make them highly attractive for monitoring stem cell therapy outcomes, although long-term retention and potential accumulation in tissues still pose safety concerns.

9.2.2 Nanomaterial-Aided Stem Cell Differentiation

Beyond tracking, nanomaterials also play a critical role in guiding stem cell fate by recreating the complex biochemical and mechanical cues of the ECM. In vivo, stem cell differentiation is regulated by ECM proteins such as collagen, fibronectin, and laminin, as well as by local mechanical stiffness and nanoscale topography. Conventional tissue culture plates fail to provide these cues, but nanomaterials through engineered scaffolds, fibers, and coatings can replicate ECM-like environments that influence stem cell adhesion, cytoskeletal tension, and lineage-specific differentiation. Nanofibrous scaffolds and hydrogels are widely employed to mimic ECM architecture. For example, neural crest stem cells cultured on nanofibrous polymer scaffolds coated with hydrogels exhibited distinct differentiation patterns: cells adjacent to the stiffer nanofibers differentiated into smooth muscle cells, while those embedded within the softer hydrogel differentiated into glial cells. Atomic force microscopy–based measurements demonstrated that stem cells respond to local stiffness gradients through integrin-mediated signaling, highlighting how nanoscale mechanics can dictate cell fate [2].

Hydroxyapatite (HAP) nanoparticles incorporated into polycaprolactone (PCL) scaffolds have been shown to promote osteogenic differentiation for bone tissue engineering [3]. Interestingly, the morphology of the HAP nanoparticles strongly influenced outcomes: needle-shaped HAP nanoparticles enhanced mechanical properties and osteoblast differentiation more effectively than spherical or rod-shaped HAP particles. This illustrates how subtle differences in nanoparticle geometry can be exploited to fine-tune stem cell responses. Titanium nanostructures provide another compelling example. When stem cells were cultured on titanium substrates with nanoscale topography, they exhibited enhanced proliferation and mineralization compared to cells grown on smooth or microstructured titanium surfaces [4]. Although both nano- and microstructured surfaces increased alkaline phosphatase activity, a marker of osteogenesis, the nanoscale features were more effective in promoting cell matrix mineralization, demonstrating the superior bioactivity of nanostructured implants for bone regeneration.

Other advanced nanomaterials, such as carbon nanotubes (CNTs), graphene oxide (GO), and black phosphorus (BP) nanosheets, are being investigated for their electrical conductivity and ability to direct neuronal differentiation, suggesting future potential in neural tissue engineering. Meanwhile, bioactive nanoparticles incorporated into hydrogels are being developed to release growth factors or signaling peptides in a controlled manner, further mimicking the dynamic functionality of native ECM. Therefore, the dual role of nanomaterials in stem cell research enables precise in vivo tracking through imaging modalities and providing biomimetic environments to regulate differentiation.

9.2.3 Targeted Delivery and Genetic Reprogramming

Lipid nanoparticles (LNPs) and functionalized polymeric carriers are examples of nanomaterials that are specifically engineered to help bypass biological barriers that usually limit genetic engineering efforts. In addition to serving as protective vehicles for fragile genetic payloads like mRNA, siRNA, or CRISPR-Cas9 ribonucleoprotein, these particles help prevent the degradation of those payloads through the actions of extracellular enzymes. Therefore, the effectiveness of these systems depends on the surface-anchored targeting ligands that enable the nanoparticles to interact through receptor–ligand recognition mechanisms with specific receptors located on the membrane of the stem cell. Because the binding of the targeting ligand to its corresponding receptor is highly specific, it allows therapeutic agents to be delivered with a high degree of precision to the target cellular population, therefore minimizing the potential for off-target effects and increasing the safety profile of the intervention.

Following internalization of the nanoparticle via endocytosis, the chemical makeup of the nanoparticle is designed in such a manner that the nanoparticle will undergo an "endosomal escape." Efficient endosomal escape is often a key determinant of successful intracellular delivery and subsequent genetic reprogramming. The delivered transcription factors or gene editing tools will allow for the "re-wiring" of the cellular circuitry. Therefore, researchers are utilizing nanotechnology to induce pluripotency in somatic cells and generate experimental, individualized induced pluripotent stem cells, as well as perform genome-specific corrections of inherited mutations. Unlike the use of traditional gene delivery (viral) vectors, these new methods promote the transient introduction of gene editing machinery to cells using a nanomaterial-based approach, thereby eliminating the risk of insertional mutagenesis. In addition, by facilitating a controlled presence of such editing machinery within cells, these methods provide the solutions needed for safe and efficient reprogramming of cell identity, forming a solid base for personalized regenerative therapies that are ethical and clinically feasible.

9.3 NANOMATERIALS IN REGENERATIVE MEDICINE

Tissue regeneration requires scaffolds that can mimic the structural and functional properties of the ECM, providing not only mechanical support but also biochemical and physical cues that guide cell attachment, proliferation, and differentiation. Nanomaterials play a pivotal role in this context, as their tunable architecture and functionalization capabilities allow the creation of scaffolds that closely replicate native tissue environments.

9.3.1 Nanofibrous Scaffold Design

Nanofibrous scaffolds are widely recognized as one of the most effective strategies for replicating ECM properties due to their nanoscale architecture, high porosity, and ability to regulate nutrient diffusion. Several fabrication techniques have been developed, including electrospinning, self-assembly, and thermally induced phase separation (TIPS), each with distinct advantages. Electrospinning has emerged as the most versatile and widely used technique for producing nanofibrous scaffolds. By applying a strong electric field to a polymer solution, ultrafine fibers with diameters ranging from tens of nanometers to a few micrometers can be deposited into a porous mat. Electrospun scaffolds exhibit high surface-to-volume ratios, tunable fiber alignment, and interconnected porosity features that closely resemble natural ECM [5]. In a recent study, electrospun PCL scaffolds have been shown to support chondrocyte proliferation and cartilage-like tissue formation, while poly(lactic-co-glycolic acid) (PLGA) nanofibers have been employed to encourage neural stem cell differentiation into functional neurons. The ability to control fiber orientation is particularly important where aligned nanofibers promote the elongation and orientation of cells such as cardiomyocytes and skeletal muscle cells, enhancing functional tissue regeneration.

Self-assembly techniques exploit the intrinsic ability of peptides, amphiphilic molecules, or block copolymers to organize into nanostructures under physiological conditions. Peptide-based self-assembling scaffolds, for instance, can form nanofibrous gels that provide biochemical signals in addition to structural support. A well-known example is RADA16-I, a self-assembling peptide that forms nanofibrous hydrogels and has been used in neural regeneration studies [6]. Such scaffolds not only mimic ECM mechanics but also present bioactive motifs that interact with cellular receptors, influencing differentiation pathways. TIPS offers another route for creating highly porous nanofibrous scaffolds. By carefully controlling solvent phase separation during cooling, interconnected networks of nanofibers are generated. TIPS-derived scaffolds have demonstrated applications in bone and cartilage tissue engineering, where high porosity and mechanical strength are required. Poly(L-lactic acid) scaffolds produced via TIPS have shown enhanced osteogenic differentiation of MSCs compared to conventional polymer foams [5].

9.3.2 Scaffold Enhancement with Nanomaterials

While nanofibrous scaffolds provide a basic structural framework, their performance can be further enhanced through the incorporation of functional nanomaterials or through structural modifications that improve mechanical, biochemical, or electrical properties. Structural modifications of nanofibrous scaffolds have been widely explored to tailor cellular responses. Aligned nanofibers have been employed to guide axonal growth in neural regeneration, while honeycomb-patterned scaffolds improve vascularization by facilitating endothelial cell migration. A particularly innovative design is the "spider-web" scaffold, where nanofibers are interwoven in a multilayered architecture, improving both mechanical stability and nutrient transport. Spider-web-like PCL scaffolds have been reported in skin tissue regeneration, where enhanced fibroblast infiltration and collagen deposition accelerated wound closure [7]. Functionalization strategies are equally critical in scaffold engineering. One approach is physical blending, where nanoparticles such as HAP, silica, or CNTs are directly incorporated into polymeric nanofibers during electrospinning. For instance, PCL-HAP nanofibers significantly improved osteogenic differentiation, while silica-incorporated fibers enhanced angiogenesis. Post-functionalization provides another route, involving surface modifications after scaffold fabrication. Techniques such as plasma treatment, peptide grafting, or coating with growth factors have been employed to improve biocompatibility and bioactivity.

A more advanced strategy is core–shell electrospinning, which allows different materials to be combined in a single nanofiber. This architecture enables the encapsulation of bioactive molecules in the fiber core while maintaining a protective outer shell for controlled release. Core–shell scaffolds have been developed for the sustained delivery of growth factors such as bone morphogenetic protein-2 or nerve growth factor (NGF), achieving localized and prolonged bioactivity that enhances tissue regeneration [8]. In neural tissue engineering, core–shell nanofibers loaded with NGF promoted neurite outgrowth and functional recovery in spinal cord injury models. By integrating structural innovations with functional nanomaterial incorporation, scaffolds can achieve multifunctionality, combining mechanical support, biochemical signaling, and controlled therapeutic delivery.

9.3.3 Nano-Architectonics for Exosome Vectorization

Regenerative medicine is transitioning away from using traditional cell-based transplants and is focusing on the development of novel approaches called "cell-free" therapies. In the case of the latter, exosomes from stem cells are being extracted and utilized as therapeutic entities and represent a significant discovery in regenerative medicine. Exosomes are nanoscale extracellular vesicles that form a major functional fraction of the stem cell secretome, encompassing diverse bioactive cargo. This biological cargo is composed of the RNA and protein molecules necessary to initiate the process of healing. However, clinical translation requires improved stability, scalable isolation, and standardized characterization, which can be achieved through nanotechnology-based strategies that protect exosomes from intrinsic fragility and address the limitations of conventional isolation methods.

Isolation of these vesicles from biological fluids represents a significant barrier to their use. Recent studies have demonstrated that magnetic-based approaches for isolating exosome populations offer advantages over older, harsher techniques such as ultracentrifugation. Research studies have created magnetic nanoparticles (MNPs) that are coated with antibodies that recognize specific markers present on the surface of the exosome populations (e.g., CD63 or CD81) [9]. By using these materials, high-purity exosome subpopulations can be captured with high purity. To facilitate ongoing progressive research around using exosomes as cellular regenerative therapies, magnetic bead isolation will be integrated into microfluidic "lab-on-a-chip" devices for continual high internal throughput processes to increase scalability and to allow for timely delivery of therapy.

The second step of this process is to preserve the therapeutic window and stability of the exosomes after they have been isolated for human use. Due to rapid enzymatic degradation by the liver, nanotechnology is being used to encapsulate exosomes in a protective "nano-shield." Exosomes are now being loaded to encase them in stimuli-responsive nanohydrogels or "cloaked" in synthetic polymers such as polyethylene glycol (PEG). The delivery systems act as a reservoir for the exosome contents while allowing for extended and controlled release of these contents at the site of injury. By combining naturally occurring exosomes with synthetic liposomes to generate hybrid vesicles, researchers are taking advantage of the biological targeting capacity of stem cell–derived exosomes while employing the superior stability of synthetic nanomaterials. In this way, the regenerative signals that the exosomes produce can be delivered to the target organs effectively.

9.4 NANOMATERIAL-ASSISTED TISSUE REGENERATION

Tissue regeneration relies on recreating microenvironments that support cell proliferation, differentiation, and integration into host tissues. Nanomaterials have emerged as powerful tools in this domain, offering structural, biochemical, and even electrical support that promote regeneration across diverse tissue types. Their tunable size, shape, and surface chemistry allow them to mimic biological architecture and actively interact with cells at the molecular level. Applications have been particularly prominent in bone, vascular, and neural tissue engineering.

9.4.1 Bone Tissue Regeneration

Bone regeneration requires scaffolds with both mechanical strength and osteoinductive properties. Traditional polymers provide the former but often lack biological activity, which nanomaterials can impart. BP nanomaterials have gained attention for their role in osteogenesis. BP nanosheets degrade into phosphate ions, which are natural components of bone mineralization. When incorporated into polymer scaffolds such as PLGA, BP not only enhances mechanical stability but also stimulates osteogenic differentiation of MSCs [5]. In vivo studies have demonstrated accelerated new bone formation in calvarial defect models treated with BP-loaded scaffolds compared to controls, highlighting their clinical potential [10]. Carbon nanomaterials such as CNTs, carbon nanofibers (CNFs), and single-walled CNTs (SWCNTs) offer another route to reinforcing bone scaffolds. Their exceptional tensile strength and ability to interact with bone cells make them ideal for load-bearing implants. CNT-reinforced HAP composites have shown improved compressive strength and higher alkaline phosphatase activity, indicating enhanced osteogenic activity. CNFs incorporated into PCL scaffolds have demonstrated improved osteoblast adhesion and mineral deposition, while SWCNTs integrated into collagen matrices promoted bone tissue regeneration with superior mechanical resilience. Noble metal nanoparticles also contribute to osteogenesis. AuNPs have been integrated into SiO_2 nanoparticle scaffolds to stimulate osteogenic signaling pathways such as ERK/MAPK [11]. These hybrid scaffolds not only enhance bone mineralization but also reduce inflammatory responses, making them promising composites for orthopedic applications. Such multifunctional nanoscaffolds represent the shift toward combining structural reinforcement with biological activity for effective bone regeneration.

9.4.2 Vascular Tissue Regeneration

Vascular regeneration is critical in tissue engineering because adequate blood supply is essential for the survival of newly formed tissues. Nanomaterials can be engineered to stimulate angiogenesis, regulate endothelial cell behavior, and provide mechanical support to vascular grafts. Electrospun tubular scaffolds have been developed to mimic the structure of native blood vessels. By incorporating bioactive nanoparticles into these scaffolds, angiogenesis can be significantly enhanced. For instance, PCL/gelatin electrospun tubes loaded with vascular endothelial growth factor (VEGF)-releasing nanoparticles promoted endothelial cell proliferation and vascular network formation in vitro [12].

Nanocatalysts such as MnO_2 nanoparticles are particularly effective in vascular applications due to their ability to modulate the cellular microenvironment. MnO_2 nanoparticles scavenge ROS while simultaneously promoting the release of oxygen, thereby improving hypoxic conditions within regenerating tissues. In ischemic models, MnO_2-loaded scaffolds accelerated neovascularization and improved tissue survival. Similarly, Fe_3O_4 nanoparticles have been used to provide magnetic stimulation, guiding endothelial cell alignment and tube formation under external magnetic fields, thereby enhancing vascular regeneration [13]. Another strategy involves nanopatterned stents and vascular grafts. By engineering nanoscale grooves, ridges, or coatings on stent surfaces, endothelialization can be accelerated, reducing the risk of thrombosis and restenosis. Titanium stents modified with nanostructured titanium dioxide coatings improved endothelial cell attachment and proliferation, while simultaneously resisting platelet adhesion.

9.4.3 Neural Tissue Regeneration

Neural tissue regeneration is one of the most challenging areas of regenerative medicine due to the limited intrinsic regenerative capacity of the central nervous system. Nanomaterials offer unique opportunities by providing scaffolds that guide axonal growth, deliver neurotrophic factors, and restore electrical communication. Various polymers have been employed in neural tissue engineering, and preclinical studies have demonstrated promising outcomes, including neural stem cell differentiation, nerve gap bridging, and enhanced neurite extension (Figure 9.3) [14]. Currently, the types of agents commonly used in nerve tissue engineering encompass polymer scaffolds, hydrogels, nanoparticles, and nerve conduits, among others. Regardless of the material utilized, it is essential to consider certain characteristics: biocompatibility,

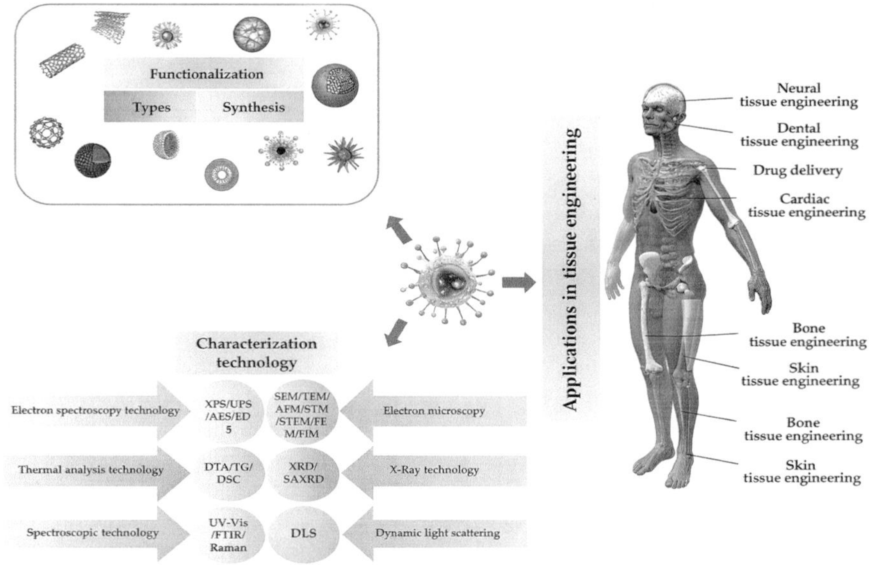

FIGURE 9.3 Illustration of the type, synthesis, characterizations, and functionalization NPs and their application for tissue engineering. (Adapted from Ref. [14] (CC BY).)

biodegradability, permeability or porosity, resistance to infection, favorable mechanical properties, and electrical conductivity. Nanofibrous scaffolds play a central role in neural repair. Biodegradable polymers such as poly(lactic acid) and peptide-based hydrogels (e.g., RADA-16 and LDLK-12 nanogels) form ECM-like structures that promote neuronal adhesion and axonal elongation. For instance, RADA-16 hydrogels have been used to repair spinal cord injuries, where they facilitated neural cell infiltration and partial functional recovery. LDLK-12 peptide nanogels provided a supportive microenvironment for neuronal survival while reducing glial scar formation, a major barrier in neural regeneration [15].

Carbon nanomaterials such as CNTs, GO, and reduced graphene oxide (rGO) have emerged as particularly promising due to their electrical conductivity [16]. CNT-based scaffolds not only support neural stem cell adhesion but also promote differentiation into neurons under electrical stimulation. GO substrates have been shown to enhance neurite outgrowth and synaptic connectivity, while rGO coatings on electrospun fibers facilitated signal transmission, improving neural network formation in vitro. More advanced systems include vertically aligned carbon nanofibers (VACNFs) and conductive nanostructures designed to restore bioelectrical signaling. VACNF arrays integrated into neural scaffolds allowed direct electrical stimulation of neurons, boosting synaptic activity and network synchronization. Conductive polymers such as polypyrrole, when combined with graphene or CNTs, created hybrid scaffolds that not only mimicked ECM mechanics but also restored lost electrophysiological functions [17]. These innovations suggest that conductive nanomaterials may one day serve as active neural interfaces for treating paralysis or degenerative neural disorders.

9.4.4 Nanomaterial-Assisted Skin Regeneration

This section focuses on electrospun nanofiber dressings for skin regeneration. These artificial dressings are made from nanofibers with diameters of 10–500 nm, and they mimic the structural complexity of natural ECM. Nanofibers provide "contact guidance" to promote migration of keratinocytes and fibroblasts across the wound bed, thus rapidly closing the wound and greatly reducing the formation of disorganized scar tissue. The porosity of nanofibers provides optimal conditions for gas exchange and moisture retention, thus creating an environment in which cells do not desiccate and in which the extruded fluids can be removed.

Nanotechnology can be applied to penetrate and eliminate bacterial biofilms that are resistant to traditional antibiotic therapy. This new generation of antibacterial agents utilizes the properties of bimetallic nanoparticles, including silver–copper alloys and silver–zinc alloy. The combined effects of these nanoparticles create a synergistic approach that can disrupt bacterial cell membranes and interfere with replication processes, prevents further division through disruption of the bacterium's internal DNA replication, and, critical to the success of this therapy, preserves the integrity of healthy host tissue. Integrating nanosensors into cyber-skin dressings is transforming wound monitoring by enabling the real-time detection of subtle changes in temperature and pH—two critical biophysical indicators of infection and tissue condition. These smart dressings can provide early warnings of complications, allowing timely intervention by healthcare professionals when necessary.

For complete tissue regeneration, the local blood supply must be restored (angiogenesis). Nanomaterials are critical because they act as stabilizing carriers for the unstable angiolytic signals (pro-angiogenic) such as VEGF or nitric oxide. In encapsulating these factors in LNPs or mesoporous silica, researchers have developed an ability to enabling sustained and localized release to stimulate the formation of new capillaries at the wound site. Moreover, metallic nanoparticles (gold and zinc oxide) have the unique ability of stimulating endothelial cells to form tubes independently [18]. Therefore, the combined use of nanotechnology for wound care is a comprehensive toolkit transitioning wound care to an integrated model of skin tissue engineering.

9.5 NANO-ENABLED THERAPEUTICS FOR NEUROLOGICAL DISORDERS

Neurological disorders such as Alzheimer's disease, Parkinson's disease, stroke, and glioblastoma remain among the most intractable medical challenges, largely due to the complexity of the brain and the protective nature of the BBB. Conventional small-molecule drugs often fail to reach therapeutic concentrations in the central nervous system, while inflammation, oxidative stress, and genetic dysregulation exacerbate disease progression. Recent advancements in gene therapy using nanocarriers (Figure 9.4) have enabled research institutions to investigate a wide range of potential treatment options [19]. The use of nanomaterials as systems for delivering genes has significantly improved the efficacy of gene therapy while minimizing the breakdown of genetic material by enzymes. In laboratory studies, it has been

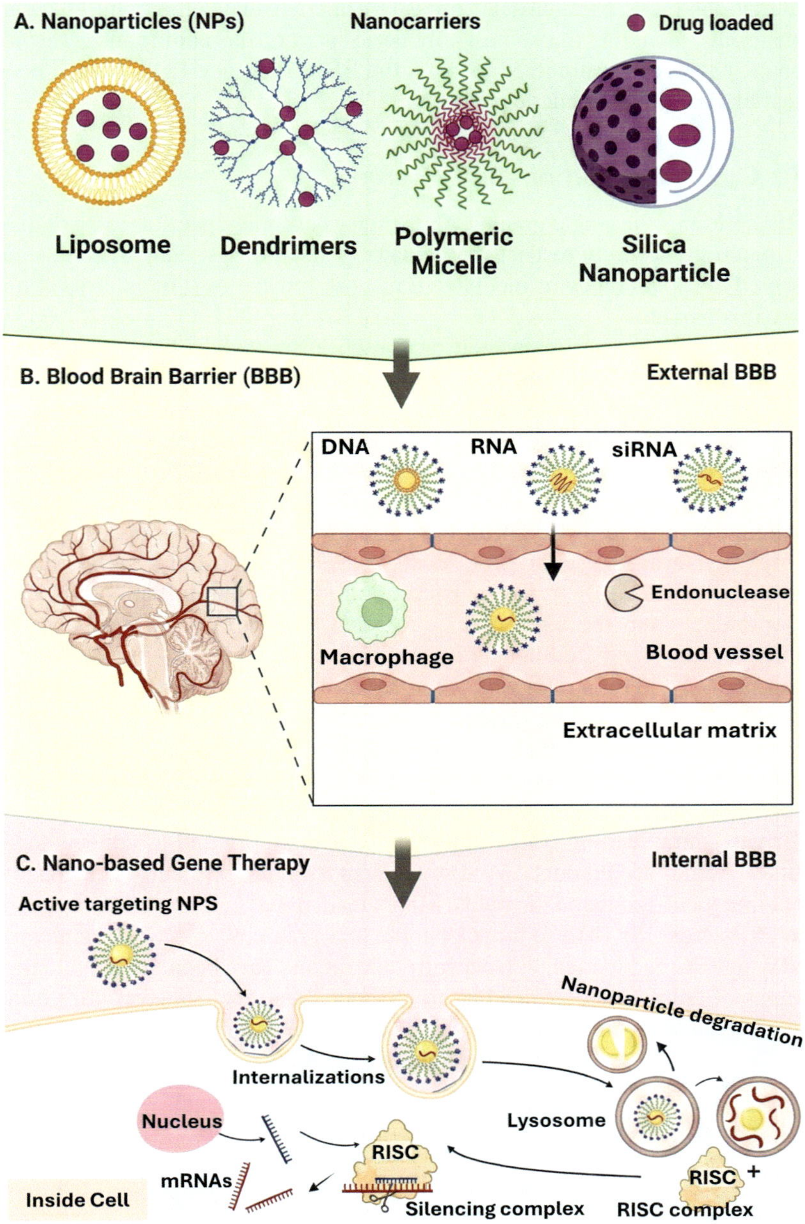

FIGURE 9.4 Nanotechnology in gene therapy and blood–brain barrier penetration for brain disorder. (a) Representation of nanoparticles, nanocarriers, and drug-loaded NPs. (b) Mechanisms of blood–brain barrier transfer. Several endogenous compounds use receptors and adsorption-mediated endocytosis and carrier-mediated pathways, which allow NPs carrying medicines to cross the blood–brain barrier and enter the brain. (c) Nano-based gene therapy in the internal blood–brain barrier. (Adapted from Ref. [19] (CC BY).)

shown that polymeric nanoparticles improve drug delivery to the brain. A variety of nanomaterials, including liposomes, polymeric carriers, inorganic nanoparticles, and exosomes, have been engineered to cross the BBB, scavenge ROS, reduce neuroinflammation, and deliver genetic payloads.

9.5.1 Crossing the Blood–Brain Barrier

The BBB presents the single greatest obstacle for neurotherapeutics, as its tight endothelial junctions severely restrict the passage of most drugs. Nanomaterials can be engineered to exploit receptor-mediated transport, transcytosis, or external stimuli to traverse this barrier.

BP nanosheets are particularly attractive because of their biodegradability and surface reactivity. BP can degrade into phosphate ions, which are biocompatible and nontoxic, while its high surface area enables conjugation with targeting ligands such as transferrin or lactoferrin to facilitate receptor-mediated transport across the BBB. In preclinical studies, BP nanosheets have successfully carried dopamine analogs to the brain for Parkinson's therapy, achieving higher drug accumulation in the striatum compared to free drug formulations. Polymeric nanoparticles, including poly(butyl cyanoacrylate) (PBCA) and polysorbate-coated systems, have also shown promise [19]. PBCA nanoparticles coated with polysorbate-80 can adsorb apolipoproteins from the bloodstream, forming a biomimetic protein corona that promotes receptor-mediated uptake by endothelial cells via low-density lipoprotein receptor pathways. This strategy has been tested in delivering analgesic peptides and anti-Alzheimer's drugs, with measurable improvements in memory function in rodent models. Liposomes, especially PEGylated and ligand-modified ones, provide another versatile platform. PEGylation prolongs circulation time, while targeting moieties such as ApoE peptides or transferrin enhances BBB penetration. Liposomal carriers of rivastigmine demonstrated improved bioavailability and prolonged cognitive benefits in Alzheimer's models. MNPs represent a unique externally guided strategy. By applying localized magnetic fields, MNPs loaded with neuroprotective agents can be directed across the BBB to target specific brain regions. Iron oxide nanoparticles coated with PEG and loaded with neurotrophic factors have been guided into the hippocampus of animal models, leading to enhanced neuronal survival after ischemic injury. This magnetically assisted approach opens the possibility of noninvasive, spatially precise delivery of drugs to deep brain structures.

9.5.2 Oxidative Stress and Inflammation Control

Oxidative stress and chronic neuroinflammation are hallmarks of most neurodegenerative diseases. Excessive ROS damages neurons, while prolonged activation of microglia and astrocytes exacerbates neuronal death. Nanomaterials can act as catalytic antioxidants or modulators of the inflammatory response. Fullerenes (C_{60} and derivatives) are powerful ROS scavengers due to their electron-rich carbon cages. They can neutralize superoxide radicals, hydroxyl radicals, and singlet oxygen, providing neuroprotection in models of Parkinson's disease and traumatic brain injury. Derivatized fullerenes with enhanced solubility have reduced dopaminergic neuron loss in toxin-induced Parkinsonism models, highlighting their therapeutic potential. BP nanosheets extend their utility beyond drug delivery by functioning as ion chelators. BP binds Cu^{2+} ions, which catalyze oxidative stress reactions via Fenton-like chemistry. In Alzheimer's models, BP nanosheets reduced Cu^{2+}-induced amyloid aggregation and oxidative neuronal death, mitigating both oxidative stress and disease pathology [20]. Cerium oxide nanoparticles (CeO_2 NPs) represent regenerative antioxidants thanks to their ability to switch between Ce^{3+} and Ce^{4+} states. This redox cycle allows continuous scavenging of ROS without being consumed, unlike traditional antioxidants. In animal models of ischemic stroke, CeO_2 NPs reduced infarct volume, decreased microglial activation, and improved neurological outcomes. Their regenerative nature makes them ideal candidates for chronic neurodegenerative conditions, where sustained antioxidant activity is required.

9.5.3 Gene Therapy and Nanomedicine

Beyond small-molecule therapeutics, nanotechnology is driving advances in gene therapy, enabling the delivery of nucleic acids that modulate disease pathways at their root. Liposomes remain a foundation of nucleic acid delivery. Cationic liposomes have been engineered to carry siRNA against beta-secretase (BACE1), a key enzyme in amyloid beta production. In Alzheimer's disease models, liposomal siRNA delivery reduced amyloid plaque burden and improved cognitive outcomes. AuNPs functionalized with siRNA or antisense oligonucleotides provide an alternative approach. Their strong surface chemistry enables dense siRNA loading, while their tunable size allows controlled biodistribution. In glioblastoma models, AuNP-siRNA systems successfully silenced oncogenes, reducing tumor progression. Similarly, Cas9 mRNA-loaded nanoparticles have been developed for in vivo gene editing, opening pathways for correcting mutations underlying Huntington's or ALS. Dendrimers, with their branched, tree-like structures, are particularly suited for carrying nucleic acids. Poly(amidoamine) dendrimers have been used to deliver siRNA targeting inflammatory cytokines in models of traumatic brain injury, reducing inflammation, and promoting recovery. Their multivalency and tunable surface chemistry enable high nucleic acid payloads and efficient intracellular delivery. Derived from stem cells or engineered cells, exosomes naturally cross the BBB and deliver RNA or proteins to specific neural cell populations. In Parkinson's models, exosomes carrying miRNA-124 promoted dopaminergic neuron survival, while in glioblastoma, exosome-based delivery of siRNA against oncogenes reduced tumor size. As "natural nanomedicine," exosomes may represent the next frontier in safe and targeted brain therapies.

9.6 NANO-ENABLED DIAGNOSTICS AND BIOSENSORS

Nanotechnology has revolutionized the field of diagnostics by enabling tools that are highly sensitive, portable, and capable of detecting diseases at much earlier stages than conventional methods. The unique optical, electronic, and catalytic properties of nanomaterials make them ideal candidates for biosensing platforms, imaging agents, and lab-on-chip devices. These innovations promise a shift from centralized laboratory testing toward rapid, decentralized, and even personalized diagnostic systems.

9.6.1 Nanosensors for Disease Detection

Bioreceptors such as nanobodies, aptamers, and DNAzymes provide high specificity toward disease biomarkers, while nanomaterials amplify the response. Carbon nanotube field-effect transistors (CNT-FETs) are widely explored for real-time biomarker detection. Their one-dimensional structure and ballistic electron transport allow them to be capable of detecting extremely low-abundance biomolecular interactions. CNT-FETs functionalized with DNA aptamers have been used to detect prostate-specific antigen at femtomolar concentrations, outperforming ELISA tests. Graphene-based biosensors similarly leverage the high conductivity and atomic thinness of graphene sheets. When decorated with AuNPs, graphene sensors have been employed for detecting cardiac troponin I, a critical marker for myocardial infarction, at clinically relevant levels within minutes. AuNPs with their strong plasmonic properties, enable colorimetric detection where binding of biomolecules induces visible color changes. AuNP-aptamer conjugates have been developed to detect thrombin, hepatitis B virus DNA, and even SARS-CoV-2 RNA in clinical samples, providing both sensitivity and ease of readout without sophisticated equipment [21]. They also help to detect very early-stage cancers by identifying rare blood proteins, often referred to as biomarkers, through the analysis of samples taken from a patient's blood (liquid biopsy). Nano-Velcro substrates made from silicon nanowires or CNTs, have functionalized surfaces that allow them to bind to cancer cells with great affinity. Superparamagnetic nanoparticles have been created to bond to the cancer cells enabling faster capture and removal from the patient using a strong external magnetic field.

Nanosensors capture not only entire living cancer cells but also fragmented tumor DNA (circulating tumor DNA), and exosomes. AuNPs have been engineered with surfaces that allow them to work based on the principle of Surface Plasmon Resonance. Additionally, QDs provide multiplexing capabilities allowing for the identification of different cancer types, thus allowing for the identification of multiple types of cancer from a single droplet of blood. The use of advanced technology such as these ultrasensitive techniques will provide the ability to identify cancers in their earliest stages, providing patients with the best chance of long-term survival.

9.6.2 Nano-Enabled Point-of-Care Devices

Nanomaterials have been integrated into POC diagnostic systems that deliver rapid results at the bedside, in clinics, or even at home. Lateral flow immunoassays (LFIAs) are the most familiar POC format, traditionally using AuNPs as colorimetric labels. Modern adaptations include fluorescent nanoparticles and QDs, which greatly enhance sensitivity. For example, QD-LFIAs have detected influenza A virus in nasal swabs at detection limits tenfold lower than conventional strips, while still maintaining the rapid visual readout.

Electrochemical sensors based on CNTs and graphene are increasingly deployed in portable, handheld devices. A CNT-modified electrode was used to detect C-reactive protein, a marker of inflammation, at nanogram-per-milliliter levels within 5 min. Similarly, graphene-based electrochemical strips have enabled glucose monitoring with greater accuracy than traditional glucometers, while offering the possibility of multiplexed detection for other metabolites in a single device. Such devices are advancing toward wearable formats, where continuous monitoring is possible. CNT-coated textiles and graphene-based patches have been trialed for detecting lactate and electrolyte levels in sweat, enabling real-time monitoring for athletes and patients alike.

Nanomaterials have also been incorporated into microfluidic lab-on-a-chip systems, enabling high-throughput, automated analysis in compact devices. MNPs are frequently used to capture and concentrate rare analytes such as circulating tumor cells or exosomes from blood. These are then directed through microfluidic channels for analysis, reducing assay times from hours to minutes. QDs provide multiplexed fluorescence signals in LOC assays. By encoding multiple colors, QD-based chips can simultaneously quantify several biomarkers from a single drop of blood, a key advance for personalized medicine. Nanoporous membranes within microfluidic chips enhance separation and enrichment of small molecules, nucleic acids, or proteins. For instance, nanoporous silicon chips have been used for ultrasensitive detection of microRNAs associated with early-stage pancreatic cancer. Such platforms are now being integrated with smartphones and portable readers, enabling personalized diagnostics at the point of care. A recent example is a graphene-integrated LOC device for multiplex detection of Zika, dengue, and chikungunya viruses in under 30 min, demonstrating the real-world potential of nanotechnology-enabled LOC systems for global health [22].

9.6.3 Imaging and Contrast-Enhancing Agents

In medical imaging, nanomaterials act as contrast enhancers, providing greater resolution and functional information compared to traditional agents. Certain iron oxide nanoparticle formulations have received clinical approval as MRI contrast agents. Their superparamagnetic properties enhance T_2-weighted imaging, making them valuable for detecting tumors, monitoring cell migration, and assessing organ function. SPIO-labeled stem cells have been tracked in vivo after transplantation, enabling real-time visualization of therapeutic cell migration in patients. AuNPs, owing to their high atomic number, provide excellent X-ray attenuation for computed tomography (CT). Targeted AuNPs conjugated with antibodies against HER2 have been used to selectively enhance CT imaging of breast cancer tumors, offering both diagnostic and therapeutic potential [23]. Development of ligand-functionalized nanoparticles have shaped the evolution of molecular imaging. Engineered nanoplatforms can localize at specific sites within the body by utilizing the specific biochemical features of diseased tissues, moving from the traditional administration method of using general contrast agents to now the targeted administration of nanoparticles that are functionalized to deliver contrast agents to specific sites. By coating the surface of the nanoparticle with high-affinity ligands, researchers are now able to provide highly selective molecular recognition of cell surface markers. One of the best examples is the use of nanoparticles that are coated with folic acid. Folic acid is a highly specific ligand for the folate receptor that is significantly increased in a variety of cancers, especially ovarian and cervical cancers, and therefore the folic acid–coated, functionalized nanoparticles can selectively label tumors with high sensitivity. Further, the use of these nanoparticles will increase the imaging signal at the specific location of the tumor and decrease background noise, thereby improving the signal-to-noise ratio in diagnostic imaging. In addition to targeting cellular receptors for metabolic processes, "general structural and vascular markers" also serve as another level of diagnostic capability. VEGF-N60-RGD-modified nanoparticles have been developed to facilitate the targeting of integrins that have high expression levels on angiogenic blood vessels, as well as allowing for more effective visualization and early detection of cancer by allowing for intervention prior to surgery. However, the real potential of these imaging agents enhanced by nanotechnology becomes apparent when they are integrated within a therapeutically diagnostic framework. By using the same targeted delivery system to provide both imaging of the disease and the delivery of an exact dose of therapeutically active agents (such as a small-molecule chemotherapeutic or an RNA molecule for silencing gene expression), the drug delivery process is streamlined. This will allow for a more personalized approach to treating diseases, with more accurate images of the disease process, and emphasize the need for a more individualized "imaging-based" approach to the development of nanomedicines.

9.7 REGULATORY CHALLENGES AND ETHICAL CONSIDERATIONS

Nanomedicine and nano-enabled diagnostics are moving out of laboratories and into hospitals but getting them approved is challenging due to the complex regulatory and ethical issues that are preventing their widespread use. The same properties that enable nanomaterials to be used in the treatment of diseases, such as their large surface area-to-volume ratio and ability to penetrate biological barriers, also create the potential for toxicity. For example, cadmium-based QDs, long, thin CNTs, and highly concentrated gold/silver nanoparticles all pose known risks for accumulation in living tissues, oxidative damage to cells, and damage to DNA. These challenges are made worse by the fact that once these particles are in living tissue, it is difficult to fully predict long-term biological effects.

The Food and Drug Administration and the European Medicines Agency are developing their own guidelines on regulating "combination products" that include nanomedicine; however, there are significant gaps in how these two agencies define standards for approving combination products as it relates to safety. Many traditional pharmaceutical products and the ways in which they are measured and reviewed do not consider, how the particulate size of a nano-formulation influences its overall safety, how each process affects how the drug is metabolized by the body, and how to assess the degree of toxicity present.

Although wearable nanosensors are an important technology for continuous monitoring in healthcare and provide patients with more individualized treatment options, they also produce new vulnerabilities in areas such as data security and privacy due to the availability of private medical information through unauthorized means. In a similar manner, the development of gene editing technologies using nanocarriers (e.g., CRISPR) may introduce the possibility of unintended consequences through gene editing advancements that could permanently change an individual's genetic makeup. Additionally, the public's view of wearable nanosensors ranges from hope and excitement to fear of the unknown. All these aspects point to the need for an open and cooperative relationship between researchers, medical professionals, government, and society to create innovative products while protecting individuals' rights to the highest standard of safety—both for themselves and for their genetic futures.

REFERENCES

1. S.F.O. Aboushoushah, Iron oxide nanoparticles enhancing magnetic resonance imaging: a review of the latest advancements, *Journal of Science: Advanced Materials and Devices*, 10(2025) 100875.
2. S.A. Maynard, A. Gelmi, S.C. Skaalure, I.J. Pence, C. Lee-Reeves, J.E. Sero, et al., Nanoscale molecular quantification of stem cell–hydrogel interactions, *ACS Nano*, 14(2020) 17321–32.
3. T.N. Pansani, C.A. de Souza Costa, L.M. Cardoso, A.M. Claro, H.d.S. Barud, F.G. Basso, Synthesis, characterization, and osteogenic ability of fibrillar polycaprolactone scaffolds containing hydroxyapatite nanoparticles, *ACS Applied Materials & Interfaces*, 17(2025) 20647–57.
4. R. Riedel, S. Pérez-Amodio, L. Cabo-Zabala, E. Velasco-Ortega, J. Maymó, J. Gil, et al., Influence of the surface topography of titanium dental implants on the behavior of human amniotic stem cells, *International Journal of Molecular Sciences*, 25(2024) 7416.
5. S. Anjum, F. Rahman, P. Pandey, D.K. Arya, M. Alam, P.S. Rajinikanth, et al., Electrospun biomimetic nanofibrous scaffolds: a promising prospect for bone tissue engineering and regenerative medicine, *International Journal of Molecular Sciences*, 23(2022) 9206.
6. X. Wu, L. He, W. Li, H. Li, W.-M. Wong, S. Ramakrishna, et al., Functional self-assembling peptide nanofiber hydrogel for peripheral nerve regeneration, *Regenerative Biomaterials*, 4(2016) 21–30.
7. M.I. Echeverria Molina, C.-A. Chen, J. Martinez, P. Tran, K. Komvopoulos, Novel electrospun polycaprolactone/calcium alginate scaffolds for skin tissue engineering, *Materials*, 16(2023) 136.
8. K.A. Blackwood, N. Bock, T.R. Dargaville, M. Ann Woodruff, Scaffolds for growth factor delivery as applied to bone tissue engineering, *International Journal of Polymer Science*, 2012(2012) 174942.
9. N. Mukerjee, A. Bhattacharya, S. Maitra, M. Kaur, S. Ganesan, S. Mishra, et al., Exosome isolation and characterization for advanced diagnostic and therapeutic applications, *Materials Today Bio*, 31(2025) 101613.
10. J.L. Cota Quintero, R. Ramos-Payán, J.G. Romero-Quintana, A. Ayala-Ham, M. Bermúdez, E.M. Aguilar-Medina, Hydrogel-based scaffolds: advancing bone regeneration through tissue engineering, *Gels*, 11(2025) 175.
11. D.H. Yang, H. Nah, D. Lee, S.J. Min, S. Park, S.-H. An, et al., A review on gold nanoparticles as an innovative therapeutic cue in bone tissue engineering: prospects and future clinical applications, *Materials Today Bio*, 26(2024) 101016.
12. K. Wang, X. Chen, Y. Pan, Y. Cui, X. Zhou, D. Kong, et al., Enhanced vascularization in hybrid PCL/gelatin fibrous scaffolds with sustained release of VEGF, *BioMed Research International*, 2015(2015) 865076.
13. R.P. Friedrich, I. Cicha, C. Alexiou, Iron oxide nanoparticles in regenerative medicine and tissue engineering, *Nanomaterials*, 11(2021) 2337.
14. X. Zheng, P. Zhang, Z. Fu, S. Meng, L. Dai, H. Yang, Applications of nanomaterials in tissue engineering, *RSC Advances*, 11(2021) 19041–58.
15. G.A. Politrón-Zepeda, G. Fletes-Vargas, R. Rodríguez-Rodríguez, Injectable hydrogels for nervous tissue repair—a brief review, *Gels*, 10(2024) 190.

16. A.B. Ganganboina, A. Dutta Chowdhury, R.-A. Doong, New avenue for appendage of graphene quantum dots on halloysite nanotubes as anode materials for high performance supercapacitors, *ACS Sustainable Chemistry & Engineering*, 5(2017) 4930–40.
17. D. Kai, M. Prabhakaran, G. Jin, S. Ramakrishna, Polypyrrole-contained electrospun conductive nanofibrous membranes for cardiac tissue engineering, *Journal of Biomedical Materials Research Part A*, 99(2011) 376–85.
18. A. Barui, V. Veeriah, S. Mukherjee, J. Manna, A. Patel, S. Patra, et al., Zinc oxide nanoflowers make new blood vessels, *Nanoscale*, 4(2012) 7861–9.
19. D. Mohapatra, M. Gopikrishnan, G.P.D. C, N. Chandrasekaran, How precise are nanomedicines in overcoming the blood–brain barrier? A comprehensive review of the literature, *International Journal of Nanomedicine*, 19(2024) 2441–67.
20. X. Shao, C. Yan, C. Wang, C. Wang, Y. Cao, Y. Zhou, et al., Advanced nanomaterials for modulating Alzheimer's related amyloid aggregation, *Nanoscale Advances*, 5(2023) 49–80.
21. S. GeGen, G. Meng, G. Aodeng, L. Ga, J. Ai, Advances in aptamer-based electrochemical biosensors for disease diagnosis: integration of DNA and nanomaterials, *Nanoscale Horizons*, 10(2025) 2668–87.
22. F. Nasrin, K. Tsuruga, D.I.S. Utomo, A.D. Chowdhury, E.Y. Park, Design and analysis of a single system of impedimetric biosensors for the detection of mosquito-borne viruses, *Biosensors*, 11(2021) 376.
23. T. Stuchinskaya, M. Moreno, M.J. Cook, D.R. Edwards, D.A. Russell, Targeted photodynamic therapy of breast cancer cells using antibody-phthalocyanine-gold nanoparticle conjugates, *Photochemical & Photobiological Sciences*, 10(2011) 822–31.

10 Nanotoxicology and Emerging Nanotechnologies in Bio-Applications

Indra Memdi Khoris and Jaebeom Lee

10.1 INTRODUCTION

Engineered nanomaterials have become central to contemporary advances in medicine and biotechnology, enabling highly precise strategies for drug delivery, molecular diagnostics, biomedical imaging, and targeted therapy. Their tunable size, surface chemistry, and multifunctional design allow interventions at cellular and even subcellular levels, offering unprecedented control over therapeutic and diagnostic processes. At the same time, these distinctive physicochemical attributes introduce complex biological interactions that demand careful safety evaluation before clinical application. A comprehensive understanding of nano–bio interfaces, encompassing cellular uptake, biodistribution, immunological responses, metabolism, and clearance, is essential for predicting both efficacy and potential adverse effects. The development of clinically viable nanomedicines therefore depends not only on performance optimization but also on rigorous toxicological assessment and risk characterization. This chapter examines the foundational principles of nanotoxicology, current in vitro and in vivo evaluation strategies, translational bottlenecks encountered during clinical development, and the evolving regulatory landscape governing nanotechnology-based therapeutics. Particular attention is given to emerging design frameworks and safety-by-design approaches that integrate material engineering with toxicological insight, aligning technological innovation with patient safety and broader public health considerations.

10.1.1 Physicochemical Properties Influencing Toxicity

Nanoparticles possess unique interfacial and quantum-scale properties that markedly increase their surface reactivity, enabling applications across biosensing, targeted drug delivery, catalysis, and environmental remediation (Figure 10.1). Yet these same physicochemical features that confer functionality can also introduce unintended biological effects. Among the various determinants of nanotoxicity, particle size plays a central role. As particle dimensions decrease, the surface area-to-volume ratio rises substantially, amplifying surface energy and chemical

DOI: 10.1201/9781003725930-10

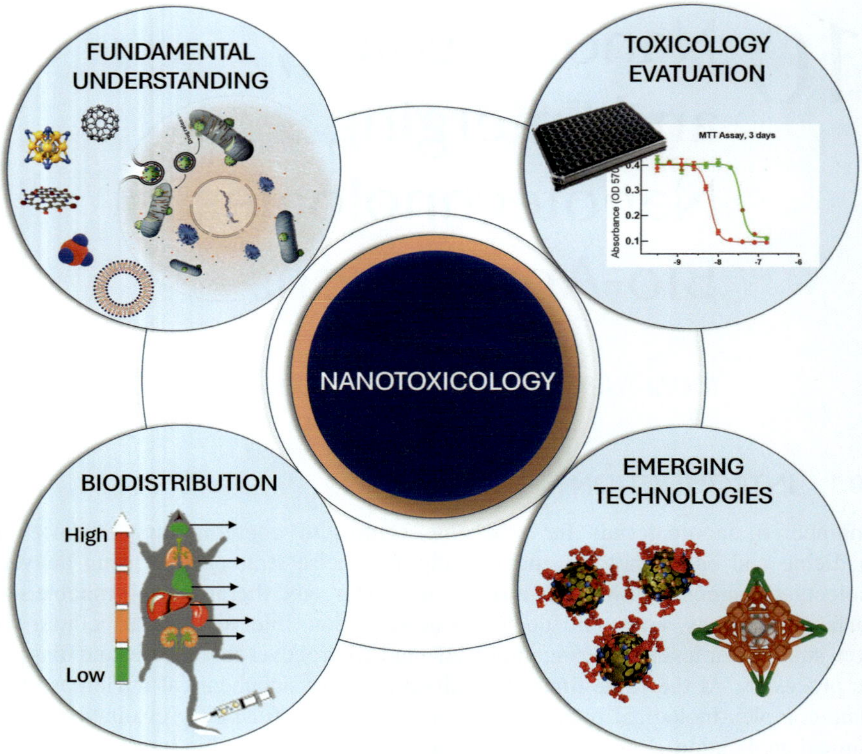

FIGURE 10.1 Overview of nanotoxicology in drug delivery, illustrating the interconnected aspects of fundamental understanding of nano–bio interactions, toxicological evaluation, biodistribution, and emerging technologies such as nanosensors, AI-assisted design, and high-throughput screening for safety assessment.

reactivity. This can promote the generation of reactive oxygen species (ROS), potentially leading to oxidative stress, inflammation, or cellular damage. Reduced particle size also influences biological transport. Smaller nanoparticles typically exhibit higher diffusion coefficients and may traverse physiological barriers, including cellular membranes, the blood–brain barrier (BBB), and intracellular organelle membranes. While such permeability can enhance therapeutic targeting and intracellular delivery, it may simultaneously intensify adverse cellular responses if exposure is not tightly regulated. Thus, miniaturization that improves performance characteristics may inadvertently elevate cytotoxic potential. Size further governs biodistribution and elimination pathways. Nanoparticles below approximately 10 nm are often cleared efficiently through renal filtration, whereas larger particles are more likely to accumulate within the mononuclear phagocyte system, particularly in the liver and spleen. Particles of intermediate size may demonstrate extended circulation times, increasing the probability of interaction with multiple tissues. These variations influence systemic exposure duration and downstream biological responses, underscoring the need to optimize particle dimensions to achieve therapeutic efficacy while ensuring safe clearance. Particle morphology is another critical variable affecting biological interactions. Nanomaterials fabricated as spheres, rods, wires, cubes, or two-dimensional (2D) sheets exhibit distinct surface geometries and mechanical behaviors. High-aspect ratio structures such as nanorods or nanowires may penetrate cellular membranes more efficiently due to their shape, but this enhanced internalization can also increase the likelihood of mechanical membrane disruption. In contrast, spherical nanoparticles often display more uniform uptake kinetics yet follow different intracellular trafficking pathways. Elongated or sheet-like materials may also trigger "frustrated phagocytosis," a phenomenon in which immune cells attempt but fail to completely engulf large or anisotropic particles, potentially leading to prolonged inflammatory responses.

Surface charge is a primary determinant of nanoparticle–cell interactions because biological membranes are predominantly negatively charged due to their phospholipid composition. Consequently, cationic nanoparticles are electrostatically attracted to cell surfaces, which can enhance cellular binding and internalization. This property is advantageous in applications such as gene delivery and intracellular imaging; however, excessive positive charge may destabilize membrane integrity, induce ion imbalance, and trigger uncontrolled permeability. Highly cationic nanomaterials are therefore frequently associated with membrane disruption and elevated cytotoxicity. In contrast, anionic or near-neutral nanoparticles generally exhibit reduced cellular uptake, which may lower acute toxicity but can also diminish therapeutic efficiency. Surface charge additionally influences colloidal behavior in physiological environments. Electrostatic interactions govern whether nanoparticles remain well-dispersed or undergo aggregation in biological fluids. Aggregated particles may display altered surface reactivity and reduced bioavailability, yet their larger effective size can contribute to vascular obstruction or preferential tissue deposition. For this reason, maintaining electrostatic stability under physiological ionic strength and pH conditions is essential for predictable in vivo performance and safety. Beyond net charge, surface chemistry plays a decisive role in defining nanoparticle biocompatibility. The nature of functional groups and surface coatings determines hydrophobicity, steric stabilization, and interaction kinetics with biomolecules. Upon exposure to biological fluids, nanoparticles rapidly adsorb proteins and other macromolecules, forming a dynamic "protein corona" that effectively redefines their biological identity. The composition of this corona governs immune recognition, opsonization, clearance pathways, and inflammatory potential. Strategic surface modification can modulate these processes. For example, grafting hydrophilic and biocompatible polymers such as polyethylene glycol (PEG) or applying silica and related coatings can reduce nonspecific adsorption, limit immune activation, and extend systemic circulation. Conversely, inadequate or unstable functionalization may enhance oxidative stress, interfere with intracellular signaling cascades, or provoke unintended immunological responses. Collectively, physicochemical parameters including size, morphology, charge, and surface composition operate in concert to shape nanoparticle biodistribution, cellular interactions, and toxicological outcomes. A mechanistic understanding of these interrelated factors enables more accurate hazard prediction and supports rational design strategies aimed at balancing functional performance with biological safety. By integrating material engineering with toxicological insight, researchers can advance nanotechnology applications while minimizing adverse effects.

10.1.2 Interaction with Biological Systems

Nanoparticles engage biological systems through a network of interrelated physicochemical and biochemical processes that govern their biodistribution, internalization, and eventual therapeutic or toxic responses. Upon entering physiological media such as blood or interstitial fluid, nanomaterials are rapidly exposed to a complex mixture of proteins and other biomolecules, leading to immediate surface adsorption events (Figure 10.2). A pivotal outcome of this exposure is the formation of a protein corona, in which biomolecules assemble on the nanoparticle surface and effectively redefine its biological identity. This adsorbed layer is dynamic and typically consists of a tightly bound "hard" corona and a more loosely associated "soft" corona, each differing in exchange kinetics and binding affinity. The composition and stability of the corona are influenced by protein concentration, binding strength, nanoparticle size, surface charge, and surface functionalization, and these factors collectively shape immune recognition, circulation behavior, and tissue distribution. In some cases, adsorption-induced conformational changes in proteins may expose hidden epitopes or alter protein structure, potentially modifying immunogenicity or triggering unintended biological responses. As a result, the protein corona serves as the principal bio–nano interface through which cells perceive and respond to nanomaterials. When corona-coated nanoparticles encounter cellular membranes, their interaction is governed by electrostatic attractions, hydrophobic forces, van der Waals interactions, and steric contributions from the adsorbed biomolecular layer. Cellular entry most commonly occurs via energy-dependent endocytic mechanisms, including clathrin-mediated and caveolae-mediated pathways, while larger aggregates may be internalized through macropinocytosis. In certain contexts, nanoparticle geometry, surface energy, or high reactivity may facilitate direct membrane translocation independent of classical endocytosis. However, excessive or uncontrolled membrane interaction, particularly in the absence of a stabilizing corona, can disrupt membrane integrity, increase permeability, and induce cytotoxic effects.

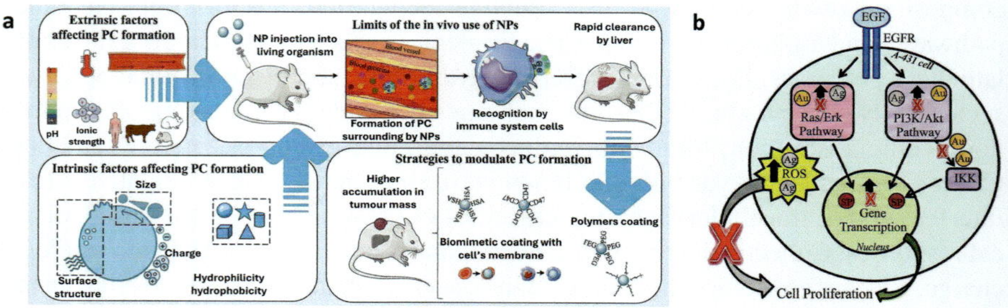

FIGURE 10.2 Schematic interaction of nanomaterials with biological systems and toxicity. (Adapted from Ref. [1] (CC BY).)

Certain nanomaterials possess physicochemical features that enable escape from endosomal compartments through pH-sensitive behavior or membrane-disruptive activity, allowing them to access the cytosol and interact with intracellular organelles. Among these, mitochondria represent a critical target due to their central role in energy metabolism and redox regulation. Nanoparticles that localize within mitochondria may interfere with components of the electron transport chain, perturb ATP production, elevate ROS levels, or induce loss of mitochondrial membrane potential, thereby activating apoptotic pathways or broader cellular stress responses. Lysosomes also play a significant role in intracellular nanoparticle processing. As acidic vesicles enriched with hydrolytic enzymes, lysosomes can partially degrade or solubilize internalized nanomaterials, potentially leading to the release of reactive intermediates, lysosomal swelling, or membrane destabilization. In gene delivery applications, extremely small nanoparticles or those engineered with nuclear localization signals may traverse into the nucleus to achieve therapeutic objectives. However, unintended nuclear accumulation raises safety concerns, including possible DNA strand damage, chromatin alterations, and disruption of transcriptional regulation. Such risks highlight the importance of controlled physicochemical design and precise surface engineering to minimize genotoxic and intracellular adverse effects while preserving functional efficacy.

To modulate nano–bio interactions, investigators implement strategic surface engineering approaches. Hydrophilic "stealth" modifications, such as PEG grafting or zwitterionic polymer coatings, are widely used to minimize nonspecific protein adsorption and extend systemic circulation [2]. Deliberate pre-coating with selected proteins can also guide the composition of the resulting corona, thereby influencing biodistribution and cellular recognition. In addition, the incorporation of pH-responsive, degradable, or stimuli-sensitive materials enables controlled intracellular release while reducing the risk of long-term tissue accumulation. Overall, nanoparticle behavior in biological environments arises from a dynamic interplay among intrinsic physicochemical characteristics, biomolecular adsorption processes, membrane interactions, and intracellular trafficking pathways. The acquired protein corona largely defines biological identity, membrane engagement governs uptake efficiency and potential cytotoxicity, and organelle-level targeting determines therapeutic performance alongside possible adverse effects. Through rational design and precise control of these interconnected factors, it is possible to enhance nanoparticle stability, improve delivery specificity, and minimize unintended toxicity. Continued advancement in this area will depend on interdisciplinary research efforts, standardized characterization protocols, and deeper mechanistic insight into nano–bio interface phenomena.

10.1.3 Mechanism of Toxicity

The toxicological behavior of next-generation nanomaterials shares core mechanistic features with traditional nanotoxicity; however, their increasingly complex architectures and multifunctional designs introduce additional layers of biological interaction. In classical nanotoxicology, parameters such as particle size, surface characteristics, and intrinsic reactivity are recognized as primary determinants of biological response. These principles remain applicable to advanced systems including doped nanoparticles, nanocomposites, and hybrid nanostructures. Nevertheless, multicomponent materials often display emergent behaviors in physiological environments because the interaction between their constituent elements can modify stability, redox activity, and cellular engagement. Accordingly, toxicity assessment must integrate established nano–bio interaction paradigms with the novel physicochemical attributes unique to contemporary engineered platforms. A central mechanism underlying both conventional and advanced nanomaterial toxicity is oxidative stress. Elevated surface area, catalytic properties, and redox-active sites contribute to the generation of ROS. In engineered systems incorporating transition metals, dopants, or hybrid architectures such as MXene-carbon dot composites, synergistic electron transfer processes may intensify ROS production beyond that observed in single-component nanoparticles. Once internalized, nanomaterials can stimulate ROS-generating enzymatic pathways, including cytochrome P450 systems, prostaglandin synthases, lipoxygenases, and NADPH oxidase complexes, leading to superoxide formation. Mitochondrial perturbation further amplifies oxidative imbalance by disrupting electron transport chains, reducing ATP synthesis, and increasing electron leakage. Superoxide is enzymatically converted to hydrogen peroxide (H_2O_2) by superoxide dismutase, and although catalase and glutathione peroxidase typically neutralize H_2O_2, excessive accumulation promotes formation of highly reactive hydroxyl radicals, frequently via Fenton-type reactions. Additional contributions from peroxisomal metabolism can compound intracellular oxidative burden when antioxidant defenses are overwhelmed. Sustained ROS elevation triggers lipid peroxidation, compromising membrane integrity; induces DNA strand breaks and chromosomal instability; and promotes protein oxidation, impairing structural and enzymatic function. While these pathways reflect canonical nanotoxicological mechanisms, the enhanced surface reactivity and composite nature of advanced nanomaterials may potentiate oxidative damage to a greater extent. Thus, oxidative stress represents a pivotal link between xenobiotic nanoparticle exposure and downstream cellular injury.

Excessive ROS accumulation produces comparable downstream effects in both conventional and advanced nanomaterial systems, including lipid peroxidation, oxidative modification of proteins, and disturbance of intracellular redox homeostasis. However, recently engineered materials may sustain ROS production for longer durations due to persistent ion leaching, slower degradation kinetics, or stable catalytic surfaces that remain reactive within biological environments. Prolonged oxidative burden can intensify membrane damage relative to simpler nanoparticles, accelerating organelle destabilization and amplifying interference with physiological signaling networks. Mitochondrial impairment represents another shared hallmark of nanomaterial-induced toxicity. Traditional nanoparticles have been associated with reduced ATP generation and loss of mitochondrial membrane potential. In contrast, hybrid constructs such as metal-carbon composites may exhibit enhanced mitochondrial accumulation owing to optimized surface functionalization and improved intracellular targeting. This preferential localization can exacerbate disruptions in oxidative phosphorylation, promote cytochrome *c* release, and activate downstream-caspase cascades, thereby facilitating apoptotic progression more rapidly than observed with less complex nanomaterials.

The molecular-level toxicity profile of nanomaterials is strongly influenced by their intrinsic chemical characteristics, including elemental composition, crystallographic structure, and surface functionalization. Reduced particle dimensions often facilitate more efficient cellular internalization, while morphological variations, such as spherical, rod-shaped, or triangular geometries govern the manner in which particles interact with lipid membranes and modulate stress-related cellular pathways. Particle agglomeration further alters biological interactions by modifying the effective surface area, sedimentation dynamics, and consequently the dose that ultimately reaches target cells. In biological environments, adsorption of proteins, lipids, and other macromolecules onto nanoparticle surfaces leads to the formation of a biomolecular corona, which redefines biological identity and plays a central role in determining biodistribution patterns and immune recognition at the tissue and organ scale. Additionally, parameters such as surface charge, hydrophobicity, and applied coatings regulate interactions with physiological barriers and cellular interfaces. Collectively, these multilevel physicochemical attributes demonstrate that nanotoxicity arises from the integrated effects of molecular structure, cellular engagement, and systemic responses, rather than from any single isolated factor, underscoring the need for comprehensive safety evaluation of engineered nanomaterials.

Inflammation represents a fundamental protective response initiated when immune cells such as macrophages, neutrophils, and lymphocytes detect harmful agents, including environmental pollutants, xenobiotics, pharmaceutical residues, or engineered nanomaterials. Activation of these cells triggers the secretion of pro-inflammatory cytokines and chemokines, among them tumor necrosis factor-α (TNF-α), IL-1β, and IL-6, which coordinate recruitment of additional immune populations to the affected site [3]. While this early inflammatory cascade is essential for host defense and tissue repair, excessive or poorly regulated activation can disrupt cellular equilibrium. Sustained release of inflammatory mediators frequently amplifies oxidative stress by promoting ROS generation, creating a self-perpetuating cycle of molecular damage. When immune stimulation persists beyond the resolution stage, a chronic inflammatory state develops, characterized by progressive structural and functional tissue impairment. Mechanisms such as fibrosis, altered signaling pathways, and induction of apoptosis or necrosis contribute to long-term pathology. Within nanotoxicology, chronic inflammation serves as a key indicator of persistent biological impact, as materials that continuously engage immune pathways may compromise organ function and increase susceptibility to disorders including malignancies, cardiovascular conditions, and neurodegenerative diseases. Therefore, detailed characterization of inflammatory processes is essential for risk assessment and for designing nanomaterials with minimized immunotoxic potential. During the acute phase following injury, neutrophils and circulating monocytes infiltrate the damaged tissue, where monocytes differentiate into classically activated (M1) macrophages. These cells release inflammatory mediators such as COX-2, PGE_2, 5-LOX-derived leukotrienes, IL-6, IFN-γ, and TNF-α to contain damage and initiate repair. If the inflammatory response proceeds appropriately, a phenotypic shift toward alternatively activated (M2) macrophages and regulatory T cells occurs. These cells secrete anti-inflammatory cytokines including IL-10, IL-3, TGF-β, and IL-33, facilitating resolution of inflammation, extracellular matrix deposition, angiogenesis, and early tissue regeneration. Successful remodeling restores structural integrity, vascular supply, and cellular organization, ultimately leading to functional recovery [4]. However, if the pro-inflammatory stage is prolonged, often beyond several weeks, the process transitions to chronic inflammation, impairing wound closure, sustaining tissue damage, and resulting in long-term functional deficits.

Genotoxicity describes the capacity of a chemical or material to damage cellular genetic material, thereby compromising genomic integrity and stability. One primary mechanism involves the induction of single- or double-strand DNA breaks when reactive agents interact with the sugar-phosphate backbone or nitrogenous bases. Certain electrophilic or chemically reactive groups present in environmental contaminants, pharmaceutical by-products, or engineered nanomaterials can bind to nucleophilic regions of DNA, leading to structural alterations and mutagenic events. In addition, genomic exposure may result in chromosomal aberrations such as deletions, translocations, or aneuploidy, which interfere with proper cell-cycle regulation and increase oncogenic risk by disrupting replication and transcription fidelity. Beyond direct chemical interactions, ROS represent a major indirect pathway contributing to genotoxic damage. Elevated ROS levels are often associated with metal-containing nanoparticles, photocatalytic nanostructures, or xenobiotic degradation can oxidize purine and pyrimidine bases, promote DNA–protein crosslink formation, and generate highly mutagenic lesions. Evaluating both direct DNA-reactive mechanisms and ROS-mediated oxidative damage is therefore essential for comprehensive safety assessment and for guiding the design of nanomaterials with reduced mutagenic potential. In parallel, nanoparticles may exert immunomodulatory effects due to their nanoscale dimensions and surface reactivity. Direct interactions with immune cells can influence cytokine secretion patterns, antigen presentation processes, and phagocytic activity. Such alterations may precipitate exaggerated immune activation, hypersensitivity reactions, or conversely, immune suppression. Overall, nanoparticle exposure has the potential to reshape immune homeostasis, either enhancing sensitivity or impairing defense mechanisms, underscoring the importance of incorporating immunotoxicity evaluation into nanomaterial development strategies.

10.2 IN VITRO AND IN VIVO TOXICITY EVALUATION

Evaluating toxicity through both in vitro and in vivo approaches is fundamental for determining the biological safety and potential health implications of emerging materials, including nanomaterials, pharmaceuticals, and environmental agents. These two strategies provide complementary perspectives: cell-based models allow controlled examination of direct cellular effects, while whole-organism studies capture systemic and long-term responses. In vitro systems enable efficient and economically feasible investigation of endpoints such as cytotoxicity, oxidative imbalance, DNA damage, and immune activation under defined experimental conditions. However, they cannot fully reproduce the complexity of physiological processes such as biodistribution, metabolism, organ-specific accumulation, and chronic exposure outcomes. In vivo studies address these limitations by incorporating integrated biological networks and organ-level interactions. Together, these methodologies form the core framework for toxicological risk evaluation, regulatory decision-making, and the rational development of safer materials for medical, industrial, and environmental applications.

10.2.1 Cell Cultures–Based Models

2D cell culture platforms, typically composed of monolayers of immortalized cell lines or primary cells, continue to serve as foundational systems in toxicological evaluation due to their capacity to quantify key cellular endpoints with precision. Standard assays such as MTT, lactate dehydrogenase leakage, and live/dead staining are routinely employed to determine cell viability, membrane integrity, and metabolic competence following exposure to test compounds. Uptake analyses using fluorescence microscopy, flow cytometry, or electron microscopy further allow assessment of nanoparticle internalization and intracellular accumulation, facilitating interpretation of dose-dependent biological effects. Moreover, 2D models support mechanistic exploration by enabling measurement of oxidative stress markers, mitochondrial impairment, activation of apoptotic signaling cascades, DNA damage, inflammatory mediator release, and shifts in gene or protein expression profiles. Although these systems lack the architectural and microenvironmental complexity of native tissues, their experimental simplicity and compatibility with high-throughput screening platforms make them highly effective for preliminary toxicity assessment and mechanistic insight.

In contrast, three-dimensional (3D) culture models including multicellular spheroids, organotypic constructs, and organoids more closely recapitulate in vivo tissue organization. These systems permit cell–cell and cell–extracellular matrix interactions that are essential for maintaining structural integrity and functional phenotype. The establishment of physiologically relevant gradients of oxygen, nutrients, and signaling molecules within 3D constructs more accurately mirrors in vivo conditions. As a result, 3D cultures enable improved evaluation of cellular proliferation, differentiation dynamics, pharmacological response, and toxicological outcomes, thereby enhancing the translational predictability of preclinical studies.

10.2.2 Animal-Based Models

Animal models ranging from rodents such as mice and rats to non-rodent species including rabbits, dogs, minipigs, and nonhuman primates play a pivotal role in preclinical evaluation of new drugs and advanced therapeutic platforms. These in vivo systems enable comprehensive assessment of systemic toxicity, biodistribution patterns, immune responses, and long-term biological consequences within an intact organism. Unlike simplified in vitro models, animal studies capture integrated physiological processes involving multiple organs, metabolic pathways, and immune regulation. Preclinical pharmacokinetic and safety investigations rely on such models to determine tissue distribution, metabolic transformation, elimination kinetics, and the potential for organ-specific accumulation, thereby informing safe and rational dose selection prior to clinical trials. Toxicological evaluation in animals encompasses both short-term and prolonged exposure paradigms. Acute studies assess immediate adverse outcomes and organ injury, whereas sub-chronic and chronic investigations identify cumulative toxicity, immunological alterations, and target-organ pathologies following repeated dosing. A concise overview of these experimental models is presented in Table 10.1.

TABLE 10.1
Summary of Model System for Nanotoxicology Evaluation

Model System	Primary Advantages	Key Limitations	Best Applications
2D cell culture	• High-throughput screening • Cost-effective • Simple protocols • Reproducible • Rapid results • Direct NP–cell interaction observation	• Overestimates toxicity for many NPs • No ECM barriers • Artificial cell morphology • Poor in vivo predictive value • Limited cell–cell interactions	• Initial screening • Mechanistic studies of NP–cell interactions • Comparative studies • High-throughput toxicity ranking
3D cell culture	• Bridges gap between 2D and in vivo • Tissue-like architecture • Physiologically relevant cell–cell contacts • Captures diffusion barriers	• More complex protocols • Lower throughput than 2D • Size heterogeneity in spheroids • Limited perfusion in large spheroids • ECM can be barrier to NP entry in some culture systems	• Intermediate screening after 2D • Mechanistic studies of NP penetration • Evaluation of tissue-level responses • Nanomedicine development
Animal models	• Complete organism responses • Biodistribution assessment • Immune system interactions • Regulatory acceptance	• Expensive • Time-consuming • Ethical concerns • Species and individuals' variability • Low throughput	• Regulatory toxicology • Safety assessment • Biodistribution and pharmacokinetics • Chronic and reproductive toxicity • Preclinical trial

10.3 BIODISTRIBUTION, METABOLISM, AND CLEARANCE

A thorough understanding of nanoparticle behavior within biological systems is essential for evaluating both their safety and therapeutic performance. From the point of administration to cellular internalization, intracellular transport, organ distribution, and final elimination, nanoparticles undergo a series of interconnected processes governed by their physicochemical characteristics and the dynamic responses of biological environments.

10.3.1 Uptake and Trafficking

Cellular internalization of nanoparticles occurs primarily via endocytosis, a collective term describing multiple uptake pathways. The principal mechanisms include phagocytosis, macropinocytosis, clathrin-dependent endocytosis, and caveolin-mediated endocytosis, as illustrated in Figure 10.3.

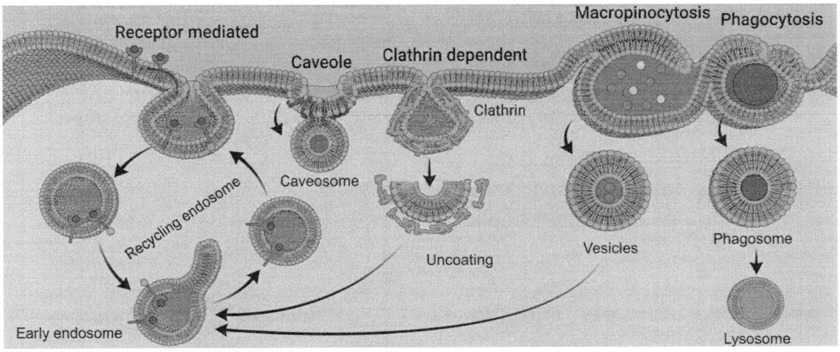

FIGURE 10.3 Schematic illustration of cellular internalization pathways of nanocarriers, including receptor-mediated endocytosis, caveolae-mediated uptake, clathrin-dependent endocytosis, macropinocytosis, and phagocytosis, followed by intracellular trafficking through early endosomes, recycling endosomes, caveosomes, and eventual lysosomal processing.

Phagocytosis is primarily performed by specialized immune cells, including macrophages, monocytes, and dendritic cells and is especially relevant for the uptake of larger particles, which are enclosed within membrane-bound phagosomes after engulfment. In contrast, macropinocytosis occurs through nonselective membrane ruffling, permitting the concurrent internalization of extracellular fluid and nanoparticles across a broad spectrum. Receptor-mediated pathways such as clathrin-dependent endocytosis generally favor smaller nanoparticles, consistent with the approximate 120 nm diameter of clathrin-coated vesicles, whereas caveolae-mediated entry involves even smaller invaginations, typically around 60 nm in size. The dominant internalization route is determined by particle attributes including size, surface charge, and chemical functionalization. For instance, cationic nanoparticles frequently engage macropinocytic mechanisms, while anionic particles are more commonly internalized through clathrin-associated processes.

Once inside the cell, nanoparticles are directed through organized intracellular trafficking pathways. The endosomal–lysosomal route represents the principal pathway, wherein particles transition from early endosomes to late endosomes and ultimately to lysosomes within a relatively short timeframe. This progression is critical because lysosomes provide an acidic, enzyme-rich environment capable of degrading internalized materials. The intracellular fate of nanoparticles strongly influences their functional outcomes; sequestration within lysosomes may limit therapeutic efficacy by promoting degradation before target engagement. Depending on their physicochemical characteristics, some nanoparticles may also be transported via endosome-to-Golgi or Golgi-to-endoplasmic reticulum pathways. During cell division, lysosome-contained nanoparticles may be distributed unevenly between daughter cells, potentially contributing to prolonged or heterogeneous cellular effects following exposure.

10.3.2 Organ Accumulation

Following systemic administration, nanoparticles exhibit nonuniform biodistribution, with predominant sequestration in the liver. The hepatic microarchitecture characterized by fenestrated sinusoids, reduced blood flow velocity, and extensive exposure of Kupffer cells to circulating blood facilitates efficient capture of nanomaterials, in some cases retaining the vast majority of injected particles. Within the first 24h post-administration, substantial hepatic accumulation is typically observed, accompanied by moderate deposition in the spleen and comparatively lower levels in other organs.

Particle size is a decisive determinant of distribution patterns. Smaller nanoparticles (approximately 10nm) tend to demonstrate reduced hepatic retention but increased renal localization, likely reflecting partial evasion of immediate uptake by the mononuclear phagocyte system and enhanced filtration through the kidneys. Meta-analytical data from animal studies indicate that particles within the intermediate size range of roughly 11–100nm show the highest degree of liver accumulation, whereas larger particles exceeding 200nm often display comparatively lower overall tissue deposition. Beyond primary organs such as the liver and spleen, nanoparticles may localize in secondary tissues including the kidneys, brain, heart, and lungs. The extent and pattern of accumulation are influenced by multiple factors, including particle size, surface properties, morphology, and route of administration.

The BBB functions as a highly selective interface that restricts the entry of most nanoparticles into the central nervous system. Its tight junction architecture and regulated transport mechanisms significantly limit passive diffusion of nanomaterials. The extent of nanoparticle accumulation in brain tissue is therefore closely associated with the integrity and permeability of the BBB, with increased permeability allowing transient passage under certain pathological or externally induced conditions, as presented in Figure 10.4. In normal physiological states, effective traversal of the

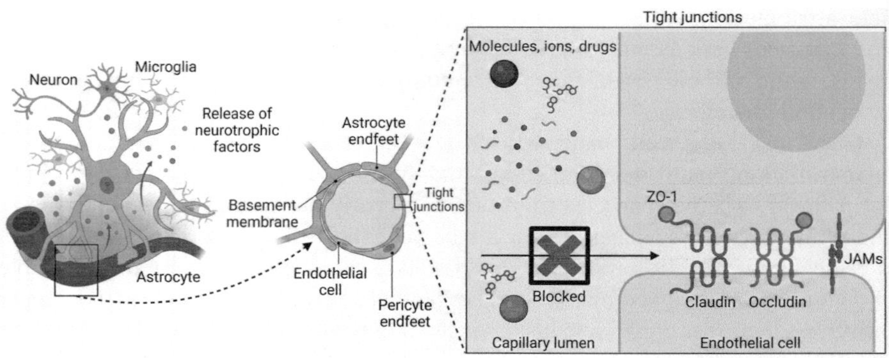

FIGURE 10.4 Structure and function of the BBB. The BBB is structurally composed of endothelial cells, the vascular basement membrane, pericytes, and astrocyte end-feet. The endothelial cells of the BBB have tight junctions that lack fenestration and pinocytic activity, thereby preventing most molecules, ions, and drugs from paracellular transport. (Adapted from Ref. [5] (CC BY).)

BBB generally requires deliberate surface engineering, such as the incorporation of targeting ligands or specific physicochemical modifications to facilitate receptor-mediated transport or other specialized translocation mechanisms.

10.3.3 Biodegradation Versus Persistence

The extent of long-term biological impact associated with nanoparticles is closely linked to their degradability within physiological environments. Biodegradable nanomaterials are designed to progressively disassemble into smaller fragments and ultimately transform into nontoxic by-products or metabolites that can be cleared from the body. Such controlled degradation is essential to prevent prolonged tissue retention and associated chronic toxicity. For instance, mesoporous silica nanoparticles can be modified to enhance degradability through strategies such as organic or metal doping, or by integrating labile bonds (e.g., thioether linkages) into their framework. These structural adaptations allow degradation to be triggered under specific biological conditions, including acidic microenvironments, intracellular reducing agents like glutathione, or enzymatic processes. Acid-sensitive nanoparticles can undergo accelerated breakdown within lysosomal compartments, producing ultrasmall fragments, typically below renal filtration thresholds that are more readily excreted.

Conversely, nondegradable or highly stable nanoparticles, such as uncoated gold nanostructures or certain metal oxide formulations, tend to persist within tissues for extended durations. Longitudinal biodistribution analyses demonstrate limited clearance of such materials over time. In prolonged studies, organ retention patterns have shown only partial reduction of hepatic accumulation, alongside increased deposition in organs such as the spleen and kidneys. Because elimination kinetics can be slow, persistent nanomaterials may remain in biological systems for years. Extrapolative modeling suggests that nanoparticles retained in animal models for several months could correspond to multi-decade persistence in human tissues, highlighting the importance of considering degradation behavior in long-term safety assessments [6,7].

10.3.4 Long-Term Effects and Chronic Responses

Persistent nanoparticle accumulation can provoke sustained inflammatory and fibrotic alterations within target organs, even when overall concentrations are relatively low. Prolonged exposure is associated with elevated production of pro-inflammatory mediators such as TNF-α and chemokine ligand 2 (CXCL2), activation of tissue-resident macrophages, and increased deposition of extracellular matrix proteins including fibronectin, an early indicator of fibrogenesis. The magnitude and progression of these responses vary among organs, reflecting differences in nanoparticle retention and tissue-specific clearance kinetics. When nanomaterials preferentially accumulate in organs such as the liver and spleen, secondary renal effects may occur, including glomerular and tubular injury accompanied by enhanced urinary albumin excretion, suggesting compromised filtration capacity. Histopathological findings often reveal expanded mesangial regions and fibronectin deposition within renal tissue, even in the absence of substantial nanoparticle burden, implying that circulating inflammatory mediators released from distal accumulation sites may contribute to kidney dysfunction. Sustained nanoparticle exposure can also initiate organ-specific fibrotic remodeling. In hepatic tissue, infiltration of mononuclear immune cells, increased extracellular matrix deposition, and activation of fibrogenic signaling pathways signal the onset of early liver fibrosis. Similarly, splenic tissue may exhibit progressive fibronectin accumulation and elevated inflammatory markers weeks after exposure, indicating a transition from acute inflammation to chronic fibrotic restructuring. Over time, these structural changes can compromise organ architecture and physiological function. Importantly, even nanomaterials generally considered biocompatible such as gold nanoparticles, may induce adverse outcomes when retained for extended periods, underscoring the need to consider long-term biodistribution and persistence in safety evaluations.

10.4 EMERGING TOOLS AND APPROACHES FOR SAFER NANOMATERIALS

The accelerated progress of nanomedicine has driven the development of sophisticated strategies and technologies designed to anticipate, minimize, and manage nanomaterial-associated toxicity before clinical application. Contemporary approaches integrate safety considerations early in the innovation process through Safe-by-Design (SbD) principles, employ artificial intelligence and machine learning (AI/ML) for rapid, data-informed toxicity forecasting, and utilize organ-on-chip (OoC) systems to generate physiologically relevant, multiparameter evaluations of nanomaterial responses. Collectively, these complementary tools form a cohesive framework that enhances translational efficiency, reduces dependence on animal experimentation, and mitigates potential human health risks during the development of nano-enabled therapeutics.

10.4.1 Safe-by-Design

SbD represents a strategic transition from post hoc hazard evaluation toward anticipatory risk minimization, embedding safety considerations at the earliest stages of nanomaterial innovation. Rather than treating safety as a downstream regulatory obligation, SbD integrates anticipated environmental and human health impacts directly into material conception, synthesis, scale-up, and application planning. The objective is to engineer nanomaterials that maintain functional performance while inherently exhibiting reduced risk profiles. Two overarching approaches underpin SbD: intrinsic hazard minimization through material modification and reduction of exposure across the product life cycle. Conceptually, SbD encompasses three interconnected pillars, safe material design, safe manufacturing, and safe end use. Safe design focuses on tailoring physicochemical attributes such as particle size, morphology, composition, surface chemistry, and functionalization to decrease reactivity, persistence, or bioaccumulation potential. Examples include decreasing the aspect ratio of fibrous nanomaterials, applying biocompatible polymer coatings to reactive metal oxides, or incorporating biodegradable linkages into silica-based systems to facilitate environmental breakdown. Drawing from green chemistry principles, multifunctional efficiency aims to maximize desired properties while eliminating unnecessary or potentially hazardous components, thereby streamlining synthesis and reducing cumulative risk.

Safe production addresses occupational exposure during fabrication through engineering controls such as closed processing systems, aerosol containment, and worker protection strategies. Safe use extends this perspective to downstream stages, including product application, recycling, and disposal, by evaluating realistic exposure scenarios. European initiatives such as NANoREG and NanoReg2 have operationalized these principles by developing structured Safety Dossiers that compile physicochemical characterization, toxicological data, and exposure assessments throughout development. This staged documentation framework supports evidence-based go/no-go decisions and fosters early dialogue between innovators and regulatory authorities, facilitating smoother approval pathways for safer nano-enabled technologies [8,9].

Effective SbD implementation depends on robust structure–activity relationship data, which are often limited for emerging nanomaterial classes. To address this gap, SbD frameworks increasingly incorporate high-throughput screening and computational modeling to rapidly assess how design modifications influence biological responses. Surface engineering strategies such as PEGylation or the introduction of zwitterionic ligands can reduce nonspecific protein adsorption, limit macrophage uptake, and decrease off-target organ accumulation and inflammation [10]. Similarly, doping metal oxides with less hazardous elements or engineering porous architectures to accelerate biodegradation can mitigate long-term persistence and chronic toxicity. Platforms such as SAbyNA provide systematic guidance by linking design parameters to safety and sustainability indicators throughout the innovation life cycle.

Despite its promise, SbD faces practical challenges. Comprehensive, high-quality datasets remain insufficient for many nanomaterial categories, and optimizing safety without compromising functionality often requires complex trade-offs. Excessive modification to enhance safety may diminish performance or complicate manufacturing scalability. Nonetheless, as regulatory bodies increasingly recognize SbD as a best-practice framework, its integration is likely to become progressively important, particularly for applications associated with significant human or environmental exposure.

10.4.2 AI/ML Applications: Accelerating Toxicity Prediction and Assessment

AI and ML are increasingly reshaping nanotoxicology by enabling the analysis of large, heterogeneous datasets to forecast nanoparticle–biological interactions. These computational strategies significantly reduce the cost, time, and animal usage associated with conventional safety assessments. Traditional experimental screening approaches are labor-intensive and often unable to match the accelerating pace of nanomaterial innovation. AI/ML methodologies help overcome this limitation by detecting complex relationships between physicochemical descriptors, such as particle size, morphology, surface charge, composition, and functionalization and biological endpoints including cytotoxicity, oxidative stress, inflammatory signaling, and genotoxic effects. This is commonly achieved through nano-adapted quantitative structure–activity relationship models (nano-QSAR), which are specifically designed to accommodate nanoscale properties.

A range of supervised learning techniques including Random Forest, Support Vector Machines, Decision Trees, Naïve Bayes classifiers, and Artificial Neural Networks have been applied successfully to nanotoxicity datasets, frequently outperforming conventional regression-based analyses [11]. Comparative evaluations of multiple classification algorithms have demonstrated that Random Forest models often provide superior predictive accuracy for nanoparticle-induced cytotoxicity. Importantly, such analyses reveal that biological context variables, such as cell type, exposure concentration, and tissue origin can be as influential as material descriptors, emphasizing the need for integrative, context-aware predictive models rather than reliance solely on physicochemical parameters.

Nano-QSAR frameworks expand traditional QSAR methodologies by incorporating nanomaterial-specific descriptors, including particle size distribution, agglomeration behavior, and detailed surface functionalization metrics. An illustrative example is the NanoToxRadar platform, a web-accessible multitarget nano-QSAR system capable of simultaneously predicting cytotoxic responses of metal-based multicomponent nanoparticles across a wide panel of cell lines (Figure 10.5). By integrating features such as electron configuration-based fingerprints and encoded biological variables, the platform achieves strong predictive performance ($R^2 \geq 0.850$) and provides researchers with a practical pre-synthesis screening tool for evaluating the safety profiles of novel nanomaterial formulations.

Similarly, ML-driven QSAR frameworks developed for mixtures of metal oxide nanoparticles have demonstrated superior predictive performance compared with conventional mixture toxicity models such as Independent Action and Concentration Addition, particularly when applied to complex binary or ternary systems [13]. Advanced deep learning architectures, including convolutional neural networks, are increasingly being employed to model nano–bio interactions by learning multilevel feature representations from large-scale imaging and spectroscopic datasets. These approaches have shown strong capability in predicting oxidative stress potential for carbon-based nanomaterials, such as fullerenes, graphene derivatives, and carbon nanotubes as well as their combinations, thereby linking structural attributes to mechanistic biological outcomes. The emergence of automated ML platforms further democratizes model development by autonomously selecting optimal algorithms and tuning hyperparameters across extensive search spaces.

Despite these advances, data-related challenges remain substantial. Many nano-QSAR models rely on relatively small and heterogeneous datasets extracted from published studies, limiting their domain of applicability and increasing the risk of overfitting. Platforms such as NanoToxRadar address this issue by explicitly defining applicability domain boundaries and flagging query nanoparticles that fall outside the training space. Broader efforts toward standardized data reporting supported by initiatives and repositories such as NanoPUZZLES and caNanoLab are essential for expanding high-quality training datasets and improving model generalizability. Rigorous validation strategies, including cross-validation and Y-randomization testing, are also critical to ensure robustness and to minimize spurious correlations.

Regulatory recognition of AI- and ML-based toxicological predictions is gradually expanding, though the framework continues to evolve. Agencies including the U.S. Food and Drug Administration and the European Medicines Agency are

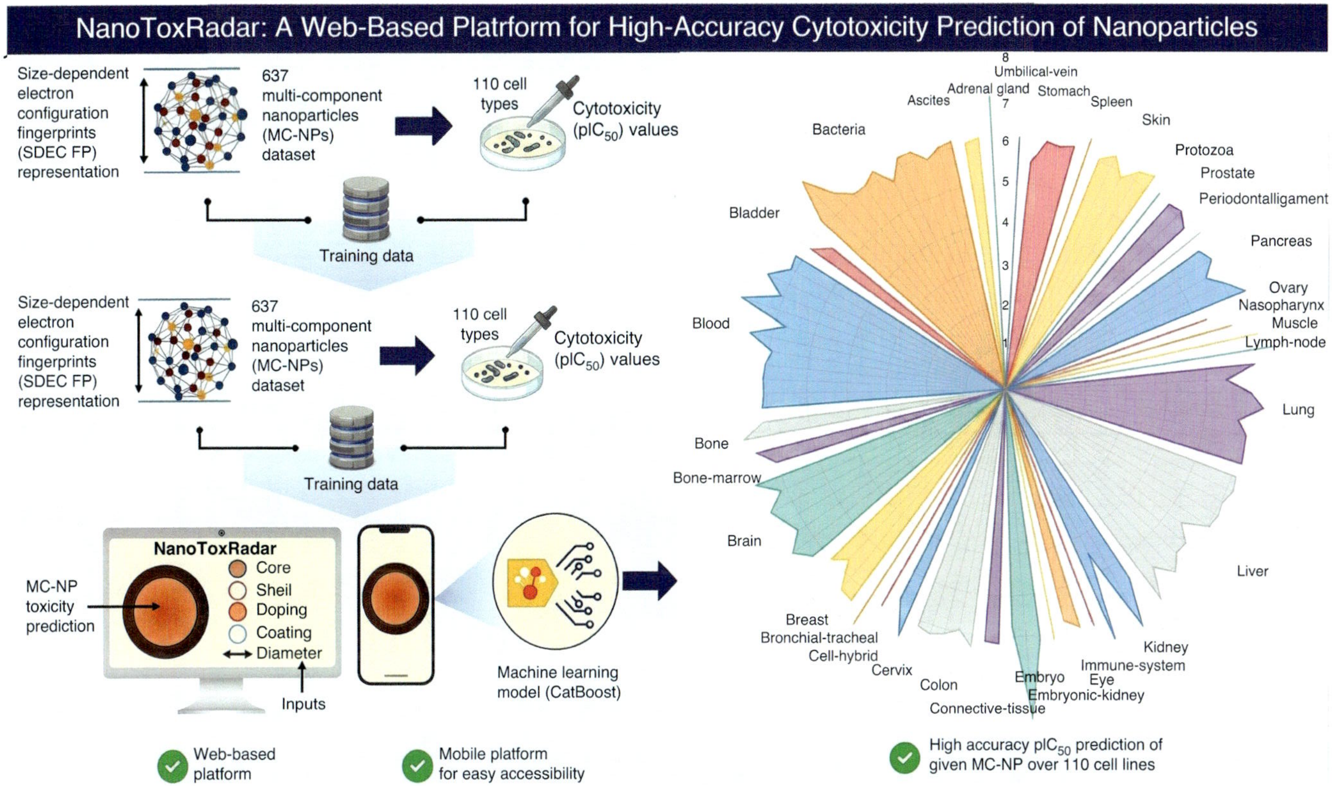

FIGURE 10.5 Schematic representation of NanoToxRadar, a web-based platform for high-accuracy cytotoxicity prediction of multicomponent nanoparticles (MC-NPs). The workflow integrates size-dependent electron configuration fingerprints (SDEC FP) and physicochemical descriptors (core, shell, doping, coating, and diameter) with cytotoxicity (pIC_{50}) data to train a CatBoost machine learning model, enabling accurate, accessible toxicity prediction via web and mobile interfaces. (Adapted from Ref. [12] (CC BY).)

increasingly considering QSAR-derived outputs within weight-of-evidence assessments, particularly during preliminary screening and prioritization stages. However, regulatory acceptance depends on thorough experimental validation and transparent documentation of model scope and limitations. Integration of ML with OoC platforms represents a particularly promising convergence: high-content data generated from microphysiological systems (MPS) can feed predictive algorithms, enabling iterative refinement of safety profiles within a closed-loop optimization framework.

10.4.3 Advanced Models: Microphysiological Systems for Human-Relevant Toxicity Prediction

OoC technologies and broader MPS represent a major advancement beyond conventional static 2D cultures, offering dynamic, organ-relevant in vitro models that replicate key aspects of human tissue architecture and function. These platforms incorporate living cells into microfluidic devices where parameters such as fluid shear stress, mechanical stimulation, and chemical gradients are tightly regulated. This design enables continuous observation of nanomaterial interactions at tissue-level resolution. A primary limitation of traditional nanotoxicity assays is the inability to capture organ-specific complexity and systemic interplay, which is therefore addressed by these systems. Individual OoC models have been engineered for critical organs including lung, liver, kidney, heart, brain, skin, and intestine, each tailored to recreate its native microenvironment [14,15]. For example, lung-on-chip systems that reproduce the alveolar-capillary interface with cyclic mechanical strain simulating respiration have demonstrated that silica nanoparticles provoke stronger inflammatory responses under dynamic mechanical conditions than in static culture, highlighting the importance of physiological forces in toxicity assessment. Similarly, liver-on-chip platforms integrating hepatocytes with resident immune cells such as Kupffer cells have shown nanoparticle-induced hepatocellular injury and cytokine production consistent with in vivo findings, supporting their utility in hepatic safety evaluation.

Expanding upon single-organ models, multi-organ-on-chip configurations interconnect multiple tissue compartments through microfluidic circulation to simulate systemic transport, metabolism, and secondary organ effects. In systems linking liver, kidney, and bone marrow modules, investigations of iron oxide nanoparticle distribution revealed metabolite-driven toxicity pathways in which inflammatory signals originating from the liver contributed to renal injury, an effect not apparent in isolated organ models. Such integrated platforms are particularly valuable for assessing systemically administered nanomedicines, as they simultaneously provide data on organ-specific accumulation, clearance dynamics, metabolic transformation, and inter-organ crosstalk [16,17].

Skin-on-chip (SoC) devices have emerged as promising tools for evaluating dermal exposure to nanomaterials in cosmetic and occupational contexts. These models replicate the stratified organization of human skin, comprising epidermal, dermal, and subcutaneous layers, while incorporating controlled perfusion and, in some designs, immune cell components (Figure 10.6). Nanomaterial penetration can occur via transcellular, intercellular, or appendageal pathways involving

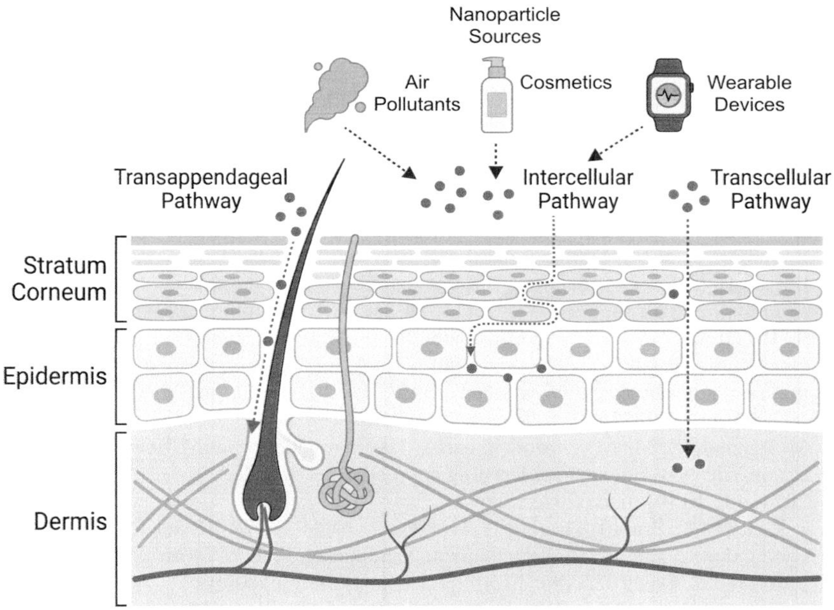

FIGURE 10.6 Conceptual overview of nanomaterial interactions with human skin, illustrating exposure routes, penetration pathways, and cellular outcomes.

hair follicles and associated glands. SoC systems allow realistic assessment of dermal permeability, sensitization potential, and inflammatory responses under mechanically and biochemically relevant conditions, offering a refined alternative to animal-based skin toxicity testing. Successful implementation depends on accurately reproducing both the structural hierarchy and dynamic functional properties of native skin tissue.

REFERENCES

1. S. Panico, S. Capolla, S. Bozzer, G. Toffoli, M. D. Bo, and P. Macor, 'Biological features of nanoparticles: protein corona formation and interaction with the immune system', *Pharmaceutics*, vol. 14, no. 12, Nov. 2022, doi: 10.3390/pharmaceutics14122605.
2. V. Torrisi et al., 'Preventing corona effects: multiphosphonic acid poly(ethylene glycol) copolymers for stable stealth iron oxide nanoparticles', *Biomacromolecules*, vol. 15, no. 8, pp. 3171–3179, Aug. 2014, doi: 10.1021/bm500832q.
3. P. Krzyszczyk, R. Schloss, A. Palmer, and F. Berthiaume, 'The role of macrophages in acute and chronic wound healing and interventions to promote pro-wound healing phenotypes', *Front. Physiol.*, vol. 9, p. 419, 2018, doi: 10.3389/fphys.2018.00419.
4. H. Zhao et al., 'Inflammation and tumor progression: signaling pathways and targeted intervention', *Signal Transduct. Target. Ther.*, vol. 6, no. 1, p. 263, Jul. 2021, doi: 10.1038/s41392-021-00658-5.
5. E. Asimakidou, J. K. S. Tan, J. Zeng, and C. H. Lo, 'Blood-brain barrier-targeting nanoparticles: biomaterial properties and biomedical applications in translational neuroscience', *Pharmaceuticals*, vol. 17, no. 5, p. 612, May 2024, doi: 10.3390/ph17050612.

6. K. Jakic et al., 'Long-term accumulation, biological effects and toxicity of BSA-coated gold nanoparticles in the mouse liver, spleen, and kidneys', *Int. J. Nanomedicine*, vol. 19, pp. 4103–4120, 2024, doi: 10.2147/IJN.S443168.
7. C. Schleh et al., 'Biodistribution of inhaled gold nanoparticles in mice and the influence of surfactant protein D', *J. Aerosol Med. Pulm. Drug Deliv.*, vol. 26, no. 1, pp. 24–30, Feb. 2013, doi: 10.1089/jamp.2011.0951.
8. B. D. Trump et al., 'Safety-by-design and engineered nanomaterials: the need to move from theory to practice', *Environ. Syst. Decis.*, vol. 44, no. 1, pp. 177–188, Mar. 2024, doi: 10.1007/s10669-023-09927-w.
9. B. Salieri et al., 'Integrative approach in a safe by design context combining risk, life cycle and socio-economic assessment for safer and sustainable nanomaterials', *NanoImpact*, vol. 23, p. 100335, Jul. 2021, doi: 10.1016/j.impact.2021.100335.
10. K. P. García et al., 'Zwitterionic-coated "Stealth" nanoparticles for biomedical applications: recent advances in countering biomolecular corona formation and uptake by the mononuclear phagocyte system', *Small*, vol. 10, no. 13, pp. 2516–2529, 2014, doi: 10.1002/smll.201303540.
11. M. Ahmadi, S. M. Ayyoubzadeh, and F. Ghorbani-Bidkorpeh, 'Toxicity prediction of nanoparticles using machine learning approaches', *Toxicology*, vol. 501, p. 153697, Jan. 2024, doi: 10.1016/j.tox.2023.153697.
12. J. Park et al., 'NanoToxRadar: A Multitarget Nano-QSAR Model for Predicting the Cytotoxicity Values of Multicomponent Nanoparticles', *ACS Nanosci. Au*, vol. 5, no. 5, pp. 344–352, Oct. 2025, doi: 10.1021/acsnanoscienceau.5c00035.
13. F. Zhang, Z. Wang, W. J. G. M. Peijnenburg, and M. G. Vijver, 'Machine learning-driven QSAR models for predicting the mixture toxicity of nanoparticles', *Environ. Int.*, vol. 177, p. 108025, Jul. 2023, doi: 10.1016/j.envint.2023.108025.
14. C. M. Leung et al., 'A guide to the organ-on-a-chip', *Nat. Rev. Methods Primer*, vol. 2, no. 1, p. 33, May 2022, doi: 10.1038/s43586-022-00118-6.
15. D. E. Ingber, 'Human organs-on-chips for disease modelling, drug development and personalized medicine', *Nat. Rev. Genet.*, vol. 23, no. 8, pp. 467–491, Aug. 2022, doi: 10.1038/s41576-022-00466-9.
16. H.-R. Moon, N. Surianarayanan, T. Singh, and B. Han, 'Microphysiological systems as reliable drug discovery and evaluation tools: Evolution from innovation to maturity', *Biomicrofluidics*, vol. 17, no. 6, p. 061504, Dec. 2023, doi: 10.1063/5.0179444.
17. T. I. Maulana et al., 'Opportunities for microphysiological systems in toxicity testing of new drug modalities', *Annu. Rev. Pharmacol. Toxicol.*, vol. 65, 2025, pp. 47–69, Jan. 2025, doi: 10.1146/annurev-pharmtox-061724-080621.

11 Translational Challenges and Safety Regulations for Bio-Applications

David Nugroho and Aphinya Thinthasit

11.1 INTRODUCTION

The clinical translation of nanomedicines has proven substantially more complicated than expectation. Unlike conventional small-molecule therapeutics or biologics, these systems are extremely responsive to even minor modifications in formulation and production parameters. Slight differences in particle size, surface characteristics, structural organization, or preparation conditions can markedly alter biodistribution patterns, immune interactions, safety outcomes, and overall therapeutic efficacy. Because of this sensitivity, many nanotechnology-based platforms that show strong preclinical promise fail to advance beyond animal studies or early-phase human trials. This translational barrier is closely linked to shortcomings in both preclinical evaluation models and existing regulatory frameworks. Although animal studies remain central to traditional drug development pathways, their predictive accuracy for nanomedicines is often limited. Pronounced interspecies variations in immune recognition, metabolic processing, biodistribution, and clearance mechanisms reduce the reliability of extrapolating animal data to human outcomes. In parallel, transitioning nanoparticle synthesis from laboratory-scale preparation to reproducible, large-scale industrial manufacturing introduces further complexity (Figure 11.1). Challenges such as maintaining strict process control, minimizing batch-to-batch variability, and ensuring rigorous quality assurance directly impact the ability to produce consistent clinical-grade materials that meet regulatory expectations.

From a regulatory standpoint, nanomedicines exist within a distinctive and continuously developing framework. At present, major authorities such as the U.S. Food and Drug Administration (FDA) and the European Medicines Agency (EMA) assess nanotechnology-enabled products under established regulatory pathways originally designed for drugs, biologics, or medical devices rather than through nanomedicine-specific legislation. This chapter explores the principal translational barriers and safety considerations that govern the advancement of nanomedicines for bio-applications. Particular emphasis is placed on three interconnected aspects. First, it discusses the technical and biological constraints that affect scalability, reproducibility, and the predictive reliability of interspecies models. Second, it highlights integrated experimental and computational strategies aimed at strengthening the connection between preclinical findings and clinical outcomes. Third, it reviews

DOI: 10.1201/9781003725930-11

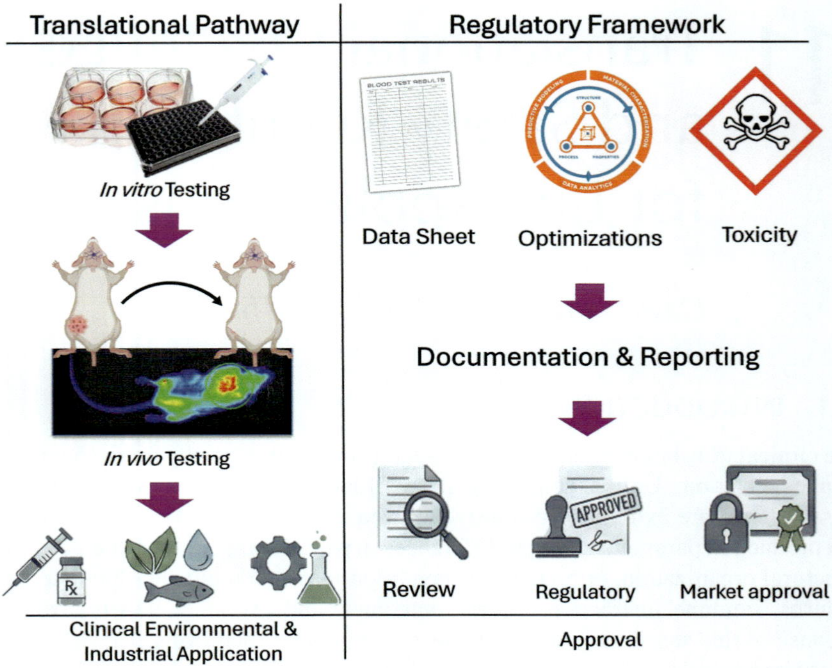

FIGURE 11.1 Translation pathway and regulatory framework for nanocarrier-based therapeutics. The regulatory framework outlines standardized testing blocks, comprehensive documentation, and safety reporting, followed by scientific review, regulatory decision-making, and market authorization.

the shifting global regulatory environment, supported by selected case examples of nanomedicine platforms that have progressed to advanced clinical stages.

11.2 TRANSLATIONAL CHALLENGES IN NANOMEDICINE

Progressing nanoparticle-based therapeutics from initial laboratory discovery to routine clinical use involves obstacles that extend beyond conventional drug development paradigms. These translational difficulties arise largely from the intrinsic structural and functional complexity of nanomaterials, the limited reliability of predicting human outcomes solely from animal models, and the technical demands associated with scaling up manufacturing processes without compromising rigorous quality and consistency standards.

11.2.1 Reproducibility and Scalability

One of the principal barriers to the clinical translation of nanomedicines is batch-to-batch inconsistency during nanoparticle synthesis, together with the technical complexity of expanding laboratory protocols to industrial production. Even when

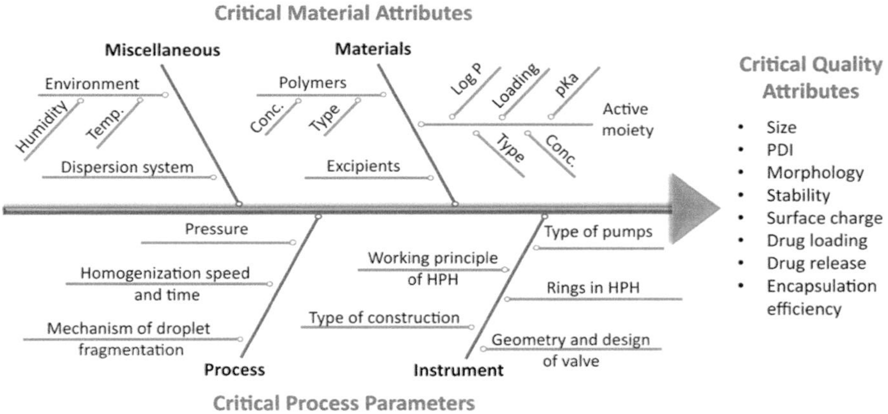

FIGURE 11.2 Representation of the critical material attributes (CMAs) and critical process parameters (CPPs) that cause discrepancy and variability of critical quality attributes (CQAs) during the rational design and production of nanomedicines. (Adapted from Ref. [1] (CC BY).)

identical synthetic routes are followed, nanoparticles often display notable variations in physicochemical properties including particle size, size distribution, surface charge, and surface chemistry, across different batches. Therefore, precise identification and control of critical quality attributes (CQAs) are essential for ensuring safety and performance during development. Among the numerous CQAs evaluated in preclinical studies (Figure 11.2), parameters such as particle size, encapsulation efficiency, polydispersity index, zeta potential, and drug release kinetics are most frequently emphasized. Evidence from a large multinational investigation involving 14 European laboratories demonstrated substantial inter-batch variability in widely used nanoparticles, including silica dioxide, zinc oxide, cerium dioxide, and titanium dioxide. Notably, nanoparticles derived from the same bulk material can exhibit markedly different biological behaviors [2]. For instance, three separate batches of cerium dioxide nanoparticles with comparable surface area and chemical composition displayed distinct protein adsorption patterns in alveolar lining fluid. Such findings underscore a critical concern: nanoparticle surface characteristics, highly sensitive to subtle changes in synthesis, directly govern biological interactions and therapeutic performance.

The root cause of this variability often lies within the synthetic methodology itself. Colloidal fabrication techniques, commonly applied to produce anisotropic plasmonic nanostructures such as gold nanorods, are particularly susceptible to reproducibility issues due to the complexity of multistep reaction schemes. Minor fluctuations in temperature, precursor concentration, or mixing dynamics can significantly influence nucleation and growth kinetics, ultimately generating batches with divergent properties. Addressing these challenges requires systematic identification and control of variability-inducing factors. Standardized process optimization strategies have improved reproducibility in polymer-based nanoparticle systems. By correlating design variables, such as polymer molecular weight and monomer composition with CQAs through predictive mathematical modeling, manufacturers can implement robust quality control frameworks. For example, reverse addition-fragmentation chain transfer (RAFT) polymerization can be optimized to achieve statistical process control with capability indices (C_{pk}) $\geq$ 1.35, indicating a stable and reliable process. RAFT maintains controlled radical polymerization behavior while offering flexibility in reaction conditions, enabling reproducible synthesis across operators, instruments, and production scales. Even diameter variations within ±5 nm may be acceptable, provided biological efficacy remains unaffected. Scaling from bench to clinical manufacturing introduces additional complexity, as increases in batch volume alter mass and momentum transfer rates, thereby affecting fluid dynamics and nanoparticle formation mechanisms. Continuous techniques such as Flash Nano-Precipitation (FNP), which employs rapid precipitation with stabilizers, have emerged as scalable solutions capable of increasing production from laboratory to pilot scale while maintaining tight control over nanoscale attributes. When integrated with downstream processes like spray drying, FNP supports continuous nanomanufacturing platforms that preserve key CQAs including particle size, polydispersity, and drug loading throughout scale-up. Such manufacturing consistency is indispensable for clinical translation since therapeutic success depends not only on preclinical efficacy but also on the ability to reproducibly produce high-quality formulations at clinically and economically viable scales.

11.2.2 Variability in Biological Responses and Species

A second critical obstacle in the translation of nanomedicines is the pronounced interspecies variability in nanoparticle processing, biodistribution, and pharmacokinetics, which limits direct extrapolation of preclinical findings to humans. Although mice and rats are the primary models used in nanomedicine research, their responses to nanoparticles often diverge significantly, not only from humans but also from each other, despite close phylogenetic relationships. Key physiological determinants of nanoparticle distribution, including organ perfusion rates, hepatic clearance efficiency, and renal filtration properties, vary considerably between rodents and larger species such as dogs and humans, resulting in distinct pharmacokinetic behaviors.

Multiple biological mechanisms underlie these species-specific differences. Variations in regional blood flow distribution influence the extent of hepatic uptake and splenic sequestration of nanoparticles. In addition, plasma protein interactions differ across species. For example, human albumin shows substantially stronger binding affinity for camptothecin (CPT), a commonly nanoparticle-conjugated payload, compared with rodent albumins. Consequently, once CPT is released into systemic circulation, its distribution and bioavailability in humans can differ markedly from that observed in rodent models due to species-dependent albumin binding. Furthermore, intracellular microenvironments, particularly lysosomal pH and enzymatic composition, are not identical across species, affecting the degradation of nanoparticles and the release kinetics of pH-responsive drug conjugates.

Importantly, recognition and quantitative correction of certain interspecies variables can improve translational predictability. A notable example is CRLX101, a polymeric nanoparticle–CPT conjugate engineered for sustained drug release followed by disassembly into renally excretable polymer fragments. When species-specific albumin binding affinities were incorporated into pharmacokinetic modeling, strong concordance was observed between animal and human data. The area under the concentration–time curve for conjugated CPT increased linearly with administered dose across rats, dogs, and humans. Moreover, differences in CPT release profiles among species could be rationalized by accounting for variations in albumin–CPT binding strength. Repeated-dose studies further demonstrated an absence of anti-nanoparticle antibody formation in both animal models and patients, indicating that multicycle preclinical data retained predictive value for human responses.

Recent methodologies have utilized physiologically based pharmacokinetic (PBPK) modeling to forecast nanoparticle behavior across various species and ultimately in humans [3]. In investigations involving dendritic nanoparticles, dose-normalized concentration–time curves measured in plasma, liver, and spleen demonstrated remarkable concordance across mice, rats, and dogs. A PBPK model constructed using murine data was able to reliably capture exposure patterns in both rats and dogs. When subsequently adapted with human-specific physiological parameters, the model generated simulated exposure profiles that closely overlaid the dose-normalized datasets obtained from the three animal species. The robustness of such PBPK frameworks relies on rigorous quantification of both the nanocarrier-bound drug fraction and the liberated drug across multiple tissue compartments. Incorporating this mechanistic resolution strengthens the ability to predict interspecies variations in release kinetics and organ distribution.

Nevertheless, even with these encouraging examples, the overall predictive capacity of animal models for complex nanomedicines remains constrained. Critical determinants of nanoparticle fate in humans, such as the degree of opsonization by plasma proteins, complement system activation, and interactions with specialized immune cell populations, often differ from those observed in preclinical species in ways that are not readily foreseeable. Moreover, conventional animal studies frequently employ single, high-dose acute exposure designs, whereas clinical regimens typically involve repeated administration at comparatively lower doses. The relevance of acute toxicity findings to long-term, chronic human exposure scenarios is therefore not fully established. Together, fundamental anatomical and physiological disparities between species, combined with the use of experimentally exaggerated dosing strategies, reduce the translational reliability of preclinical toxicity data for nanomedicine applications.

11.2.3 Bridging Preclinical and Clinical Evidence: Integrated Approaches

Bridging the disconnect between preclinical observations and human outcomes requires coordinated integration of complementary experimental and computational strategies. During a multidisciplinary workshop involving regulatory authorities, academic investigators, and industry representatives, consensus emerged regarding the essential infrastructure and methodological priorities necessary to strengthen nanomedicine translation. A key conclusion was that conventional regulatory tools developed for small molecules or biologics may not adequately capture the structural complexity and functional behavior of nanomedicines, thereby underscoring the need for more tailored evaluation approaches.

To address these concerns, a structured translational framework termed DELIVER has been introduced to guide preclinical development with a focus on improving clinical predictability. This model emphasizes early-stage design considerations that incorporate scalability and manufacturability as foundational criteria rather than afterthoughts. It also calls for rigorous experimental standards, including the use of well-characterized reference materials, systematic validation against appropriate positive and negative controls, and independent replication of pivotal findings. From a production standpoint, the framework integrates principles aligned with good manufacturing practices and process analytical technologies to ensure quality consistency. Equally important is proactive alignment with regulatory guidance throughout development. Rather than promoting universally applicable nanoparticle platforms, the DELIVER strategy advocates for disease-oriented design, generating robust and context-specific preclinical datasets that more accurately forecast therapeutic performance in defined patient populations [4].

Compared with conventional two-dimensional cell cultures or single-species animal experiments, advanced cellular and tissue-engineered platforms offer improved translational relevance. Three-dimensional tissue constructs and organ-on-a-chip technologies better recapitulate key features of human physiology, including native tissue architecture, multicellular complexity, and dynamic microenvironmental conditions relevant to nanoparticle exposure. When carefully selected and validated using appropriate positive and negative control nanoparticles, these platforms can achieve meaningful in vitro-to-in vivo correlation (IVIVC) for acute toxicological endpoints such as hemolysis, complement activation, pyrogenicity, and cytokine release (Figure 11.3). Establishing robust IVIVC through such physiologically

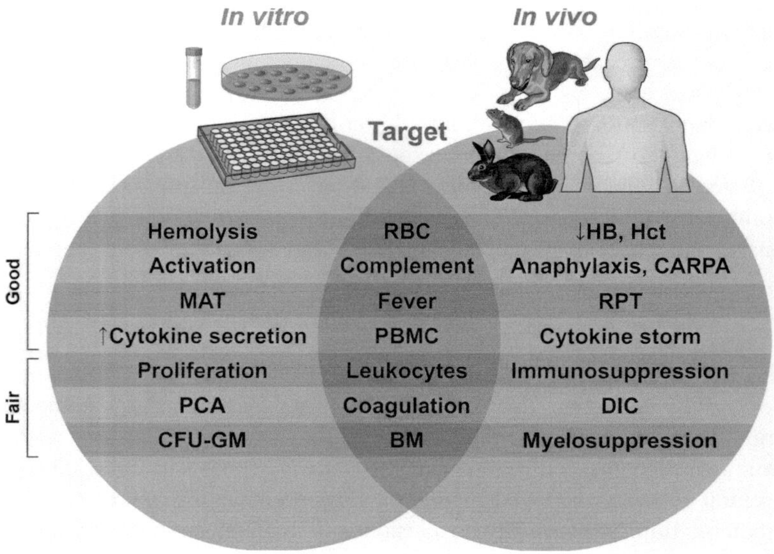

FIGURE 11.3 Correlation between in vitro and in vivo immunological tests for nanoparticle characterization. (Reprinted from Ref. [5] with permission from Elsevier.)

representative systems has the potential to substantially reduce reliance on animal models while enhancing the accuracy of predicting human biological responses to nanomedicines.

Ensuring translational reproducibility in nanomedicine research depends heavily on the standardization and rigorous quality control of reference materials. The National Institute of Standards and Technology maintains well-characterized libraries of reference nanoparticles with precisely defined physicochemical properties. Benchmarking experimental outcomes against such validated standards, along with performing independent replicate analyses, strengthens data reliability and interlaboratory comparability. In parallel, the International Organization for Standardization (ISO) has established globally recognized guidelines for assessing both the material characteristics and biological interactions of nanoparticles. These internationally harmonized standards provide methodological frameworks that enhance consistency across laboratories and support more reproducible and transparent nanomedicine development [5].

Multi-institutional preclinical investigations generally offer greater translational robustness than studies conducted within a single laboratory. By engaging independent research groups, such collaborative efforts allow systematic evaluation of reproducibility across sites and help uncover methodological or biological sources of variability that could later affect clinical performance. When findings are independently replicated and remain consistent across multiple centers, the evidentiary foundation supporting progression to clinical trials becomes substantially stronger. Transparency can be further improved through preregistration of experimental protocols before study initiation. In this approach, detailed study designs are peer reviewed and provisionally accepted for publication prior to data collection, clearly distinguishing predefined hypotheses, and analyses from post hoc exploratory evaluations. This practice reduces bias and enhances confidence in the reported outcomes.

Large-scale collaborative initiatives, including EUNCL (European Nanomedicine Characterisation Laboratory) and REFINE (Regulatory Science Framework for Nanomedicines), are actively advancing regulatory science in this domain. These programs focus on developing, validating, and harmonizing characterization methodologies that directly support regulatory decision-making. In addition, they are building decision support systems that integrate scientific and regulatory evaluation tools, guiding users toward the most appropriate and reliable testing strategies based on the specific attributes and intended clinical application of each nanomedicine. Through coordinated, science-driven testing frameworks, combined with cross-sector training and knowledge exchange among regulators, academia, and industry, the translational pathway from preclinical innovation to clinical implementation is becoming progressively more structured and reliable [6].

11.3 REGULATORY FRAMEWORKS AND GUIDELINES

At present, most nanomedicines are regulated within the broader legal frameworks established for pharmaceuticals and chemical products. However, scientific and regulatory bodies have introduced more specialized guidance documents addressing nanomaterial-specific aspects such as physicochemical characterization, toxicological evaluation, and quality assurance. Despite these efforts, the absence of a universally harmonized definition of "nanomaterial" continues to complicate regulatory alignment across countries and across different product categories. Regulatory pathways may also vary depending on the formulation and intended application. For instance, liposomal drug formulations and nanoparticle-based vaccines are often assessed under distinct approval routes, reflecting differences in their composition, mechanism of action, and regulatory classification [7].

11.3.1 International Guidelines and Oversight Framework

11.3.1.1 FDA in the United States

The U.S. FDA oversees nanomaterial-containing products primarily under existing statutory frameworks governing drugs, biologics, medical devices, and cosmetics, rather than establishing a separate regulatory classification for nanotechnology. To address nano-specific considerations, the agency issues targeted guidance documents that clarify expectations for safety evaluation and product characterization. For example, in the context of cosmetics, the FDA emphasizes comprehensive physicochemical characterization of nanomaterials, including detailed assessment of composition, particle size and distribution, morphology, aggregation or agglomeration state, surface chemistry, impurity profile, stability, and behavior in biologically relevant media. Where conventional toxicological assays are insufficient to capture nano-related properties, testing strategies may need adaptation or redevelopment, with particular attention to toxicokinetics, absorption, distribution, metabolism, and excretion (ADME).

Within pharmaceuticals and biologics, the FDA's established risk-based framework for chemistry, manufacturing, and controls (CMC), nonclinical safety, and clinical evaluation generally remains applicable to nanomaterial-containing products. Nevertheless, such products often require more extensive physicochemical profiling, tailored toxicity studies, and heightened oversight of manufacturing consistency. Specific guidance for liposomal drug products highlights the necessity of stringent control over parameters such as particle size distribution, lamellarity, encapsulation efficiency, in vitro release characteristics, and the identification of empty or partially loaded vesicles as impurities. These CQAs must be systematically correlated with clinical performance and maintained under tight control throughout the product lifecycle [8]. In all these documents, FDA emphasizes that "nanomaterial" is used descriptively and does not constitute a binding regulatory definition, enabling flexibility as scientific understanding evolves.

11.3.1.2 EMA in the European Union

Within the European Union (EU), nanomedicines are regulated under the overarching legislative framework applicable to medicinal products. At the same time, the EMA has issued dedicated reflection papers and guidance documents addressing specific nanotechnology-enabled platforms, including liposomal formulations, block-copolymer micelles, and iron-based colloidal systems. In its horizon-scanning assessments of nanotechnology-based medicinal products, the EMA reiterates that standard requirements for quality, nonclinical testing, and clinical evaluation remain applicable. However, these documents also outline heightened expectations regarding detailed nanoform characterization, stability in biological environments, immunogenic potential, and biodistribution profiling [9]. Beyond pharmaceuticals, the EU Medical Device Regulation (MDR) introduces Rule 19, which specifically addresses devices incorporating nanomaterials. This rule upgrades device classification according to the likelihood of nanoparticle exposure and internalization within the human body, thereby imposing stricter conformity assessment procedures where risk is greater. The MDR also references internationally recognized ISO standards for physicochemical characterization and toxicological evaluation. Across the EU, regulatory frameworks for chemicals, food products, biocides, cosmetics, medical devices, and medicinal products operate under distinct legal instruments. While efforts are underway to harmonize nano-specific data requirements and testing expectations across these sectors, meaningful differences in definitions, risk assessment approaches, and documentation standards persist and continue to require alignment.

11.3.1.3 OECD Test Guidelines and Mutual Data Acceptance

The OECD Working Party on Manufactured Nanomaterials, together with the OECD Test Guidelines Programme, has played a central role in establishing internationally harmonized tools for evaluating the hazards and risks associated with nanomaterials. Through coordinated efforts among member countries, these initiatives aim to ensure consistency in safety assessment approaches across jurisdictions. The OECD Council Recommendation on the Safety Testing and Assessment of Manufactured Nanomaterials affirms that existing chemical safety assessment frameworks are generally applicable to nanomaterials, provided that appropriate test methods are selected, and nano-specific physicochemical attributes are adequately characterized. In this context, numerous OECD Test Guidelines (TGs) addressing physicochemical characterization, ecotoxicology, environmental fate, and human health effects have been systematically reviewed and, where necessary, adapted to account for nano-relevant considerations such as dispersion stability, dose metrics, and particle tracking. In addition, new TGs and supporting guidance documents are being developed to address endpoints particularly pertinent to nanomaterials. A key objective of these efforts is to ensure that nano-specific studies generate data compliant with the principle of Mutual Acceptance of Data, thereby allowing results from a single high-quality study to be recognized for regulatory decision-making across multiple countries.

11.3.1.4 ISO Standards

Regulatory authorities and industry stakeholders widely rely on standards and technical reports issued by the ISO, particularly those developed by technical committees dedicated to nanotechnologies and the biological evaluation of medical devices. These documents provide detailed guidance on terminology, measurement of particle size and morphology, determination of specific surface area, zeta potential analysis, assessment of dissolution or solubility, and nano-specific toxicological evaluation strategies. For instance, ISO/TR 10993-22 outlines recommendations for the physicochemical characterization and release-related toxicokinetic assessment of manufactured nano-objects used in medical applications. The report addresses critical aspects such as sample preparation procedures, identification, and quantification of released species, and evaluation of ADME profiles. In many cases, OECD guidance documents either directly reference ISO methodologies or adapt them to meet regulatory testing requirements. As a result, ISO standards serve as a foundational technical framework underpinning internationally harmonized nano-safety evaluation and regulatory decision-making [10].

11.3.2 Difficulties with Definitions and Harmonization of Rules

Although there has been increasing alignment in testing methodologies, a globally harmonized regulatory definition of "nanomaterial" is still lacking, and this inconsistency continues to hinder coordinated international oversight. The European Commission issued a 2011 recommendation defining a nanomaterial primarily on the basis of a number-based particle size distribution, specifying that 50% or more of particles should fall within the 1–100 nm range. However, applying this definition consistently across regulatory sectors has proven challenging, especially for complex, heterogeneous, or highly polydisperse materials. Ongoing efforts within the EU seek to refine and stabilize this definition by maintaining the 50% threshold, thereby reducing discrepancies where a material may qualify as a nanomaterial under one regulatory framework but not under another. Nevertheless, significant technical difficulties persist, particularly in accurate particle counting, distinguishing primary particles from aggregates or agglomerates, and accounting for matrix-related interferences during measurement [11].

Regulatory approaches to defining nanomaterials vary considerably across jurisdictions. In Canada, a working definition emphasizes intentional manufacture at the nanoscale and the presence of novel size-dependent properties. This approach has been aligned in part with U.S. authorities through the Canada–United States Regulatory Cooperation Council to improve cross-border consistency. By contrast, several countries in the Asia-Pacific region incorporate nano-specific considerations into existing chemical or product-based legislation but apply different size thresholds or regulatory triggers depending on the sector. In the United States, the U.S. FDA does not rely on a rigid size-only definition. Instead, it applies a functional, risk-based perspective, assessing whether materials with dimensions in the 1–100 nm range or even slightly larger, exhibit altered physicochemical or biological properties that are relevant to safety, quality, or effectiveness.

These definitional differences have important practical implications.

- Manufacturers must navigate divergent registration procedures and data requirements across markets, often repeating similar studies to satisfy region-specific criteria. This duplication increases development costs and complicates global commercialization strategies.
- Variability in thresholds and classification criteria affects labeling, product traceability, and exposure assessment, limiting the comparability of production volumes, environmental releases, and risk evaluations between countries.
- Regulatory authorities face ongoing challenges in categorizing borderline or structurally complex materials, such as nanoplastics or hybrid and hierarchical nanostructures where functional behavior, rather than particle size alone, may be the primary determinant of risk.

11.3.3 Case Studies: Approval Pathways for Nanomedicine

Regulatory standards and practical expectations for nanomedicines are reflected in the clinical authorization of several established platforms including liposomal formulations, nanoparticle-based vaccines, iron oxide nanoparticles, and gold nanoparticle systems, while the continued developmental difficulties associated with quantum dots (QDs) highlight persistent translational and safety challenges. Together, these examples demonstrate both meaningful regulatory progress and the unresolved scientific and clinical barriers that continue to shape the pathway from innovation to approved medical application.

11.3.3.1 PEGylated Liposomal Doxorubicin and Other Liposomal Drugs

Polyethylene glycol (PEG)ylated liposomal doxorubicin (PLD), marketed as Doxil in the United States and Caelyx in the EU, became the first nanomedicine approved by the U.S. FDA in the mid-1990s and remains a landmark product in the field. This formulation incorporates doxorubicin within PEG-coated liposomes, thereby altering the drug's pharmacokinetic profile, tissue distribution, and toxicity characteristics relative to conventional free doxorubicin [12]. The development and management brought up several regulatory:

- For PLD products such as Doxil and Caelyx, regulatory authorities imposed stringent control over multiple CQAs. Parameters including liposome size distribution, PEG surface density, encapsulation efficiency, and in vitro drug release profiles were tightly regulated and explicitly correlated with clinical safety and efficacy outcomes—particularly cardiotoxicity and palmar–plantar erythrodysesthesia.
- Manufacturing changes and supply disruptions later exposed vulnerabilities in global production networks, including challenges in scale-up and product comparability. In response, the U.S. FDA issued detailed guidance and subjected process modifications to rigorous review through prior-approval supplements, emphasizing the importance of maintaining consistency throughout the product lifecycle.
- The introduction of generic or follow-on versions of liposomal doxorubicin further highlighted regulatory complexities. These products contributed to the recognition of "complex generics," which require substantially more comprehensive comparative quality assessments, nonclinical evaluations, and, in some cases, clinical data than conventional small-molecule generics. Consequently, the FDA developed product-specific guidance for doxorubicin HCl liposome abbreviated new drug applications, outlining detailed expectations for demonstrating equivalence.

Similarly, the EMA has authorized multiple liposomal and nanoparticle-based formulations, including Myocet, Mepact, and Vyxeos. The EMA has consistently emphasized that non-biological complex drugs cannot typically establish therapeutic equivalence solely through standard bioequivalence studies, underscoring the necessity for comprehensive, multiparameter comparability evaluations. These regulatory experiences have directly shaped current EMA and FDA expectations for liposomal products. Contemporary guidance requires validated in vitro release assays capable of discriminating clinically meaningful differences, robust process validation demonstrating scalability and ongoing process verification, and extensive stability programs, encompassing physical, chemical, and microbiological stability, including in-use stability after dilution.

11.3.3.2 RNA Therapies Based on Lipid Nanoparticles

The approval of Onpattro (patisiran) in 2018 for hereditary transthyretin-mediated amyloidosis represented a landmark achievement as the first RNA interference therapy and among the earliest lipid nanoparticle (LNP)-based therapeutics to receive global marketing authorization. Its regulatory evaluation established important precedents for LNP-formulated drugs. The review process involved comprehensive physicochemical characterization of the LNP components, including ionizable lipids, helper lipids, and PEGylated lipids. Authorities required detailed assessment of lipid purity, polymorphic forms, impurity profiles, and degradation pathways. Because certain lipid excipients had not previously been listed in inactive ingredient databases, additional safety justification was necessary, sometimes supported by proprietary Drug Master Files. Regulators also conducted an extensive evaluation of biodistribution patterns, hepatic accumulation, innate immune activation, and complement responses. This reflected broader concern regarding potential class-specific effects of LNP systems that might extend beyond the individual siRNA payload.

The relatively rapid approvals by agencies such as the U.S. FDA, EMA, and Medicines and Healthcare products Regulatory Agency demonstrated regulatory openness to accelerated and orphan-designated pathways for nanomedicines when supported by robust CMC data and compelling clinical evidence. At the same time, the review process highlighted nuanced differences among agencies in how LNP components are categorized whether as part of the active substance or as excipients illustrating ongoing regulatory evolution in the classification of complex nanomedicine platforms.

11.3.3.3 LNP-mRNA COVID-19 Vaccines and Platform Regulation

The emergency and conditional approvals of the LNP-mRNA vaccines BNT162b2 (Comirnaty) and mRNA-1273 (Spikevax) for COVID-19 mark a turning point in the regulation of nanomedicine [13]. Based on their functional components, they can be grouped into three main categories: viral, nucleic acid–based, and protein-based. Nanocarriers mostly have the same structural components, such as cholesterol, structural lipids, PEG lipids, and ionizable lipids, which then form nanoparticles measuring 50–150 nm. These products use LNPs to protect and deliver mRNA that codes for the spike protein of SARS-CoV-2 [14].

Key regulatory consequences emerging from large-scale deployment of LNP-based products include several transformative developments. First, unprecedented real-world safety and effectiveness datasets for LNP formulations have provided regulators with substantial evidence to evaluate potential class-related risks, including rare anaphylactic reactions, myocarditis signals, and other uncommon immune-mediated events. Such pharmacovigilance data have strengthened the scientific basis for ongoing benefit–risk assessment.

Second, authorities now expect rigorous, high-throughput analytical characterization of nanoparticle attributes, including particle size distribution, polydispersity index, encapsulation efficiency, residual solvent content, and RNA integrity. In addition, validated potency assays are required to establish a meaningful link between in vitro protein expression and observed clinical immunogenicity, ensuring that analytical metrics correlate with therapeutic performance.

Third, stringent oversight of cold-chain logistics and stability has become essential, as mRNA/LNP formulations are highly sensitive to temperature fluctuations, mechanical stress, and freeze-thaw cycles. This sensitivity drives regulatory demands for stability-indicating analytical methods and comprehensive in-use stability studies following thawing and dilution.

The global response to the COVID-19 pandemic significantly accelerated regulatory innovation. In the United States, the U.S. FDA has introduced a Platform Technology Designation Program, enabling certain well-characterized platforms, such as LNP-mRNA systems to benefit from streamlined review processes based on prior knowledge of quality, manufacturing, and safety. Similarly, the EMA and other regulatory bodies increasingly recognize LNPs as platform technologies for vaccines and gene therapies. This evolving perspective is shaping new guidance on how previously established CMC and nonclinical data can be leveraged to support subsequent products targeting new antigens or therapeutic indications.

11.3.3.4 Iron Oxide Nanoparticles: Therapeutic and Diagnostic Applications

Iron oxide nanoparticles represent one of the most clinically mature categories of nanomedicine, with several products demonstrating both therapeutic and diagnostic (theranostic) applications. Nevertheless, regulatory scrutiny has at times resulted in market withdrawals and strengthened safety warnings, reflecting ongoing concerns regarding hypersensitivity and risk management.

A representative example is Ferumoxytol, approved by the U.S. FDA in 2009 for the treatment of iron deficiency anemia in adults with chronic kidney disease [15]. The formulation consists of superparamagnetic iron oxide cores coated with a carbohydrate shell that stabilizes bioactive iron until uptake by macrophages within the reticuloendothelial system. Approval was supported by three randomized, open-label clinical trials demonstrating superior hemoglobin increases compared with oral iron therapy. The recommended dosing schedule involves two intravenous injections of 510 mg administered 3–8 days apart. In 2019, the FDA broadened the indication to include adults with iron deficiency anemia who are intolerant of, or unresponsive to, oral iron preparations, based on comparative safety data indicating that rates of hypersensitivity were similar to other parenteral iron formulations. Beyond its hematologic indication, ferumoxytol's superparamagnetic properties have enabled off-label use as a magnetic resonance imaging (MRI) contrast agent for vascular and oncologic imaging. Investigational studies have explored its application in brain and head-and-neck tumor imaging, including orphan-designated research programs. However, post-marketing surveillance identified 79 cases of anaphylactic reactions associated with therapeutic use, prompting the FDA to issue a boxed warning. Clinicians are therefore advised to carefully weigh potential risks and benefits, particularly in elderly individuals and patients with prior hypersensitivity to iron products. Controlled safety evaluations have indicated that moderate to severe reactions occur in fewer than 1% of treated patients within five weeks of administration, but vigilant monitoring remains essential [16]. This shows how hard it is to balance risk–benefit profiles for different uses and how post-market safety signals can affect exploratory uses.

There are five types of superparamagnetic iron oxide that have been designed and clinically approved, but only Resovist (ferucarbotran) is available in some countries for use as contrast agents in liver MRI scans. Meanwhile, the other four types have been withdrawn from market [17]. Later, there is another superparamagnetic iron oxide agent, Feraheme (ferumoxytol) that is clinically approved for the treatment of adult chronic kidney disease patients and as potential agent for imaging certain liver tumors [15]. Resovist, which has particles that are about 60 nm in size, could be given as a quick bolus, which would allow for both dynamic and delayed-phase imaging. Feridex, on the other hand, needed to be slowly infused and could only be used for delayed-phase imaging. Feridex also presents safety concerns, including severe back pain, which limits its administration as an intravenous bolus injection. Resovist is still sold in Japan, but Feridex is no longer sold. This shows how commercial viability and pharmacovigilance can affect the long-term success of nanomedicine even after it has been approved by regulators. Ferumoxtran-10 (Combidex/Sinerem), a dextran-coated ultrasmall iron oxide, was created to find lymph node metastasis [16]. Although phase II studies in prostate cancer demonstrated improved visualization of lymph node involvement, a false-positive rate of approximately 24.1% resulted in unnecessary surgical interventions. Owing to concerns that the diagnostic accuracy did not translate into sufficient overall clinical benefit, the U.S. FDA declined approval in 2005. The product was subsequently authorized in Europe under the name Sinerem; however, its risk–benefit evaluation has remained complex. In the case of diagnostic nanomedicines, regulatory standards are particularly stringent, as false-positive findings can directly influence treatment decisions and expose patients to avoidable procedures [18]. These instances demonstrate that regulatory approval does not ensure commercial success, and that post-market surveillance, pharmacovigilance, and comparative effectiveness significantly influence the lifecycle of iron oxide nanomedicines.

11.3.3.5 Gold Nanoparticles: Platforms for Photothermal Therapy and Drug Delivery

Gold nanoparticles represent a distinctive class of nanomedicines that have progressed into early-phase human clinical trials, although most proposed applications still require full regulatory authorization. In the United States, clinical development has generally proceeded through the Investigational New Drug (IND) pathway under the oversight of the U.S. FDA, reflecting their classification as drug or combination products depending on intended use. Their biomedical interest stems largely from unique physicochemical properties, particularly optical behavior and surface plasmon resonance, which enable light absorption and scattering at tunable wavelengths. These characteristics support applications in imaging and light-activated therapies (Figure 11.4a) [19]. Beyond conventional chemical synthesis, gold nanoparticles can

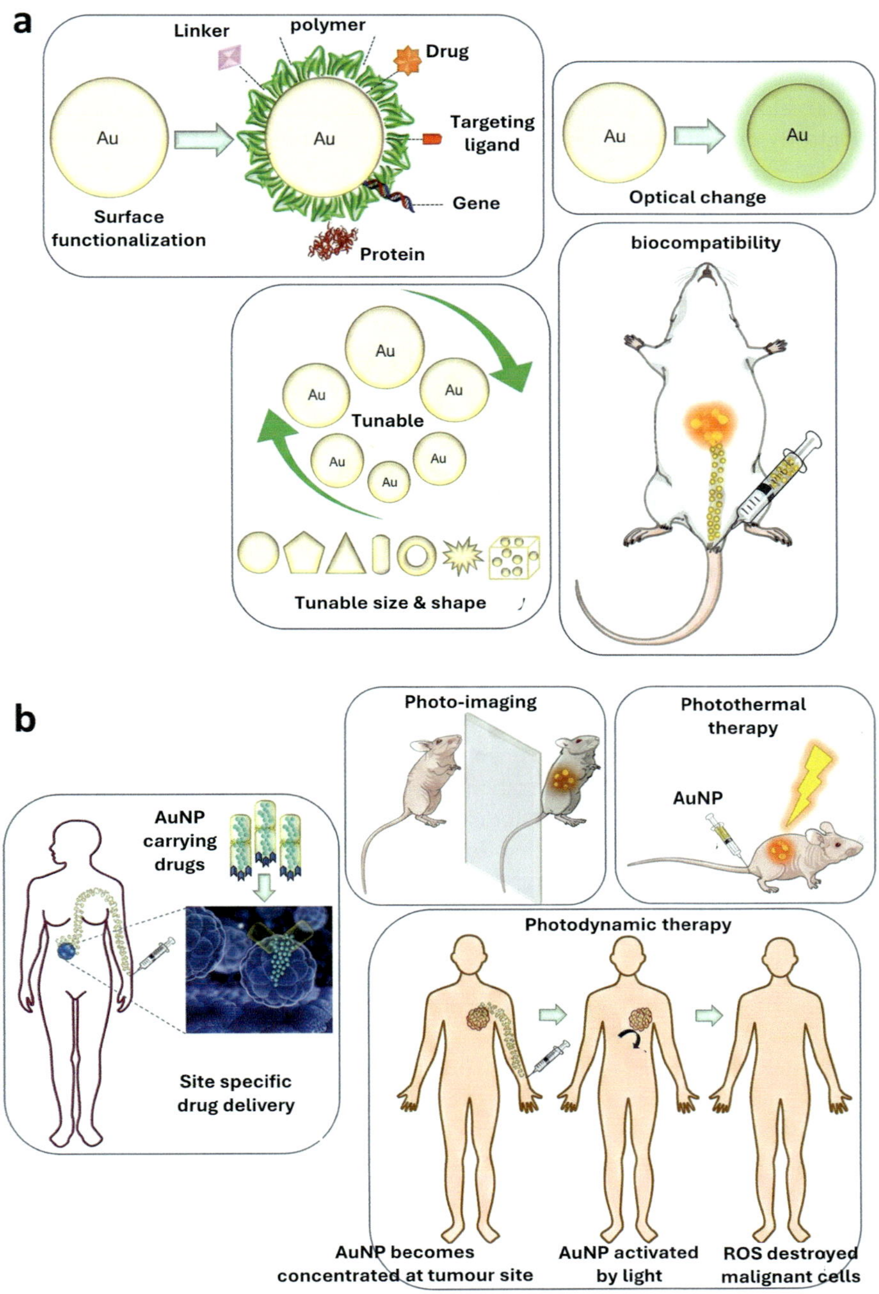

FIGURE 11.4 Important properties of gold nanoparticles; different approaches of gold nanoparticles in cancer diagnosis and treatment. (Adapted from Ref. [19] (CC BY).)

also be produced via biological routes. Numerous plant extracts have been shown to rapidly reduce gold salts to stable nanoparticles, sometimes within seconds. Likewise, certain microorganisms are capable of adsorbing gold ions and promoting nanoparticle formation through enzymatic reduction mechanisms. Such "green" or biologically mediated synthesis approaches are often highlighted for their potential biocompatibility and scalability, although regulatory evaluation still requires rigorous characterization of purity, reproducibility, and residual biological contaminants. As a result of their tunable size, surface chemistry, and optical properties, biologically and chemically synthesized gold nanoparticles are being explored as multifunctional platforms for biosensing, immunoassays, targeted drug delivery, photoimaging, photothermal therapy (PTT), and photodynamic therapy (PDT). Despite this promise, translation to routine clinical use continues to depend on comprehensive data addressing biodistribution, long-term clearance, immunogenicity, and manufacturing consistency (Figure 11.4b).

Among gold-based nanotherapeutics, Nanospectra Biosciences' AuroShell® platform (gold–silica nanoshells) represents one of the most clinically advanced approaches. Structurally, these particles consist of a silica core coated with a thin gold layer, engineered to absorb near-infrared laser light, and convert it into localized heat for photothermal tumor ablation. The U.S. FDA authorized AuroShell particles for human investigation under IND applications, including trials such as NCT00848042 and NCT01679470 in head and neck cancers and primary or metastatic lung tumors. This positioned them among the few inorganic nanomaterials cleared for clinical PTT studies.

Before entering clinical trials, AuroShell underwent extensive ISO-aligned preclinical safety testing. These assessments included bacterial reverse mutation (Ames) testing, in vitro chromosomal aberration assays, in vivo mouse micronucleus studies, hemocompatibility evaluations, cytotoxicity assays, and 28-day repeated-dose systemic toxicity studies in rodents and dogs. No mutagenic, hemolytic, or overt cytotoxic effects were observed at therapeutic dose ranges, and no consistent dose-related abnormalities emerged in hematology, serum chemistry, or histopathology. However, a 10-month chronic toxicity study in beagle dogs revealed pigment deposition in organs such as the liver, spleen, and lymph nodes, consistent with long-term tissue sequestration [20]. These findings underscore the regulatory emphasis on biodistribution, persistence, and chronic safety, particularly for indications that may require prolonged or repeated exposure. Early human studies suggested potential utility in localized prostate cancer. In a small pilot cohort, tumor-targeted hyperthermia was achieved with minimal systemic toxicity. Nevertheless, technical limitations in laser delivery prevented completion of photothermal treatment in some cases. Importantly, subsequent salvage brachytherapy following nanoshell administration was performed without major complications, indicating compatibility with conventional radiation modalities. The possibility of radiosensitization, however, remains an area requiring further mechanistic and clinical clarification [21]. A second platform, Aurimune (CYT-6091), developed by Cytimmune Sciences, completed Phase I evaluation under FDA oversight. This system employs PEGylated gold nanoparticles to deliver recombinant human tumor necrosis factor alpha selectively to tumors, leveraging enhanced permeability and retention effects to mitigate systemic toxicity. While Phase I data demonstrated acceptable safety and evidence of tumor localization, the program has not yet advanced to Phase II trials, illustrating the lengthy and uncertain progression from early clinical feasibility to full marketing authorization [22,23]. From a regulatory standpoint, gold nanoparticles present several ongoing challenges. Although gold-containing therapeutic agents have previously been approved for other medical uses, there is limited nano-specific regulatory guidance. Consequently, developers are expected to provide

- comprehensive physicochemical characterization, including particle size distribution, morphology, surface chemistry, aggregation behavior, and batch-to-batch reproducibility;
- robust toxicological assessment covering genotoxicity, immunotoxicity, and long-term organ accumulation, particularly in the liver, spleen, and kidneys; and
- a clear and indication-specific risk–benefit justification, especially where established therapeutic alternatives already exist.

As of 2026, no gold nanoparticle therapeutic has received full marketing authorization from the U.S. FDA. Despite promising preclinical and early clinical findings, the absence of approval reflects the stringent evidentiary standards applied to novel nanomedicines, particularly regarding long-term safety and biodistribution. These experiences also reinforce an important scientific and regulatory insight: the perceived chemical inertness of noble metals at the bulk scale does not necessarily translate to biological neutrality at the nanoscale.

11.3.3.6 Quantum Dots: Problems with Development and Concerns about Toxicity

QDs are semiconductor nanocrystals with size-tunable optical properties, which generate substantial interest for imaging, diagnostics, and PDT because of their unique fluorescence spectrum, making it an optimal fluorophore for biomedical imaging. However, QD-based products have not achieved full marketing authorization yet due to persistent toxicity concerns and regulatory uncertainty in vivo applications. Cadmium-based QDs (CdSe, CdTe) can release toxic Cd^{2+} ions upon degradation, and surface coatings may not fully prevent dissolution in acidic lysosomal compartments or under oxidative stress (Figure 11.5). Studies on animals show that systemic administration can cause liver damage, kidney damage, and immune system damage, with dose-dependent inflammatory responses and organ accumulation.

QDs are semiconductor nanocrystals characterized by size-dependent optical properties, which allow precise tuning of their emission wavelength. Owing to their narrow emission spectra, high brightness, and photostability, QDs have attracted considerable interest in biomedical imaging, diagnostics, and photodynamic applications, where they function as highly efficient fluorophores. Despite this promise, QD-based products have not yet received full marketing authorization from major regulators such as the U.S. FDA or the EMA. The primary obstacles remain unresolved safety concerns and regulatory uncertainty regarding long-term in vivo behavior. A major issue involves cadmium-containing QDs, such as CdSe and CdTe nanocrystals. Upon degradation,

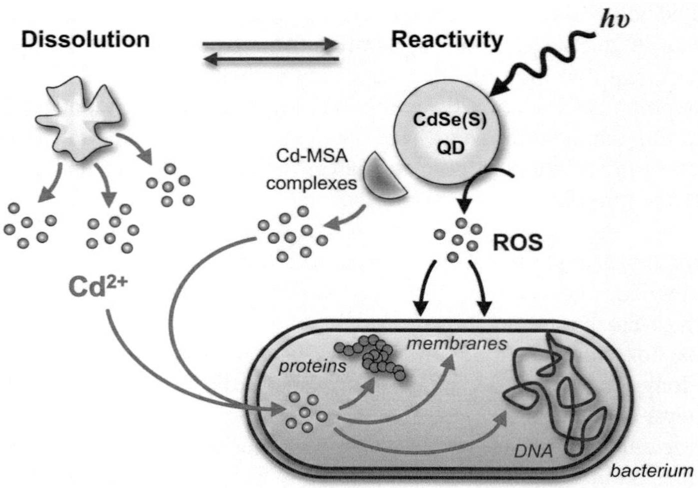

FIGURE 11.5 The schematic overview of cellular mechanisms in cells treated with Cd containing QDs [24].

these materials may release toxic Cd^{2+} ions. Although surface coatings (e.g., polymer or silica shells) are designed to improve stability and reduce ion leakage, they may not fully prevent dissolution under biologically relevant conditions, particularly within acidic lysosomal compartments or in environments characterized by oxidative stress.

Preclinical animal studies have reported dose-dependent accumulation in the liver, spleen, and kidneys following systemic administration. Observed toxicities include hepatocellular injury, renal impairment, and immune activation, often accompanied by inflammatory responses. Persistent organ retention and uncertain clearance kinetics further complicate risk assessment, especially for diagnostic applications where the clinical benefit must clearly outweigh potential long-term harm. From a regulatory perspective, these findings raise critical questions regarding biodegradation, chronic toxicity, immunogenicity, and environmental persistence. Consequently, QDs illustrate a recurring theme in nanomedicine regulation: highly advantageous optical or functional properties must be balanced against rigorous demonstration of long-term safety before clinical translation can proceed to full approval.

11.4 CONCLUSION

The trajectory of nanotechnology from experimental innovation to clinically approved and commercially viable bio-applications has been marked by both scientific breakthroughs and persistent translational challenges. While laboratory advances continue at a rapid pace, large-scale manufacturing variability, limited batch-to-batch reproducibility, and interspecies differences in biological responses complicate reliable prediction of human safety and therapeutic performance. These realities underscore the necessity for evaluation frameworks that move beyond traditional toxicological models toward more integrated, mechanism-informed, and nano-specific assessment strategies.

Regulatory authorities, including the U.S. FDA and the EMA, have progressively adapted existing medicinal product frameworks to address nanomedicines. Nevertheless, the continued absence of a universally harmonized definition of "nanomaterial" and fully aligned global testing requirements remains a structural barrier to regulatory convergence. Comprehensive physicochemical characterization, encompassing particle size distribution, morphology, surface chemistry, colloidal stability, and functional performance, remains fundamental to regulatory decision-making. Yet, the pace at which new multifunctional nanoplatforms are being developed frequently exceeds the scope of current guidance documents.

Recent experience with nano-enabled rapid-response technologies, particularly LNP-based mRNA vaccines, demonstrates that when safety evaluation, regulatory preparedness, and scalable manufacturing are integrated early in development, translational timelines can be significantly shortened without compromising oversight. These examples illustrate that regulatory agility is achievable when supported by robust prior knowledge, platform characterization, and coordinated international review mechanisms. Looking forward, sustained commitment to embedding safety-by-design principles throughout the research and development pipeline will be essential. Early hazard identification, standardized testing methodologies, transparent data sharing, and international harmonization efforts will collectively determine whether nanotechnologies can fully realize their promise in enhancing patient outcomes and strengthening global public health systems.

REFERENCES

1. S. Đorđević et al., 'Current hurdles to the translation of nanomedicines from bench to the clinic', *Drug Deliv. Transl.* Res., vol. 12, no. 3, pp. 500–525, Mar. 2022, doi: 10.1007/s13346-021-01024-2.
2. S. Mülhopt et al., 'Characterization of nanoparticle batch-to-batch variability', *Nanomaterials*, vol. 8, no. 5, May 2018, doi: 10.3390/nano8050311.
3. C. Vasalou, J. Harding, R. D. O. Jones, N. Hariparsad, and D. F. McGinnity, 'Interspecies evaluation of a physiologically based pharmacokinetic model to predict the biodistribution dynamics of dendritic nanoparticles', *PLoS One*, vol. 18, no. 5, p. e0285798, May 2023, doi: 10.1371/journal.pone.0285798.
4. P. Joyce et al., 'A translational framework to DELIVER nanomedicines to the clinic', *Nat. Nanotechnol.*, vol. 19, no. 11, pp. 1597–1611, Nov. 2024, doi: 10.1038/s41565-024-01754-7.
5. M. A. Dobrovolskaia and S. E. McNeil, 'Understanding the correlation between *in vitro* and *in vivo* immunotoxicity tests for nanomedicines', *J. Controlled Release*, vol. 172, no. 2, pp. 456–466, Dec. 2013, doi: 10.1016/j.jconrel.2013.05.025.
6. B. Halamoda-Kenzaoui et al., 'Bridging communities in the field of nanomedicine', *Regul. Toxicol.* Pharmacol., vol. 106, pp. 187–196, Aug. 2019, doi: 10.1016/j.yrtph.2019.04.011.
7. J. Allan et al., 'Regulatory landscape of nanotechnology and nanoplastics from a global perspective', *Regul. Toxicol.* Pharmacol., vol. 122, p. 104885, Jun. 2021, doi: 10.1016/j.yrtph.2021.104885.
8. Y. Wang and D. W. Grainger, 'Regulatory considerations specific to liposome drug development as complex drug products', *Front. Drug Deliv.*, vol. 2, Apr. 2022, doi: 10.3389/fddev.2022.901281.

9. E. A. J. Bleeker et al., 'Towards harmonisation of testing of nanomaterials for EU regulatory requirements on chemical safety – a proposal for further actions', *Regul. Toxicol.* Pharmacol., vol. 139, p. 105360, Mar. 2023, doi: 10.1016/j.yrtph.2023.105360.
10. K. Rasmussen, P. Sayre, A. Kobe, M. Gonzalez, and H. Rauscher, '25 years of research and regulation: Is nanotechnology safe to commercialize?', *Front. Toxicol.*, vol. 7, Jul. 2025, doi: 10.3389/ftox.2025.1629813.
11. J. Wang et al., 'A journey of challenges and victories: a bibliometric worldview of nanomedicine since the 21st century', *Adv. Mater.*, vol. 36, no. 15, p. 2308915, 2024, doi: 10.1002/adma.202308915.
12. A. A. Gabizon, S. Gabizon-Peretz, S. Modaresahmadi, and N. M. La-Beck, 'Thirty years from FDA approval of pegylated liposomal doxorubicin (Doxil/Caelyx): an updated analysis and future perspective', *BMJ Oncol.*, vol. 4, no. 1, Jan. 2025, doi: 10.1136/bmjonc-2024-000573.
13. L. Milane and M. Amiji, 'Clinical approval of nanotechnology-based SARS-CoV-2 mRNA vaccines: impact on translational nanomedicine', *Drug Deliv. Transl.* Res., vol. 11, no. 4, pp. 1309–1315, Aug. 2021, doi: 10.1007/s13346-021-00911-y.
14. G. Guerrini, D. Magrì, S. Gioria, D. Medaglini, and L. Calzolai, 'Characterization of nanoparticles-based vaccines for COVID-19', *Nat. Nanotechnol.*, vol. 17, no. 6, pp. 570–576, Jun. 2022, doi: 10.1038/s41565-022-01129-w.
15. Y. Huang, J. C. Hsu, H. Koo, and D. P. Cormode, 'Repurposing ferumoxytol: diagnostic and therapeutic applications of an FDA-approved nanoparticle', *Theranostics*, vol. 12, no. 2, pp. 796–816, 2022, doi: 10.7150/thno.67375.
16. H. E. Daldrup-Link, 'Ten things you might not know about iron oxide nanoparticles', *Radiology*, vol. 284, no. 3, pp. 616–629, Sep. 2017, doi: 10.1148/radiol.2017162759.
17. Y.-X. J. Wang, 'Current status of superparamagnetic iron oxide contrast agents for liver magnetic resonance imaging', *World J. Gastroenterol.*, vol. 21, no. 47, pp. 13400–13402, Dec. 2015, doi: 10.3748/wjg.v21.i47.13400.
18. Y.-X. J. Wang, 'Superparamagnetic iron oxide based MRI contrast agents: current status of clinical application', *Quant. Imaging Med. Surg.*, vol. 1, no. 1, pp. 35–40, Dec. 2011, doi: 10.3978/j.issn.2223-4292.2011.08.03.
19. P. Singh, S. Pandit, V. R. S. S. Mokkapati, A. Garg, V. Ravikumar, and I. Mijakovic, 'Gold nanoparticles in diagnostics and therapeutics for human cancer', *Int. J. Mol. Sci.*, vol. 19, no. 7, p. 1979, Jul. 2018, doi: 10.3390/ijms19071979.
20. S. C. Gad, K. L. Sharp, C. Montgomery, J. D. Payne, and G. P. Goodrich, 'Evaluation of the toxicity of intravenous delivery of auroshell particles (gold-silica nanoshells)', *Int. J. Toxicol.*, vol. 31, no. 6, pp. 584–594, 2012, doi: 10.1177/1091581812465969.
21. A. R. Rastinehad et al., 'Gold nanoshell-localized photothermal ablation of prostate tumors in a clinical pilot device study', *Proc. Natl. Acad. Sci. USA*, vol. 116, no. 37, pp. 18590–18596, Sep. 2019, doi: 10.1073/pnas.1906929116.
22. D. Sung, A. Sanchez, and J. D. Tward, 'Successful salvage brachytherapy after infusion of gold auroshell nanoshells for localized prostate cancer in a human patient', *Adv. Radiat. Oncol.*, vol. 8, no. 4, Jul. 2023, doi: 10.1016/j.adro.2023.101202.
23. A. R. Hajrasouliha, B. McCall, Y. Gao, S. L. Gong, K. Robinson, and A. Izadian, 'Toxicity analysis of gold nanoparticle formulations used for intraocular applications', *Sci. Rep.*, vol. 15, no. 1, p. 19606, Jun. 2025, doi: 10.1038/s41598-025-03804-z.
24. F.-A. Kauffer, C. Merlin, L. Balan, and R. Schneider, 'Incidence of the core composition on the stability, the ROS production and the toxicity of CdSe quantum dots', *J. Hazard. Mater.*, vol. 268, pp. 246–255, 2014.

Abbreviations

ABC	Accelerated Blood Clearance
AD	Applicability Domain
ADME	Absorption, Distribution, Metabolism, Excretion
AFM	Atomic Force Microscope
Ag	Silver
AgNP	Silver Nanoparticle
AI	Artificial Intelligence
ANDA	Abbreviated New Drug Application
ASTM	American Society for Testing and Materials
ATMP	Advanced Therapy Medicinal Product
ATP	Adenosine Triphosphate
Au	Gold
AUC	Area Under Curve
AuNP	Gold Nanoparticle
AutoML	Automated Machine Learning
BACE1	Beta-Secretase 1
BBB	Blood-Brain Barrier
BMP-2	Bone Morphogenetic Protein-2
BNP	B-type Natriuretic Peptide
BP	Black Phosphorus
CD	Cluster of Differentiation
CdSe	Cadmium Selenide
CDT	Chemodynamic Therapy
CdTe	Cadmium Telluride
CEN	European Committee for Standardization
CeO_2 NP	Cerium Oxide Nanoparticle
CFU	Colony Forming Unit
CMC	Critical Micelle Concentration
CNF	Carbon Nanofiber
CNN	Convolutional Neural Network
CNS	Central Nervous System
CNT	Carbon Nanotube
CNT-FET	Carbon Nanotube Field-Effect Transistor
COF	Covalent Organic Framework
COPD	Chronic Obstructive Pulmonary Disease
COX-2	Cyclooxygenase-2
Cpk	Capability Index
CPP	Critical Process Parameter
CPT	Camptothecin
CQA	Critical Quality Attribute
CQD	Carbon Quantum Dot

CRLX101	Polymeric Nanoparticle Camptothecin
CRP	C-Reactive Protein
CT	Computed Tomography
CTC	Circulating Tumor Cell
Cu	Copper
CXCL2	C-X-C Motif Chemokine Ligand 2
DDS	Drug Delivery System
DENV	Dengue Virus
DOX	Doxorubicin
DSS	Decision Support System
ECM	Extracellular Matrix
EFSA	European Food Safety Authority
EIS	Electrochemical Impedance Spectroscopy
ELISA	Enzyme-Linked Immunosorbent Assay
EMA	European Medicines Agency
EPR	Enhanced Permeability and Retention
ERK	Extracellular Signal-Regulated Kinase
EU	European Union
EuMOF-FITC	Europium MOF with Fluorescein Isothiocyanate
EUNCL	European Nanomedicine Characterisation Laboratory
FA	Folic Acid
FAO	Food and Agriculture Organization
FDA	Food and Drug Administration
Fe_3O_4	Iron(II, III) Oxide
FET	Field-Effect Transistor
FGF	Fibroblast Growth Factor
FNP	Flash Nanoprecipitation
FR	Folate Receptor
FRET	Förster Resonance Energy Transfer
GMP	Good Manufacturing Practice
GO	Graphene Oxide
GQD	Graphene Quantum Dot
GSH	Glutathione
H_2O_2	Hydrogen Peroxide
HAP	Hydroxyapatite
HBV	Hepatitis B Virus
HER	Hydrogen Evolution Reaction
HNT	Halloysite Nanotube
HOF	Hydrogen-Bonded Organic Framework
HPV	Human Papillomavirus
HSV	Herpes Simplex Virus
IAEA	International Atomic Energy Agency
IFN	Interferon
IL	Interleukin
IND	Investigational New Drug
IONP	Iron Oxide Nanoparticle

IoT	Internet of Things
iPSC	Induced Pluripotent Stem Cell
ISO	International Organization for Standardization
ISO/TR	ISO Technical Report
IVIVC	In Vitro–In Vivo Correlation
LDH	Lactate Dehydrogenase
LDL	Low-Density Lipoprotein
LET	Linear Energy Transfer
LFA	Lateral Flow Assay
LFIA	Lateral Flow Immunoassay
Ln-MOF	Lanthanide-Based Metal-Organic Framework
LNP	Lipid Nanoparticles
LOC	Lab-on-a-Chip
LOD	Limit of Detection
LOX	Lysyl Oxidase
LSPR	Localized Surface Plasmon Resonance
MAD	Mutual Acceptance of Data
MAPK	Mitogen-Activated Protein Kinase
MDR	Medical Device Regulation
MHRA	Medicines and Healthcare Products Regulatory Agency
MIP	Molecularly Imprinted Polymer
ML	Machine Learning
MMT	Montmorillonite
MNC	Metallic Nanocarrier
MNP	Magnetic Nanoparticle
MOBO	Multi-Objective Bayesian Optimization
MoC	Multi-Organ-on-Chip
MOF	Metal-Organic Framework
MPc	Metal Phthalocyanine
MPor	Metal Porphyrin
MPS	Microphysiological System
MRI	Magnetic Resonance Imaging
mRNA	Messenger RNA
MSC	Mesenchymal Stem Cell
MTT	Tetrazolium Assay
MWCNT	Multi-Walled Carbon Nanotube
NADPH	Nicotinamide Adenine Dinucleotide Phosphate
Nano-QSAR	Nano Quantitative Structure–Activity Relationship
NC	Nanocarrier
NCP	Nanoscale Coordination Particle
NGF	Nerve Growth Factor
NIR	Near-Infrared
NIST	National Institute of Standards and Technology
NLC	Nanostructured Lipid Carrier
NLS	Nuclear Localization Signal
NP	Nanoparticle

OECD	Organisation for Economic Co-operation and Development
OFET	Organic Field-Effect Transistor
OoC	Organ-on-Chip
ORR	Oxygen Reduction Reaction
PA	Polyacetylene
PAA	Poly(acrylic acid)
PAMAM	Poly(amidoamine)
PANI	Polyaniline
PBCA	Poly (butyl cyanoacrylate)
PBPK	Physiologically Based Pharmacokinetics
PCL	Poly (ε-caprolactone)
PCR	Polymerase Chain Reaction
Pd	Palladium
PDGF	Platelet-Derived Growth Factor
PDT	Photodynamic Therapy
PE	Polyethylene
PEDOT	Poly (3,4-ethylenedioxythiophene)
PEG	Polyethylene Glycol
PEI	Polyethyleneimine
PET	Positron Emission Tomography
PET (Polymer)	Polyethylene Terephthalate
PGE_2	Prostaglandin E_2
PL	Photoluminescence
PLA	Polylactic Acid
PLD	Pegylated Liposomal Doxorubicin
PLGA	Poly (lactic-co-glycolic acid)
PLLA	Poly (L-lactic acid)
PNIPAAm	Poly (N-isopropylacrylamide)
POC	Point-of-Care
PP	Polypropylene
ppb	Parts Per Billion
PPI	Poly(propylene imine)
ppm	Parts Per Million
ppt	Parts Per Trillion
PPy	Polypyrrole
PSA	Prostate-Specific Antigen
Pt	Platinum
PTh	Polythiophene
PTT	Photothermal Therapy
PVA	Polyvinyl Alcohol
QbD	Quality by Design
QCM	Quartz Crystal Microbalance
QD	Quantum Dot
R&D	Research and Development
RAFT	Reversible Addition–Fragmentation Chain Transfer
REFINE	Regulatory Science Framework for Nanomedicines

RES	Reticuloendothelial System
RGD	Arginine-Glycine-Aspartic Acid
rGO	Reduced Graphene Oxide
rhTNF-α	Recombinant Human TNF Alpha
RME	Receptor-Mediated Endocytosis
RNAi	RNA Interference
ROS	Reactive Oxygen Species
SAbyNA	Safe by Design of Nanomaterials and Nano-enabled Products
SARS	Severe Acute Respiratory Syndrome
SARS-CoV-2	Severe Acute Respiratory Syndrome Coronavirus 2
SAW	Surface Acoustic Wave
SbD	Safe-by-Design
SERS	Surface-Enhanced Raman Spectroscopy
siRNA	Small Interfering RNA
SIRT	Selective Internal Radiation Therapy
SLN	Solid Lipid Nanoparticle
SoC	Skin-on-Chip
SOP	Standard Operating Procedure
SpC	SpyCatcher
SPECT	Single-Photon Emission Computed Tomography
SPIO	Superparamagnetic Iron Oxide
SPION	Superparamagnetic Iron Oxide Nanoparticle
SPR	Surface Plasmon Resonance
SpT	SpyTag
STM	Scanning Tunneling Microscope
SVM	Support Vector Machine
SWCNT	Single-Walled Carbon Nanotube
TB	Tuberculosis
$\mathbf{T_c}$	Phase Transition Temperature
TDD	Targeted Drug Delivery
TG	Test Guideline
TGF	Transforming Growth Factor
TIPS	Thermally Induced Phase Separation
TMD	Transition Metal Dichalcogenide
TME	Tumor Microenvironment
TNF	Tumor Necrosis Factor
TNF-α	Tumor Necrosis Factor Alpha
TNT	2,4,6-Trinitrotoluene
TPP	Triphenylphosphonium
TRT	Targeted Radionuclide Therapy
VACNF	Vertically Aligned Carbon Nanofiber
VAMAS	Versailles Project on Advanced Materials and Standards
VEGF	Vascular Endothelial Growth Factor
VLP	Virus-Like Particles
VOC	Volatile Organic Compound
WPMN	Working Party on Manufactured Nanomaterials

Index

H

I

L

N

O

P

Q

R

S

W

Z

For Product Safety Concerns and Information please contact our EU representative GPSR@taylorandfrancis.com Taylor & Francis Verlag GmbH, Kaufingerstraße 24, 80331 München, Germany